Fluid, Electrolyte and Nutrient Therapy in Surgery

Fluid, Electrolyte and Nutrient Therapy in Surgery

EDWARD E. MASON, M.D., Ph.D.
Professor of Surgery
University of Iowa College of Medicine

Staff
Department of Surgery
University Hospitals
Iowa City, Iowa

LEA & FEBIGER • 1974 • Philadelphia

Library of Congress Cataloging in Publication Data

Mason, Edward Eaton, 1920—
Fluid, electrolyte and nutrient therapy in surgery.

1. Therapeutics, Surgical, 2. Fluid therapy, 3. Electrolyte therapy. I. Title. [DNLM: 1. Body fluids. 2. Electrolytes. 3. Surgery. 4. Water-electrolyte balance.
WD220 M398f 1974]
RD51.M37 1974 617'.91 73-8805
ISBN 0-8121-0447-1

Published in Great Britain by Henry Kimpton Publishers, London

PRINTED IN THE UNITED STATES OF AMERICA

Preface

This book was written over several years after twenty years of practical experience with patients and students of the subject. The chapters were given headings and subheadings which indicate a variation in specific emphasis, but the approach is more holographic than such headings might suggest. For example, the whole forest is viewed in Chapter 1. Relationships between total body sodium plus total body potassium and total body water are discussed from different vantage points in Chapters 2 and 3. Chapter 3 contains important information about the prevention and treatment of shock even though Chapter 9 is specifically designated as a review of shock and its treatment. In a hologram the superimposition of the entire picture from multiple vantage points provides maximum clarity and depth. The objective is to promote optimum patient care and to stimulate a curiosity to learn more than is presented, or presently known, about this fascinating and rewarding subject.

The emphasis has been dictated by the background, interest and opportunities of the author. Parathyroid disease has displaced thyroid disease in importance in current surgical practice as is explained in Chapter 11. Nutrition has always been of central importance in the successful practice of surgery, but the use of complete central venous nutrient solutions has reached a new prominence and, properly used, saves life and reduces complications (Chapter 7). Chapter 8 marks a new concern of surgeons. Extreme obesity is now recognized as a disease with such risk to life and comfort as to warrant operative treatment. Gastric bypass is presented as the procedure of choice. Intestinal bypass poses certain risks of fluid and electrolyte imbalance. Ileal bypass is used for treatment of hyperlipidemia. Even the obese need intravenous glucose to prevent thromboembolic complications from excessive elevation of plasma free fatty acids.

Chapter 12 was written by a friend and colleague and serves as a final summary of many of the concepts of current management of fluids, electrolytes and nutrition in the patient with severe trauma; in this instance thermal trauma.

I cannot begin to acknowledge all of the help from many people over the lifetime that this material has accumulated. I would like to thank Mrs. Pat Piper for her typing and medical student John Hoines for assistance in reading, reacting and gathering together the many bits and pieces that get misplaced in the struggle towards completion. Finally, R. T. Tidrick deserves credit for getting this book started when he asked Ed Wickland, Jr., Editor for Lea & Febiger, to consider the author and the subject. My fellow Department members and Chairman, S. E. Ziffren, have given a helpful push whenever it was needed.

Iowa City, Iowa EDWARD E. MASON

Contents

Chapter

1

A Surgeon's Viewpoint

Surgeons are physicians who operate. The balancing of fluids and electrolytes requires the use of the same basic principles which are used by physicians in other specialties. The difference between a surgeon's approach and that of an internist is dictated by the types of patients that are cared for. Every patient who has a major operation receives parenteral fluids for at least a brief period of time. Many patients are unable to use their digestive tracts for a longer period of time because of the disease or the operative procedure. Whatever the patient cannot provide for himself must be provided by the physicians and nursing staff.

A surgeon must order fluids so often and for so many different types of patients in varying degrees of illness that he would do well to adopt a system which would provide quick and simple answers for the patients whose requirements are easy to meet but would still call attention to the detailed analyses that are required for those occasional complicated patients. The following approach is not original, but I have found it efficient and effective. Each patient's daily fluid requirements can be divided into three major portions:

1. Maintenance fluids
2. Repacement of current abnormal loss
3. Restoration requirements for
   a. Volume abnormalities
   b. Tonicity and chemical composition deviations
   c. Acid-base imbalance

MAINTENANCE FLUIDS

For the average patient in a modern air-conditioned hospital, 2 liters a day of 5% glucose will provide the fluid necessary for replacement of insensible loss, evaporation from the skin and lungs, and water sufficient for excretion of the daily solute load. The fluid which is lost from the skin and lungs contains no electrolytes. Of course if the patient is sweating, salt will be lost, but this is not insensible. The maintenance fluid volume should be increased by 15% for each degree Celsius of body temperature elevation. If no sodium chloride is provided, the kidneys are normally capable of conserving body sodium. It is common practice, however, to provide 500 ml of isotonic saline solution or, in other words, 4.5 gm of sodium chloride since about this much salt is lost in the urine when patients are in fluid and electrolyte balance. The kidneys do not conserve potassium even when the body is deficient in this cation, and therefore 40 mEq or 3 gm of potassium chloride are usually added to the glucose solution. Forty mEq can be placed in 1 liter or 20 mEq of potassium chloride in each of the 2-liter bottles of 5% glucose. Potassium should not be added if the patient has an elevated serum potassium level or is oliguric, but these are special situations which will be covered later.

Intravenous fluids should never be ordered without thinking about their caloric value. The available glucose stores in the body are limited to about 200 gm which means, at 4 calories per gram, that there are only 800 calories available in body stores. When these are used up, glucose can only be derived from the breakdown of protein, and energy requirements are also met by the mobilization of fat. This has certain undesirable aspects and, as a matter of fact, may even be hazardous as will be pointed out later. If all of the 2500 ml of metabolic fluids ordered are provided as 5% glucose, this will provide 125 gm of glucose or 500 calories. If the 2 liters of nonelectrolyte solution are given as 10% glucose and the 500 ml of saline are provided as 5% glucose, the patient will then receive 900 calories, which is sufficient to prevent the burning of body protein for energy and will provide enough glucose to permit use of some of the fat stores without hazard to the patient from excessive elevation of plasma fatty acids. If the patient is malnourished and is to receive intravenous fluids for more than a few days and cannot take nourishment by mouth, then consideration should be given to the use of a central venous nutrient solution. For most patients, however, the above fluids will take care of metabolic needs.

ABNORMAL FLUID LOSS

The most common fluid loss which the surgeon must replace is that which comes from nasogastric suction. In a hospital where the suction bottles are emptied at midnight, the amount of fluid in the suction bottle at the time of morning rounds will approximate one-third of the patient's requirements for replacement on that day. The fluid lost by nasal gastric suction has the same strength as body fluids. The composition can be estimated by checking the pH of the fluid with pH paper. If the patient has lost 500 ml of acid gastric juice by 8:00 A.M., then he will need 1500 ml of isotonic saline replacement for the day. If this is given as a 5% glucose in saline solution, the patient will receive 300 calories in addition to calories provided in the metabolic fluids. It may be possible to supply the daily caloric needs with 5% glucose in all fluids which is less irritating to veins than the use of more concentrated glucose solutions. Gastric juice contains around 10 mEq/l of potassium. If the patient's serum potassium is not elevated and his urinary output is satisfactory, 40 mEq of potassium as potassium chloride are added to each liter of electrolyte solution given as replacement for fluids lost from the gastrointestinal tract. This is a generous replacement and empirical. The fluid from a small bowel fistula may contain as much as 40 mEq/l of potassium, but most digestive tract loss is lower than this. Lans et al. recommended 40 mEq/l for gastrointestinal juices replaced in addition to 40 mEq of potassium in the metabolic fluids. If renal function is normal and there is no other cause for an elevation of serum potassium, this replacement recommendation will prevent development of hypokalemia and is a reasonably safe dose when spread out in the day's fluid prescription.

If the pH of the gastric aspirate is neutral, then it should be replaced with an isotonic electrolyte solution more closely simulating extracellular fluid composition. Lactated Ringer's is often used. A mixture of 4 parts isotonic saline and 1 part 1/6 molar sodium lactate would provide about the same proportion of chloride and bicarbonate (the lactate is metabolized to bicarbonate) as is found in extracellular fluid. This would indicate ordering 1200 ml of saline and 300 ml of 1/6 molar sodium lactate. Since such exactness is not required the order is usually rounded to the nearest 500 ml, and the order would likely be written for the administration of a liter of saline and 500 ml of 1/6 molar sodium lactate. If the gastric aspirate is alkaline in pH, the replacement solution should be 2 parts saline and 1 part 1/6 molar sodium lactate.

Notice the simplicity of the solutions which suffice for replacement (Fig. 1-1). Isotonic saline has 155 mEq/l of sodium and 155 mEq/l of choloride. In comparison to body fluids, it has an excessive amount of chloride and tends to produce a hyperchloremia and acidosis. One-sixth molar sodium lactate has 166 mEq/l of sodium and 166 mEq/l of lactate. Since extracellular fluid contains only 24 mEq/l of bicarbonate, this solution has a considerable excess of bicarbonate (lactate) and is five times as effective in changing the body pH as isotonic saline. All of these solutions have approximately the same ionic strength as body fluids.

Gastric juice aspirated from the stomach is most likely to be acid and to require replacement with saline. Bile or pancreatic juices

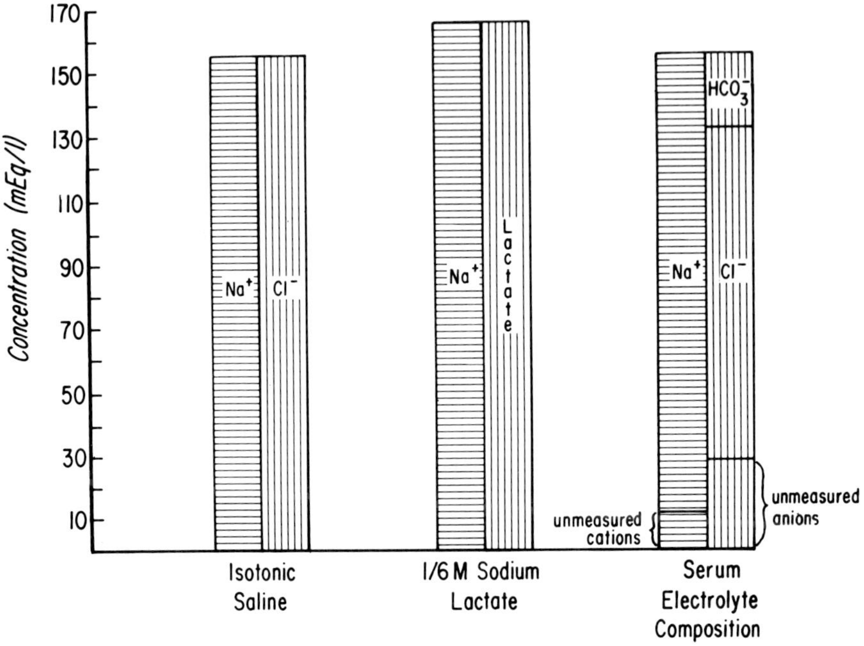

Figure 1-1. Isotonic solutions of saline and sodium lactate given in a proportion of 4:1 will replace loss of extracellular fluid. The proportions are modified to provide replacement for more acid or more alkaline fluid loss.

lost from a duodenal fistula will be alkaline and require more of the 1/6 molar sodium lactate. The pH of the fluids being replaced is a guide to the proportions of saline and sodium lactate to be used. My Scottish ancestors would be pleased to know that I always recommend that, after testing the pH of the gastric aspirate, the other end of the piece of pH paper be dipped in the urine, which provides another index of the appropriateness of replacement. The loss of an acid gastric juice will leave behind an alkalosis, and the patient's urine should be alkaline. However, if the replacement is appropriate, with the proper amount of saline, the urine will be slightly acid.

If the patient is losing an alkaline intestinal juice, he will tend to become acidotic and his urine more acid. The urine pH is normally slightly acid. Serial checks of the pH of the urine will help to guide the replacement of abnormal body fluid loss. Intestinal fluids may contain as much as 60 mEq/l of potassium. I have followed the recommendation of Lans et al. of giving 40 mEq of potassium for each liter of digestive tract fluids replaced. This is in some instances generous but is well tolerated providing the patient's kidneys are functioning normally and the serum potassium level is not elevated.

The greater the gastrointestinal fluid loss, the more that has to be replaced and the greater the opportunity to provide calories by ordering all of this replacement solution as 5% glucose in addition to the electrolyte. Such a solution is slightly hypertonic. The higher the tonicity of the fluids given intravenously into peripheral veins, the greater the incidence of phlebitis. The combination of 5% glucose and isotonic electrolyte solution, however, is usually tolerated almost as well as 5% glucose alone. There may be some irritation from addition of 40 mEq/l of potassium. If this seems to cause pain along the vein, the potassium can be reduced to 20 mEq/l and the total dose of potassium spread out over a larger number of bottles.

EVALUATION OF DATA

The surgeon's most valuable aid in maintaining fluid balance is the record of intake and output. If this is carefully kept and frequently examined, the patient will usually remain in balance. Whenever a patient seems to be suffering from some imbalance of fluid or electrolytes, a tabulation of the intake and output for the previous few days will frequently reveal a likely cause for the patient's difficulty. The joke is made that a consultant is one who does a rectal examination, but in the case of managing a patient's fluids the consultant is often the physician who takes the time to tabulate the urines for each day, the volumes of various abnormal fluids lost, and the totals of electrolyte and nonelectrolyte solutions that have been provided. An educated guess must be made about the patient's insensible loss over the selected period of time. The probable accuracy of these records needs to be considered. The patient's imbalance may occur because no one has paid attention to the intake and output records or because the records are inadequate. Regardless of the patient's disease process, the patient can be maintained in balance if his fluid and electrolyte losses are accurately replaced in volume and composition. The mere presence of imbalance indicates a failure in management. This may be a sin of omission rather than commission as, for example, when a patient first comes under the care of a physician.

The second most important source of information is the patient himself, through the history, physical examination, and laboratory tests. A patient who has been vomiting should be questioned as to the number of episodes, the quantity of the vomitus, and its characteristics. Quantitative estimates may be obtained which will fairly accurately indicate the volume of electrolyte solution lost. The current composition is estimated by the simple expedient of measuring the pH by indicator paper. The pH of the urine also indicates the type of fluid which should be replaced.

A part of extracellular fluid is the plasma volume so that pulse rate, blood pressure, urinary output, warmth of skin, rate of refill of the capillary bed beneath the nails, alertness, thirst, and other signs and symptoms can be used to help estimate any deficit of extracellular fluid. A low-grade fever may accompany hypernatremia from depletion of total body water. Disturbances in alertness are found in patients in whom there is either desiccation or overhydration.

Muscle weakness without loss of deep tendon reflexes may suggest a total body potassium deficit. Such patients are likely to have ileus and abdominal distention. Muscular weakness is also seen occasionally when serum potassium is elevated.

The apathy, tiredness, depression, and listlessness which are frequently observed in hypercalcemia are often attributed to some neurotic tendency. These patients are irritable and sometimes paranoid. Loss of appetite, nausea, and vomiting accompanied by abdominal pain may mislead the surgeon into a suspicion of some abdominal emergency when the actual problem is hyperparathyroidism.

In contrast to the nonspecific nature of most of the signs and symptoms of fluid and electrolyte imbalance, the signs of hypocalcemia are almost pathognomonic. The patient has increased irritability of his nervous system with tingling about the mouth, fingers, toes; muscle spasm and the presence of Chvostek's sign (contraction of the facial muscles upon tapping over the facial nerve). Excessive magnesium levels are depressive. Abnormally low magnesium may lead to confusion, irritability, loss of appetite, seizures, trembling of the hands, increased deep tendon reflex, and clonus.

Abnormalities of acid-base balance come under suspicion whenever breathing is abnormal. So-called Kussmaul breathing, which is deep and increased in frequency, strongly suggests metabolic acidosis and usually is due to uncontrolled diabetes. It represents an increase in the rate of excretion of CO_2 and a lowering of body carbonic acid so as to produce a respiratory alkalosis in compensation for a nonrespiratory acidosis. The lungs must be examined to make sure that the patient is not attempting to compensate for primary pulmonary disease. Consideration should also be given to the possibility that the disease process is primary in the central nervous system, driving the respiratory center and causing the patient to blow off CO_2 and to develop a primary respiratory alkalosis.

Body weight is one of the most neglected and valuable measurements in medicine. Bedside scales are available for weighing patients who are helpless. Rapid changes in body weight are due to changes in body water. Serial measurements of body weight complement serial debit and credit balances calculated from the intake and output records. A serious discrepancy requires both reweighing the patient and reviewing the most recent treatment while it is still fresh in the minds of those who measured and recorded the fluids given and carried away from the patient's bedside. Depending upon the severity of the illness, the weight of the patient, and the caloric intake provided by intravenous fluids, a patient may lose as much as 0.5 to 1.0 kg a day from metabolism of body fat. Where large tissue masses, ascites, or other sequestered fluids are removed, as during an operative procedure, the patient should be weighed immediately before and after the procedure. Daily weights are usually sufficient but if a patient has had a large volume of ascites removed, and reformation of that fluid is anticipated, it may be helpful to weigh the patient more than once a day during the period of fluid reaccumulation. Serial measurements of abdominal girth should be recorded as well.

There is a great tendency to rely upon expensive laboratory analyses in the hospital chemistry laboratory and to neglect the simple bedside observations that can be made, such as the rate of urine formation, urine specific gravity, and pH, as determined by indicator paper. Serial measurements are more valuable than just single checks. The changes observed indicate the effects of loss of various fluids upon the composition of remaining body fluid. For example, a patient who is losing acid gastric juice should have a more alkaline urine or, if kidney function is normal, the patient who is dehydrated should have a urine of high specific gravity. One of the advantages of repeated testing is to determine whether the kidneys are functioning as normal excretory organs and are varying the specific gravity of the urine appropriate with the needs of the patient or whether the kidneys are so abnormal as to continually form a urine of approximately the same specific gravity as body fluids (isosthenuria). If it is known that the patient has recently been able to form a concentrated and/or a dilute urine and that at the present time his specific gravity is in the range of body fluids (1.008 to 1.010), this is an indication that the patient is receiving appropriate amounts of fluids such as to allow excretion of the solute load with a minimum of osmotic work. Do not be lulled into an unwarranted sense of security regarding the patient's state of hydration merely by the fact that he is passing a liter or more of urine per day. A high specific gravity accompanying such a volume of urine may indicate that the patient is undergoing osmotic diuresis and becoming increasingly dehydrated because obligatory urine loss is in excess of water intake.

In 1936, Bernard Fantus wrote about the experience during the first year after opening an intravenous fluid production laboratory at Cooke County Hospital. Among other things Fantus called attention to the implications of varying concentrations of chloride in the urine. The extremes of values observed for urinary chloride were shown to correlate with an increased mortality. The Fantus test is not of particular use in trying to determine what fluids to give for the day, but it is of value as an index of abnormal function which may be primary in the kidney or due to electrolyte imbalance or the consequence of disturbed hormonal function. The implication was that if urinary chloride concentration was either extremely high or extremely low, then probably the sodium was also varying in the same direction.

If all of the above recommendations are carefully followed, electrolyte determinations upon serum will be required only occasionally to confirm a suspected diagnosis of imbalance. Actual measurement of electrolytes in body fluids and urine will be required infrequently. The surgeon would do well to diagram or write down his diagnosis in the patient's chart regarding suspected fluid and electrolyte imbalance and to indicate the abnormalities which he expects to find before requesting analysis of serum. This is the scientific method. On the basis of the information available, an hypothesis (diagnosis) is stated, and then the chemical analyses are run to help test the hypothesis. The surgeon should demand this kind of record keeping for himself just as he should demand good intake and output records from his nursing staff. When such information is recorded in graphs or statements in the record, it is then possible to go back over these in a self-audit and to learn from both one's achievements and failures.

When data come back from the chemistry laboratory, they must be evaluated for internal consistency before any interpretation is made about the patient (Fig. 1-2). Chemistry laboratories are also run by human beings. The results are accurate only to a certain degree, and in any batch of data there will be some results that are obviously erroneous. For example, the rule of electrical neutrality says that there should be the same concentration of anions and cations in an electrolyte solution. The excess of sodium concentration over chloride concentration is sometimes referred to as a fixed cation excess or a fixed anion deficit. If this discrepancy is larger than normal, it indicates an increase in the concentration of unmeasured anions or laboratory error (Fig. 1-3). An excess of measured anions ($Cl^- + HCO_3^-$) as compared with sodium indicates laboratory error. Since sodium is the chief cation in blood plasma and since other cations such as calcium, magnesium, and potassium cannot vary more than a few milliequivalents per liter without causing death, it should be evident that a set of data indicating that the CO_2 is 24, chloride 103, and sodium 120 mEq/l contains a laboratory error; therefore, this set of data cannot be used to diagnose or confirm the diagnosis of a fluid or electrolyte imbalance in the patient.

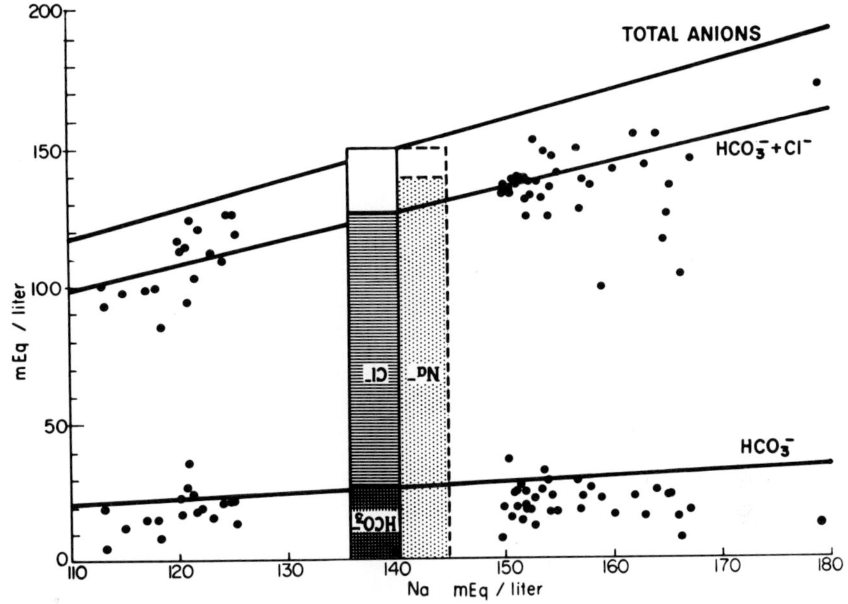

Figure 1-2. Shows data from patients whose serum sodium concentrations were abnormal and shows a correlation between anion and sodium concentration. There are patients with an accumulation of unmeasured anions so that the HCO_3 + Cl concentration falls below the predicted level. There are other sets of data in which there must have been a laboratory error because the measured anions are so numerous as sodium. The usual bar graph introduced by Gamble has been inverted in order to allow a plot of bicarbonate and chloride plus bicarbonate and to show the unmeasured anions as an addition which must be related to both concentration of measured anions and concentrations of sodium. (From Mason, E. E., and Dryer, R. L.: The implications of abnormal sodium concentrations. Surg. Gynec. Obstet. *105*:273, 1957.)

This set of data is unbelievable because the measured anions, CO_2 and chloride equal 127 mEq/l which is more than the concentration of the major cation sodium. Looked at as a bar graph with cations on one side and anions on the other side, there is not enough room for the unmeasured anions such as protein (Fig. 1-3). In the other direction, a set of data indicating that the concentration of CO_2 plus chloride is much lower than the concentration of

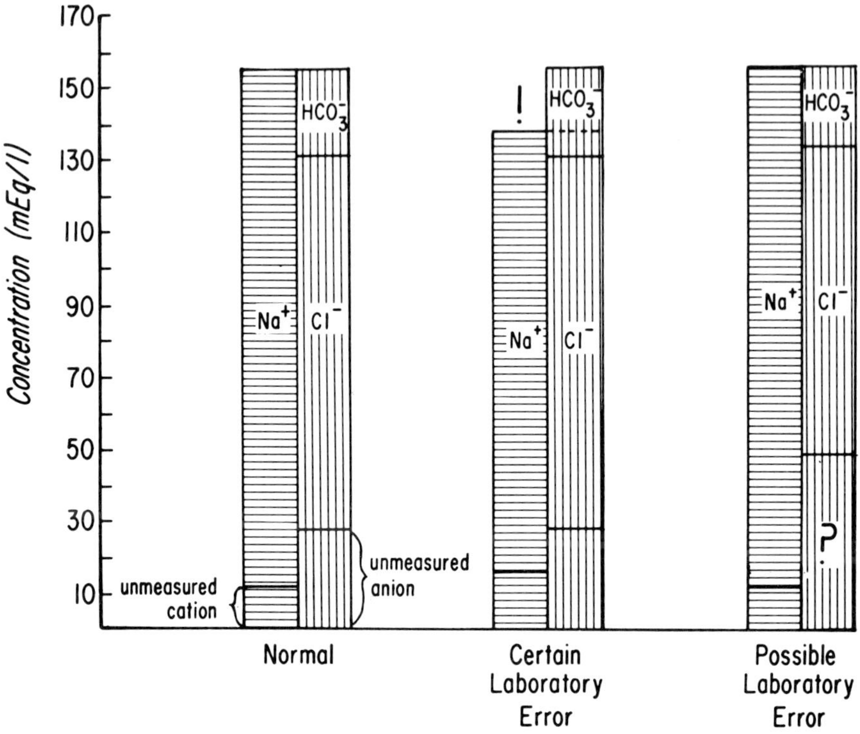

Figure 1-3. The rule of electrical neutrality. The Gamble bar graph can be used to determine if a laboratory error has been made. If the unmeasured anion is decreased, there has been a laboratory error. If the unmeasured anion is greatly increased, there might have been a laboratory error. $[Na^+] - ([Cl^-] + [HCO_3^-])$ = UMA; normal, 143 − (103 + 24) = 16; certain error, 120 − (103 + 24) = −7; possible error, 143 − (87 + 22) = 34.

sodium implies that there should be an increase in concentration of unmeasured anions. This may be due to diabetic acidosis, uremia, lactic acidemia, or some other condition which is known to cause an increase in unmeasured anions. If such a condition is not present, then this set of data is also suspect.

DIAGRAMS

There are three well-known diagrams that are used to teach fluid and electrolyte balance but are infrequently used by physicians in the patient's record. These diagrams should be mastered and used whenever a patient has any significant analytical problem in fluid and electrolyte balance. They require a real understanding of the patient's problem. They commit the surgeon to a definite estimate about each of the three aspects of body composition. They provide a basis for specific treatment which will be appropriate both in quantity and quality. These diagrams are (1) the diagram of health; (2) a bar graph of extracellular fluid composition after Gamble; and (3) a graph of acid-base balance. I will present these diagrams in the forms which I have found most useful. You may wish to make modifications. For example, instead of a plot of pH and P_{CO_2} for analysis of the patient's acid-base balance, you may wish to plot bicarbonate against pH or some other combination of two of the three variables in the Henderson-Hasselbalch equation. After collecting a data base (from the history, physical examination, laboratory data, and review of the patient's intake and output records), if it is felt that the patient is in a state of fluid and electrolyte imbalance, then a summary set of appropriately modified diagrams should be drawn in the patient's record.

Many surgeons are not particularly happy with mathematical equations or diagrams. If you are one of these persons, I beg your indulgence and promise that if you follow the next brief argument, you will be amply rewarded in your ability to manage patients. Figure 1-4 shows Cartesian coordinates with a plot of an equation $K = XY$. The curved line indicates the constant K and also indicates that there is an inverse relationship between X and Y. An increase in X requires a decrease in Y and vice versa. It should be evident that the curved line for total body solute (TBS), Figure 1-5, is a small portion of the curved line depicted in Figure 1-4.

Let me diverge in another direction and suggest that you consider a glass of isotonic saline which contains a certain quantity of solute (sodium and chloride). This glass we will use to represent the body, and the total sodium and chloride can be referred to as the total body solute. If water is allowed to evaporate from the glass over a period of time, the total body solute remains constant; but because of the decrease in volume of fluid, the measured concentration of sodium will increase. On the other hand, if distilled water is poured into the glass, the concentration of sodium will fall, simply because the volume has increased. The sodium concentration is, therefore, an index of the relationship of total body water and total body solute, and changes in the concentration of sodium can be used to indicate changes in total body water. This is a keystone to Chapters 2 and 3. The inverse relationship between volume and concentration assumes that there is no gain or loss of solute. The use of sodium concentration as an index of total body solute concentration can be justified only when it is reasonably certain that there is no accumulation of nonelectrolyte solute, such as glucose or urea.

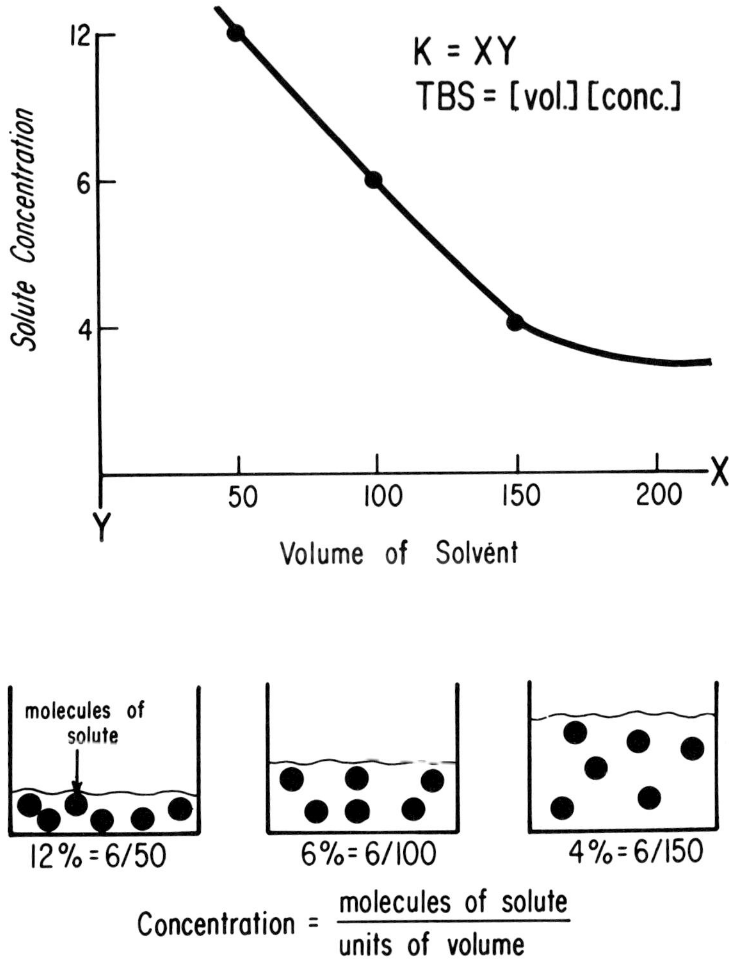

Figure 1-4. The interrelationships of volume and concentration are used so extensively in the analysis of fluid and electrolyte balance abnormalities that special study of this simple equation is warranted. For example, this principle can serve to explain the use of a change in sodium concentration to determine a change in total body water, provided total body solute remains constant.

Diagram of Health

Figure 1-5 shows the Cartesian coordinates of concentration and volume which should be used to represent the normal patient and the deviations from normal which are hypothesized to exist at the moment in the patient under consideration. Volume is plotted on the abscissa or X axis and is divisible into extracellular, or sodium-containing, fluid and intracellular, or potassium-containing, fluid as indicated by ECF and ICF. In addition to the fluids of the body, there are solids and a variable amount of fat. The patient

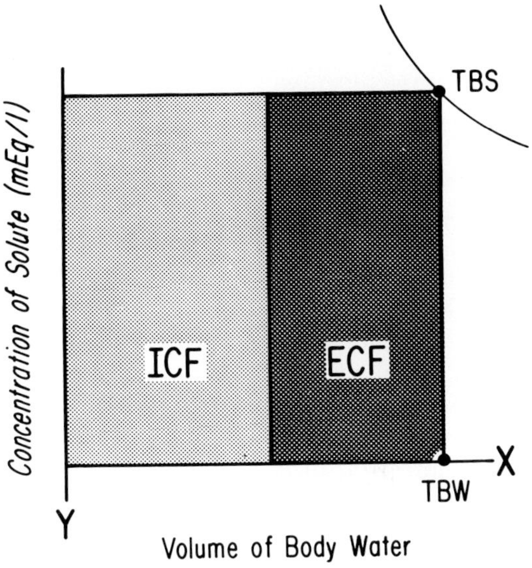

Figure 1-5. The basic diagram of health in which intracellular fluid (ICF) and extracellular fluid (ECF) are shown in terms of volume and concentration of solute. Total body solute (TBS) is the product of volume and concentration.

should be weighed to give a figure for the total volume of the patient, and then an estimate has to be made as to the degree of obesity and therefore how much of the body weight comprises body fluid. Women, in general, have a greater proportion of fat than men. In the extremely obese, it is necessary to estimate a lean, non-fat, ideal weight to use in plotting and planning treatment. Lean tissues are approximately 60% water whereas fat is less than 30% water. In a lean man weighing 70 kg, there are normally an estimated 42 liters of total body water. This can be roughly subdivided into 40% of total body weight which is intracellular and 20% of body weight which is extracellular fluid (or 28 liters of intracellular and 14 liters of extracellular fluid.)

Actual determination of the patient's intracellular fluid would require the use of a trace substance which would distribute in the intracellular fluid and by dilution allow determination of the volume of that space. Extracellular fluid is determined by the distribution of thiocyanate, bromide, or some other anion that is distributed approximately as is the anion chloride or the cation sodium. Total body water is determined by the use of heavy water, antipyrine, or some other trace substance that will diffuse throughout the body water. Even though the clinician does not have these more accurate methods available for day-to-day use, he should estimate volumes of body fluids; lines should be drawn on the basic diagram to show the deviations which he believes have occurred as a result of loss of extracellular fluid through vomiting or gastric drainage; or loss of total water by desiccation and solute diuresis.

The ordinate or Y axis of the Cartesian diagram is used to depict an estimate of concentration of electrolytes in the body fluids. An actual measurement of concentration of total solute can be obtained by requesting a determination of the freezing point which indicates the serum osmolality. The normal middle range value is about 280 milliosmoles per liter. In most instances, since the osmolality of body fluids is related to the relative amounts of total body water and total body electrolyte, it is possible to determine the osmolality simply by measuring the concentration of sodium in plasma. The total anion concentration will be approximately equal to the sodium concentration in view of the rule of electrical neutrality for electrolyte solutions. Osmolality of intracellular fluid will always be equal to the osmolality of extracellular fluid, since water diffuses freely across cell membranes. This equality of the strength of the solution outside and inside cells is sometimes referred to as *the rule of osmotic equilibrium.* There are nonelectrolyte solutes, such as glucose and urea, which if elevated must be taken into consideration in estimating osmolar strength or tonicity of body fluids. For example:

mOsm/l = 2 (sodium + potassium + magnesium + calcium) + (glucose/18) + (urea/2.8); serum electrolytes in mEq/l; glucose and urea in mg percent.

The majority of students of these problems find the use of sodium concentration as an index of concentration of total body solute difficult to grasp because sodium is restricted to extracellular fluid. How could a change in sodium concentration indicate a change in concentration of potassium in intracellular water? There are two spaces with regard to localization of potassium and sodium, but there is only one total body water space. When measuring relative amounts of water and solute one takes what one can. It is inconvenient to aspirate cellular fluid.

Attention should be called to a further subdivision of body water: about one-fourth of the extracellular fluid is located in the vascular space and comprises the plasma volume. Just as the total body sodium controls the size of the extracellular fluid space, so does the availability of albumin influence plasma volume. In the intracellular section of the diagram of health (Fig. 1-5), one might divide off another segment representing red blood cell volume. The fact that the red cells circulate in plasma which in turn is a part of extracellular fluid makes it possible to use changes in the hemoglobin concentration and hematocrit as an index of changes in volume of extracellular fluid. Concentration alone does not indicate volume, but if it is known that there is no gain or loss of red blood cells and yet a change in concentration of red cells occurs, this signifies an inverse change in volume of extracellular fluid and/or of plasma volume.

Gamble Bar Graphs

The second diagram to be drawn in the chart when analyzing the data from a patient during an attempt at diagnosis of suspected fluid and electrolyte imbalance is the bar graph popularized by Gamble. This can conveniently be drawn to the left of the diagram of health so that any changes in concentration of sodium due to changes in total body water or total body solute will be shown to have an effect upon all major components of the bar graph. If the surgeon develops the habit of always drawing these diagrams in the same way, he will no longer need to label them and can simply record his estimate of what the values ought to be or what they have been reported to be by the laboratory.

A normal average value for sodium is 143 mEq/l. Of course, this value can vary above and below the average by 2 standard deviations for a given laboratory and still remain within the expected levels of 95% of the normal population. On the right side of the bar graph, bicarbonate is depicted as an average normal of 24 mEq/l at the upper end of the bar. Below this, chloride is shown as having a value of 103 mEq/l. Space is left for the unmeasured anions below. The discrepancy between commonly measured anions and cations would be indicated by variation in the height of the unmeasured anions.

In evaluating a set of data from the laboratory, there are two steps. One of these, mentioned previously, consists of ruling out laboratory error. If the data appear to be internally reasonable, then the second interpretation has to do with *tonicity* and *chemical composition* in that order. Tonicity means the strength of the solution and indicates the concentration of solutes in water. Abnormalities in tonicity are evidenced by changes in concentration of all of the ions. Since sodium is the only cation in major concentration in plasma, the concentration of sodium is used as an index of tonicity. Once the *concentration of water in sodium* has been determined, it is then possible to say something about chemical composition.

The importance of evaluating tonicity before thinking about chemical composition is illustrated in Figure 1-6, where three different patients are represented, all with the same approximately "normal" concentration of CO_2 but with different concentrations of sodium. A normal value for sodium concentration indicates a normal relationship between total body water and total body solute, and in such a situation a CO_2 content of 24 is, in fact, normal. If, however, the sodium concentration is high, indicating a total body water deficit in relation to total body solute, then the CO_2 of 24 represents a low value and should be interpreted as evidence of a nonrespiratory acidosis. If the concentration of sodium is low, then a CO_2 of 24 is relatively high and indicates a nonrespiratory (metabolic) alkalosis in a patient whose total body water is in excess of total body solute.

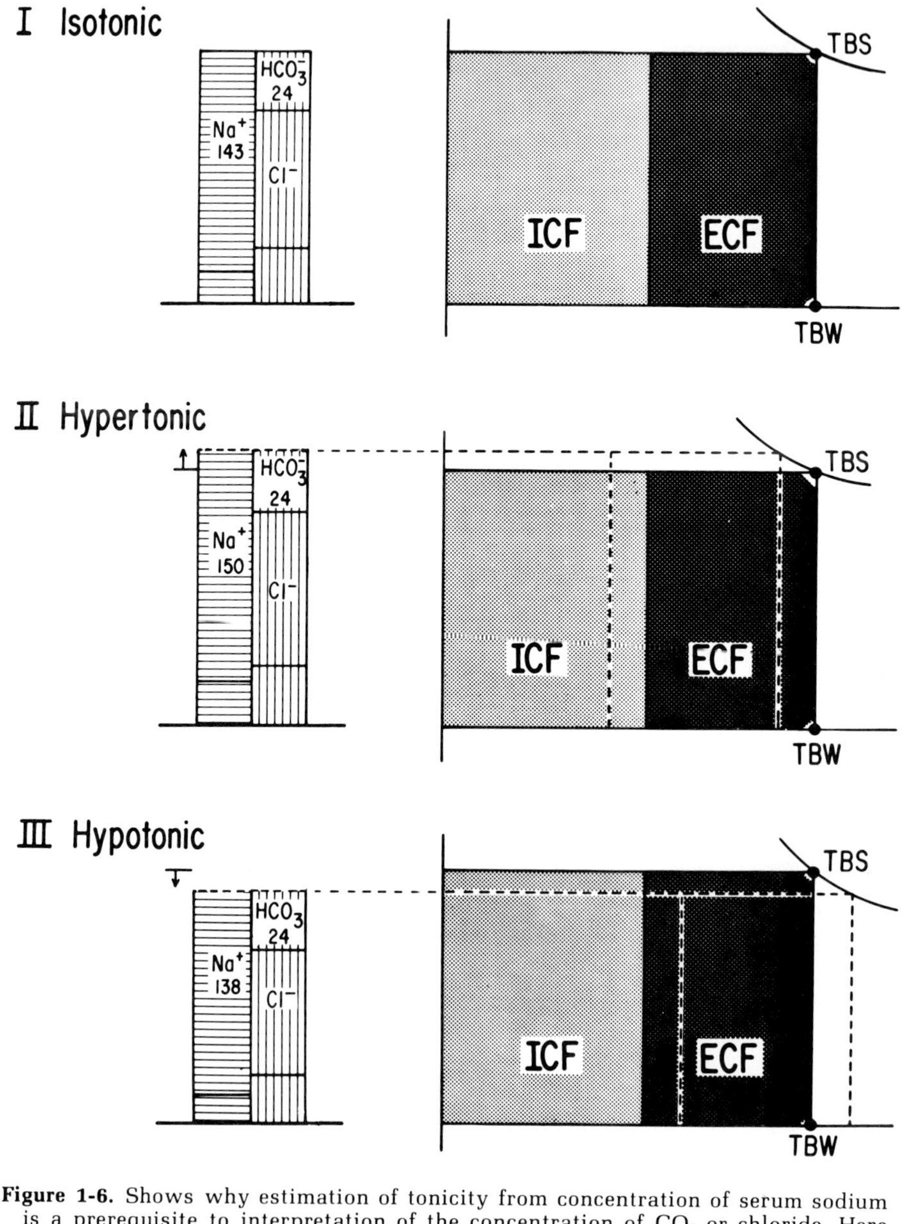

Figure 1-6. Shows why estimation of tonicity from concentration of serum sodium is a prerequisite to interpretation of the concentration of CO_2 or chloride. Here are three patients all having the same CO_2 content in serum but with varying tonicity. Bicarbonate concentration is normal in I, indicates metabolic acidosis in II, and metabolic alkalosis in III.

I recommend that you run through the last paragraph again, substituting "chloride" for "CO_2" and deciding what interpretation should be made about a serum chloride which is always of the same "normal" concentration but at different times is observed in relation to an abnormally high or abnormally low concentration of sodium. If there is still confusion in your mind about the interpretation of the concentration of serum sodium, refer back to Figure 1-4 and consider again the inverse relationship between total body water and concentration of sodium in water (but the interpretation is actually the concentration of water in total body solute). The only reason it is sodium that is measured and not potassium is because the fluid sample comes from the extracellular fluid space. If it were possible to sample intracellular fluid, then the concentration of potassium could be used to determine the relative amounts of water in the body solute.

There is a reciprocity between CO_2 (content) and chloride concentration. The rule of electrical neutrality requires that for a given concentration of sodium, the increase in concentration of one anion requires a decrease in concentration of other anions. Thus, if the patient retains chloride and has an increasing concentration of chloride it is necessary that bicarbonate be converted to CO_2 which in turn is excreted through the lungs. On the other hand, if the patient loses chloride as from the loss of acid gastric juice, this requires an expansion of some other anion. Bicarbonate is always available because of the continual production of CO_2. There are other ions which are in such low concentration that they are not influenced significantly by changes in total body water. I examined data from patients selected from our laboratory whose serum sodiums were extremely high or extremely low and found no relationship between the concentration of sodium and potassium.

I have placed great emphasis so far and will continue to use the concept of interrelationships between total body solute and total body water. I present these ideas as gospel and of great use but take no responsibility for either their conception or proof. For the skeptics and unusually interested persons who are not familiar with this concept, the work of Edelman et al. should be consulted. By the use of trace substances for estimation of total body sodium, total body potassium, and total body water, they have shown a high correlation for the following equation:

$[Na^+]_S = 1.11\ (Na_e + K_e)/TBW - 25.6;$

$[NA^+]_S$ = sodium concentration in serum;
$Na_e + K_e$ means total Na and K in the body *exchangeable* with the trace elements used.
TBW = total body water.

Their data are shown in Figure 1-7.

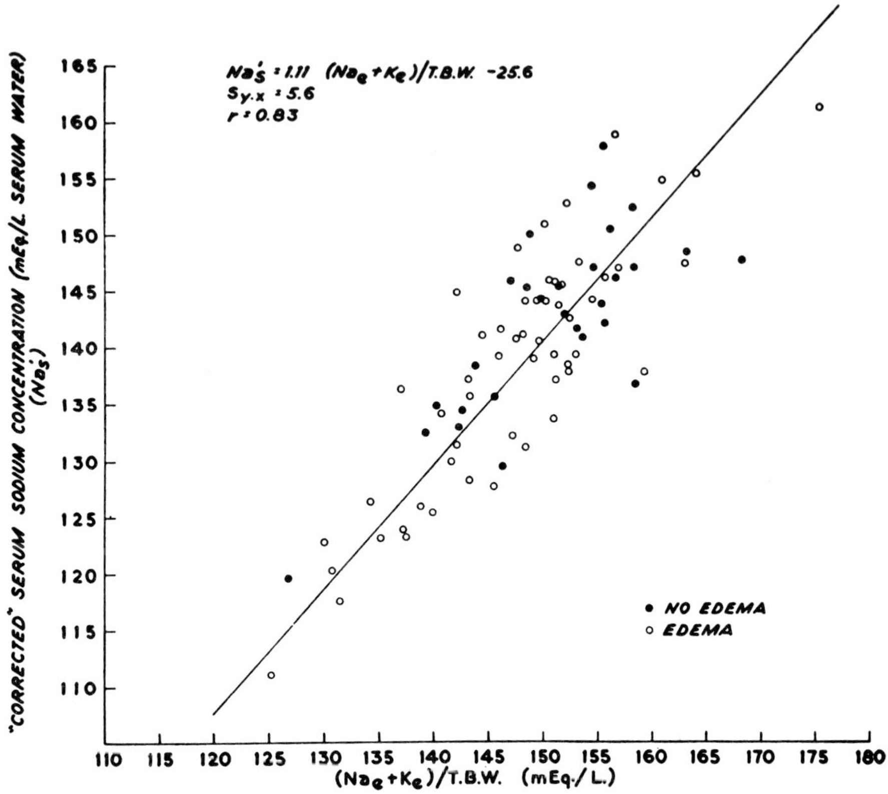

Figure 1-7. Shows the relation between concentration of serum sodium and the ratio of (Na_e + K_e/TBW). "Corrected" serum sodium concentration means the ratio of sodium concentration to measured water content of serum in order to eliminate spurious effects of high lipid content. (From Edelman, I. S., Leibman, J., O'Meara, M. P., and Birkenfeld, L. W.: Interrelations between serum sodium concentration, serum osmolarity and total exchangeable sodium, total exchangeable potassium and total body water. J. Clin. Invest. 37:1236, 1958.)

Figure 1-8 shows that there also is a high correlation between changes in serum sodium concentration and changes in the ratio of (Na_e + K_e)/total body water, when serial sets of data are obtained in patients in whom the change in sodium concentration exceeds 3 mEq/l. The contribution that Edelman and coworkers made was to take this very logical concept and prove that it really was so. My task is to convince you that it is not necessary to have available these elaborate techniques for measuring exchangeable potassium, sodium, and water in order to make a fairly reliable guess as to how the concentration-volume diagram should be modified in a given patient's problem. Chapters 2 and 3 will go into this in greater detail with regard to the effect of changes in water and the effect of changes in the various body solutes.

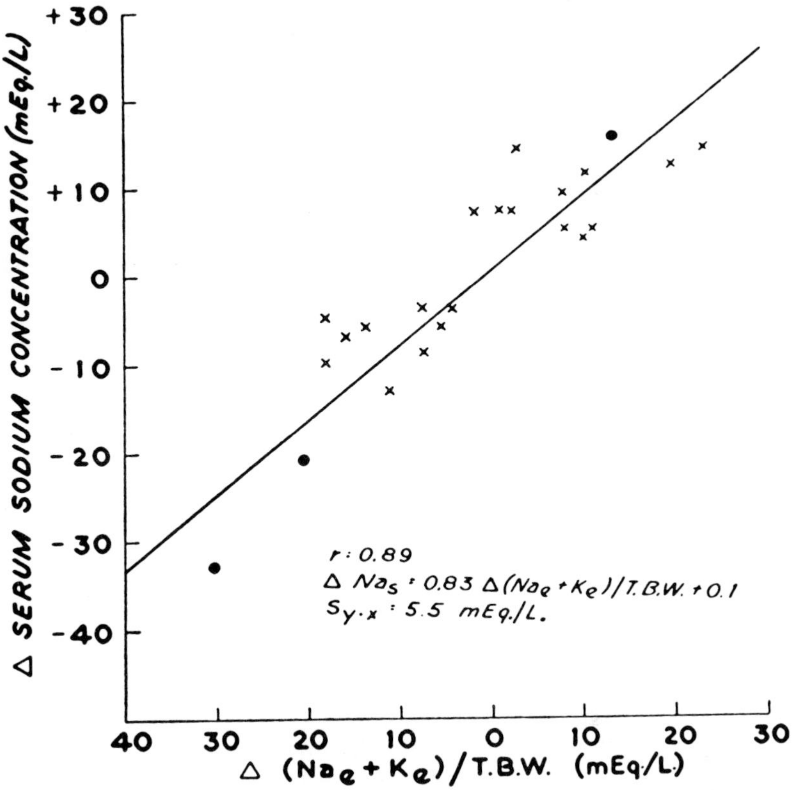

Figure 1-8. Shows the correlation between a change in serum sodium concentration and a change in the ratio of (Na_e + K_e/TBW) for individual patients studied before and again after operations on the mitral valve (x) and for serial studies in three groups of patients (•). (From Edelman, I. S., Leibman, J., O'Meara, M. P., and Birkenfeld, L. W.: Interrelations between serum sodium concentration, serum osmolarity and total exchangeable sodium, total exchangeable potassium and total body water. J. Clin. Invest. 37:1236, 1958.)

Hydrogen Ion Concentration

You should memorize the diagram in which P_{CO_2} is plotted against pH, as shown in Figure 1-9. Siggaard-Andersen has published a similar diagram so that it faces a diagram of plasma bicarbonate plotted against pH on the opposite page. These two diagrams look somewhat similar, and although either one can be used they should not be confused. The advantage of working with the P_{CO_2}-pH diagram is that each of these variables defines an item of direct clinical interest. The normal P_{CO_2} is 40 mm Hg. An elevated level indicates that the patient has retention of CO_2 and therefore has a respiratory acidosis. A P_{CO_2} below 40 mm Hg indicates that the patient is blowing off CO_2 in amounts which are creating a respiratory alkalosis. Having determined from P_{CO_2} the patient's respiratory acid-base status, the next question is with regard to interpretation of pH. A normal pH of 7.4 indicates that the patient has a normal concentration of hydrogen ions but does not necessarily indicate that the patient has normal respiratory and nonrespiratory acid-base balance function. For example, a patient with chronic lung disease may retain CO_2 and have a chronic elevation of P_{CO_2}, a respiratory acidosis; but because of his renal excretion of chloride and the creation of a hypochloremic, nonrespiratory alkalosis his pH may be 7.4. (Take several deep breaths, and you will correct any impending CO_2 narcosis. More important, put the book aside, and draw a short arrow on the P_{CO_2}-pH graph which you memorized. This is what should go into the notes you write in the patient's record.)

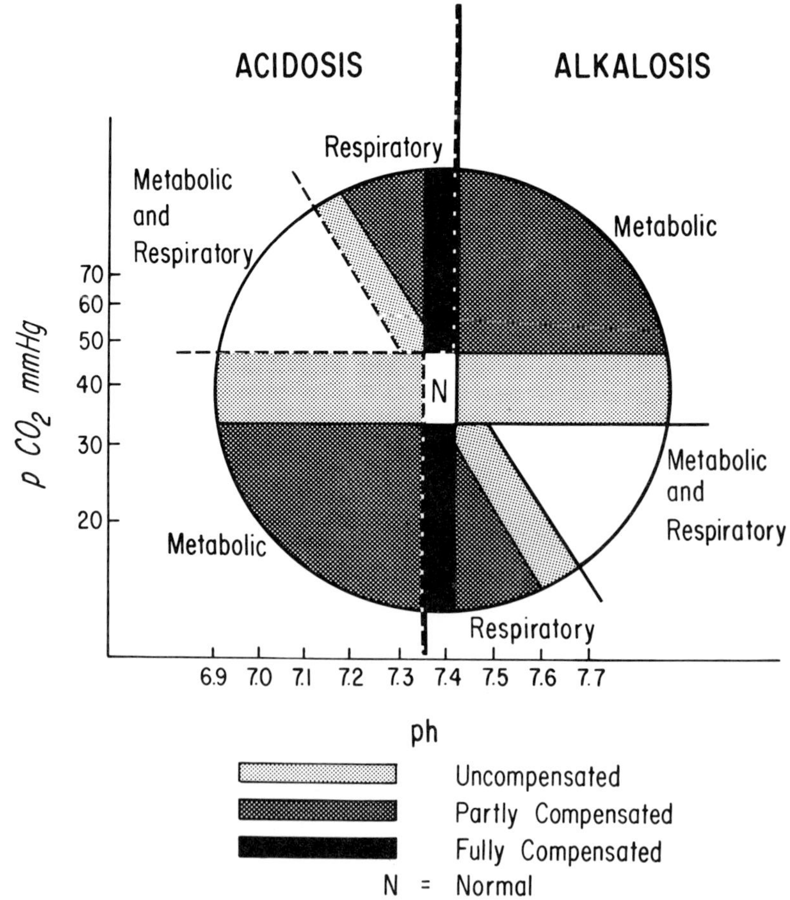

Figure 1-9. Shows the important features of the relationship between P_{CO_2} and pH. (Modified from Siggaard-Andersen)

Much of the confusion about acid-base balance is related to the difference in terminology between clinicians and chemists. A generally accepted definition of acidosis for the chemist is a pH below 7.0 and for alkalosis a pH above 7.0. The clinician is interested in mechanisms. When he talks about alkalosis he is talking about a *mechanism* which will tend to raise the pH or, in other words, lower the hydrogen ion concentration. The clinician talks about a respiratory mechanism which causes acidosis and the compensatory or perhaps unrelated nonrespiratory mechanism which tends to create an alkalosis. These terms do not in themselves indicate what the actual hydrogen ion concentration might be. One of the advantages of Figure 1-9 is that it helps to separate the various mechanisms which are influencing hydrogen ion concentration and to indicate as well the actual observed pH at any time. By sequential plotting of data, it can be observed that a single patient may pass through a variety of pure, mixed, or compensatory acid-base abnormalities.

Attempts have been made to have clinicians use the terms "acidemia" and "alkalemia" to indicate the actual change in pH from a normal of 7.4. As far as the chemist is concerned, almost all patients are in a state of alkalosis all of the time since they seldom have a pH below 7.0. What the clinician means by acidosis, or even acidemia, is a *reduction* of pH and by alkalemia an *elevation* in pH. Chapters 5 and 6 will serve to elaborate upon the role of hydrogen ions in surgery.

COLLATION

A patient's problem is analyzed into component parts on the basis of the data obtained from history, physical findings, and laboratory analyses. Conclusions are reached regarding the patient's possible abnormalities in terms of (1) *fluid volume*, (2) *tonicity and chemical composition*, and (3) *acid-base balance*. Each of these is derived from a separate analysis, but the conclusions reached in the analysis of fluid volumes have implications with regard to tonicity and chemical composition; these in turn suggest certain expectations with regard to acid-base balance.

For example, a patient with a decrease in total body water is expected to have an increase in tonicity and an increase in concentration of chloride. The increase in chloride concentration, however, is interpreted as a consequence of the decrease in total body water and not as hyperchloremia. The expected abnormality of hydrogen ion concentration in such a situation would be a slight increase above normal as a result of dehydration and extrarenal azotemia. Can you diagram such a patient's abnormalities of fluid volume, tonicity, chemical composition, and acid-base balance?

To take another example, a patient who has been vomiting large volumes of acid gastric juice over a few hours might be expected to have a decrease in extracellular fluid volume and a decrease in total body solute but probably no detectable change in tonicity. Because of the hypochloremic alkalosis the bicarbonate would be expected to be high, and the plot of P_{CO_2} and pH should show a shift of the buffer curve to the right, or in other words, a metabolic alkalosis with possibly some mild compensatory respiratory acidosis. Do not peek before you do your homework, but the diagrams that should be in the patient's chart for these two examples are shown as Figures 1-10 and 1-11.

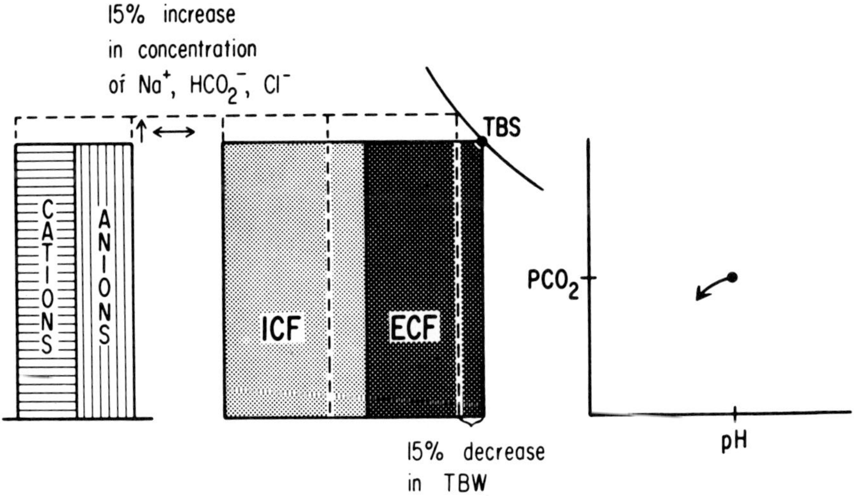

Figure 1-10. Shows how the loss of total body water would increase the concentration of all major ions. The measured anions should be increased by the loss of body water, and they may be altered also by the retention of unmeasured anions from poor kidney function. The CO_2 content (HCO_3-) would be less elevated than predicted from the sodium concentration and might be lower than normal. There is a decrease in pH from the mild metabolic acidosis and there should be a compensatory decrease in P_{CO_2}.

Chapters 2 and 3 will amplify the specific problems that are encountered. I merely use the above illustrations to call your attention to the obvious, that although the analysis of the problem is broken up into three parts and three different digrammatic representations are used in the analysis, each of these has implications for the other two. It is not infrequent after completion of these three separate parts of the analysis of the patient's problem to become aware of certain discrepancies between the conclusions reached with regard to, say, the *volume* abnormalities and abnormalities in *tonicity and chemical composition.* Such discrepancies when found should lead to a review of the data base from which the analysis was begun and the logic of the interpretation of the

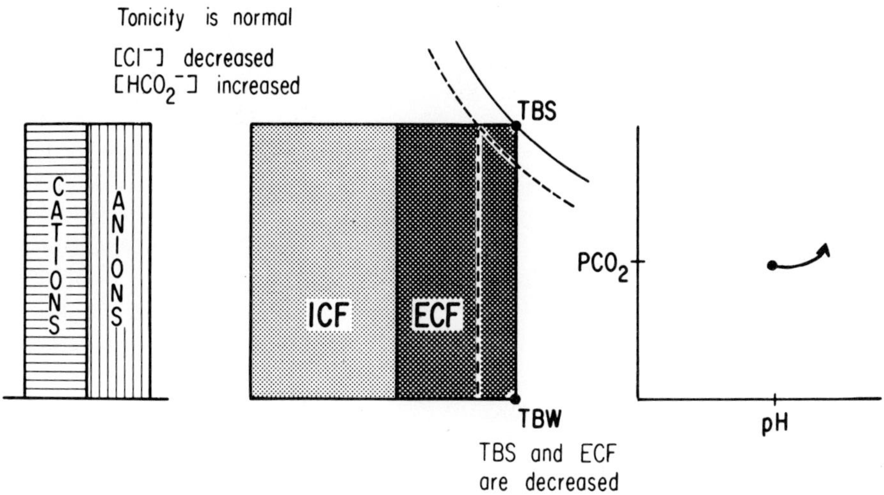

Figure 1-11. Loss of gastric juice does not change the tonicity but would change the ratio of the two major anions. The hypochloremia should increase pH, and P_{CO_2} is likely to be mildly increased. You may wish to predict specific values for these data and compare these predictions with what is reported later from the laboratory.

data. Questions raised about the accuracy of the data may lead to a repeat of chemical analyses or reexamination of the patient or attempts to obtain more information from the patient's relatives and nursing staff. It is the ultimate consistency of conclusions and the cohesiveness of the various components of the analysis that allow a final synthesis of the problem which is likely to be reliable in spite of the fact that much of the data used in the development of the final diagnosis is incomplete and inexact.

ACTION

The surgeon should have his diagnosis diagramed in such a way that both quantity and quality of derangements are defined. Even, as unfortunately is so often the case, the diagnosis regarding fluid and electrolyte imbalance is only in the surgeon's mind (and not diagramed in the progress notes), a commitment to paper has to be made in the writing of a prescription for the patient's daily fluid order. A tabulation may also be useful and can be included in the bedside notes with the diagrams:

Fluids needed	Volume	Sodium	Potassium	Chloride	Bicarbonate
Metabolic					
Replacement					
Correction					
Total					

In addition to prescribing fluids, the surgeon should decide the number of calories to be given and whether or not the patient should receive any amino acids. With a list of the available fluids from the hospital pharmacy, an order can be written instructing the nurse to give the patient a series of bottles of either 500 or 1000 ml volume containing all of the tabulated solutes and including nutrients. The exact squence and the rate at which the fluids are to be administered should be indicated. The various types of solute should be spread out so that the patient does not receive all of his calories during a brief portion of the day and all of the fluids which might cause a change in acid-base balance during another portion of the day. There may be certain priorities to consider in the sequence; for example, if a patient has marked oliguria, the potassium will usually be withheld during the early infusions. If a patient has severe acidosis, the indicated sodium lactate might be given early during the treatment.

I like to specify the rate of the infusion by drops per minute, calculating that each milliliter of fluid contains approximately 16 drops and that each 24-hour day has 1440 minutes. If, for example, the patient is to receive 3500 ml in 24 hours, this approximates 40 drops per minute. You should also request that the nursing staff keep records of urine volume, specific gravity, pH, and semi-quantitative urinary glucose at intervals appropriate to the problem which the patient presents.

REACTION

When the patient is first seen there may be a number of desired pieces of information that are totally lacking so that educated guesses must be made about the probable volume and type of fluid lost, the approximate sizes of the various body fluid compartments, and the probable concentration of hemoglobin and various electrolytes prior to the onset of the patient's illness. The data obtained come from procedures that require a number of steps, and in each of these there is variation. The diagnosis should be looked upon as a tentative working diagnosis. It is the best estimate of the type and quantity of fluid needed. As treatment is administered and subsequent observations are made, it may become evident that a patient's requirements are somewhat different than anticipated in quantity and occasionally even in ionic composition of fluid. Such discrepancies again indicate that efforts should be made to obtain additional information about the earlier course, to repeat the electrolyte analyses, or to obtain new estimates of intake, output, and body weight, in order to try to determine any errors in either data or logic. With continued observation and serial measurements of body weight, urine volume, specific gravity, and other studies and with repeated modifications of estimates of the patient's daily insensible loss and requirements for excretion of the daily solute load at a reasonable specific gravity of urine and with accurate measurements of the daily loss of fluid from gastric suction, the diagnosis is refined to an accuracy which is much greater than its many components.

CALCULATIONS

The concentration-volume diagram for body fluids has been recommended for incorporation in the progress notes in the patient's chart. It should be labeled with estimates of the patient's normal fluid volumes calculated on the basis of the patient's ideal lean body weight. Sixty per cent of this weight is a rough but sufficiently accurate estimate of total body water with 40% of the lean weight as intracellular fluid and 20% extracellular fluid. One-fourth of the extracellular fluid or 5% of the body weight approximates the plasma volume. The normal blood volume is estimated to be about 8% of a lean person's body weight. This leaves 3% for red blood cell mass, which is slightly low, and would estimate the hematocrit at 38%.

These are crude estimates designed to keep one's thinking in the approximately correct range. The estimates are modified slightly by taking into consideration the greater amount of fat in women than in men and the increasing fat with increasing age in most individuals. The absolute extracellular fluid volume tends to remain fairly constant with age whereas the intracellular fluid volume decreases. There is circulation of blood, extracellular fluid, and some cellular supporting tissue in fat so that as much as 30% of the fat can be considered as water. Extremely obese patients can be adequately treated by calculating their normal body water compartments on the basis of the maximum ideal weight for that individual's height.

I recommend the memorization of the three diagrams. The surgeon will find it worthwhile to memorize the atomic weights of a few of the electrolytes so that he can convert grams per cent to milliequivalents per liter. Approximate weights are sufficiently accurate, such as 23 for sodium, 39 for potassium, 35 for chloride, 12 for carbon, 16 for oxygen, and 1 for hydrogen. How many milliequivalents of sodium are there in 1 liter of 0.9% sodium chloride? You should come up with the answer 155 and, since there are also 155 mEq of chloride, giving 310 mOsm/l. The atomic weight of sodium lactate is not required to determine the number of milliequivalents of bicarbonate that will be derived from the administration of 1 liter of 1/6 molar sodium lactate. A molar solution by definition has one molecular weight of a substance in a liter of solution or 1000 mM, and 1/6 of that is equal to 166.

Estimates of daily caloric intake are indicated, especially when patients are receiving their nourishment entirely by way of intravenous fluids. Five per cent glucose solution contains 50 gm of glucose in a liter and there are 4 calories per gram, making a total of 200 calories. The caloric value of amino acids is also 4 per gram and fat contains approximately 9 calories per gram. Alcohol has 7½ calories per gram. A few memorized values are essential if the patient's requirements for the day are to be calculated and ordered while making rounds.

REFERENCES

Edelman, I. S., Leibman, J., O'Meara, M. P., and Birkenfeld, L. W.: Interrelations between serum sodium concentration, serum osmolarity and total exchangeable sodium, total exchangeable potassium and total body water. J. Clin. Invest. *37*:1236, 1958.

Fantus, B.: Fluid postoperatively: a statistical study. J.A.M.A. *107*:14, 1936.

Gamble, J. L.: *Clinical Anatomy, Physiology, and Pathology of Extracellular Fluid.* Cambridge: Harvard University Press, 1950.

Lans, H. S., Stein, I. F., and Meyer, K. A.: Diagnosis, treatment and prophylaxis of potassium deficiency in surgical patients. Surg. Gynec. Obstet. *95*:321, 1952.

Mason, E. E., and Dryer, R. L.: The implications of abnormal sodium concentration. Surg. Gynec. Obstet. *105*:273, 1957.

Siggaard-Andersen, O. C.: *The Acid-Base Status of the Blood.* Baltimore: Williams & Wilkins Co., 1964.

Chapter

2

Water Balance

SERVOMECHANISMS

Daily variations in normal water balance are less than 1%. Servomechanisms are involved. These include sensors, transfer of signals, and responders organized so as to provide a closed-loop negative feedback. For example, in the Hickey–Hare test for the differential diagnoses between diabetes insipidus and psychogenic polydypsia, a patient who is well-hydrated is given an infusion of hypertonic saline. This increases the osmolality of intracellular fluid. Water is therefore withdrawn osmotically from cells, including the cells of the hypothalamus where the supraoptic nucleus is located. An increased production of antidiuretic hormone and release of that hormone from the neurohypophysis result, and the rate of urine excretion decreases. Other neurons in adjacent areas in the hypothalamus are influenced by change in osmotic pressure, as with hypertonic saline injections, so that the individual becomes aware of thirst.

The system of supraoptic nucleus, posterior pituitary, antidiuretic hormone, and collecting tubule of the kidney has both fine and coarse adjustments as has been demonstrated by Ukai et al. The fine adjustment responds to changes in the tonicity of extracellular fluid, giving rise to maximum antidiuresis at antidiuretic hormone levels of 6 uU/ml of serum. Impulses from left atrial stretch receptors which pass through the vagus nerve and which are activated by changes in position can produce up to 60 uU/ml of antidiuretic hormone. Such concentrations are of an order of magnitude higher than is required for antidiuretic effects and bring into play vasopressor actions.

A sudden decrease in arterial blood pressure activates baroreceptors from the carotid sinus and from other large vessels which transmit nerve impulses to the supraoptic nucleus. There follows release of antidiuretic hormone to the extent of producing concentrations as high as 600 uU/ml. According to Silva and Rosenberg the baroreceptor-mediated response is a transient effect which comes more from the change in blood pressure than from the low, absolute, mean blood pressure. A more sustained release of vasopressor is mediated by a decrease in firing of sensors in the left atrium when atrial distention is decreased following hemorrhage. When normal blood pressure is restored and the volume of blood and extracellular fluid provides sufficient venous return to normally distend the left atrium, antidiuretic hormone decreases and the system returns to its fine adjustment based on variations in osmolality.

Surgeons have the potential to override the system by producing pain impulses which induce a release of antidiuretic hormone. This may be completely inappropriate as far as water balance is concerned. The relationship of release of adrenocorticotropic hormone, growth hormone, and antidiuretic hormone mediated by hypothalamic neurohumoral mechanisms is thought to have permitted our ancestors to survive, whereas without these mechanisms some of the similarly injured but more chaotically designed must have failed to pass the test.

The surgeon who performs operations on the stomach causes intraoperative pain impulses which travel through the posterior roots between T_4 and L_5 and, in spite of a general and effective anesthesia, these impulses reach the hypothalamus through the anterolateral spinothalamic tract. Ukai et al. have shown that posterior rhizotomy blocks the excessive antidiuretic hormone release which otherwise occurs during gastric resection. Vagotomy does not block this response.

At low concentrations, antidiuretic hormone regulates water excretion by the kidney. At high concentrations, it may cause ischemic injury to the kidney. During and immediately after a major operation, the excretion of water is related to renal blood flow and solute load, and the fine adjustments mediated by antidiuretic hormone are inoperative. If the blood pressure is low, there may be no formation of urine. If the solute load is high or total body water low and the blood pressure is in the normal range, then the solute load controls urine volume.

The final site of action of antidiuretic hormone is in the kidney. With a normal glomerular filtration rate, approximately 20% of the cardiac output passes through the kidneys. Eighty per cent of the filtered fluid is reabsorbed in the proximal convoluted tubule as an isotonic fluid. The remaining filtrate passes through the loop of Henle where, in the ascending limb, some of the remaining sodium is actively transported out of the lumen into the surrounding tissue. This countercurrent mechanism produces a high concentration of solute in the medullary portion of the kidney. The remaining fluid in the tubule lumen which reaches the distal convolution is hypotonic. Modification of the composition of the filtrate also occurs in the distal convoluted tubule under the influence of aldosterone. Aldosterone stimulates the exchange of potassium with sodium in the filtrate, providing there is any sodium remaining in the filtrate at this level of the nephron.

It is in the lower nephron, or collecting tubules, where antidiuretic hormone is thought to increase the size of the pores so that under the influence of hypertonic medullary interstitial fluid, there is diffusion of the water from the more dilute fluid in the lumen thereby concentrating the urine. The degree of urine concentration under the influence of a strong antidiuretic hormone stimulus is dependent upon all those factors which lead to a countercurrent concentration of solutes in the medullary part of the kidney. If the patient's blood volume or extracellular fluid volume is decreased so that glomerular filtration is low, all of the sodium may be reabsorbed in the proximal convoluted tubule and sodium will not be available for countercurrent action. When concentration of solutes does not occur in the medulla of the kidney, then variations in concentration of antidiuretic hormone will have no influence upon the concentration of urine. Under such circumstances the urine volume will depend upon the amount of solute being excreted.

WATER INTOXICATION

The dangers of excessive administration of nonelectrolyte solution to the traumatized patient are evident from what has already been reviewed regarding the regulation of water balance and the effects of hemorrhage and pain in overriding the normal finely adjusted controls of water balance. There have been many contributors to our knowledge of fluid balance in patients undergoing major operative procedures. I was fortunate to have trained at the University of Minnesota with a group of trainees that included Bernard Zimmermann, who made an early declaration of interest in the metabolic response to trauma and was following patients with eosinophil counts, measurements of potassium and sodium in the urine, and other potential indices of altered hormonal activity. Many of these patients were under the care of Owen Wangensteen, who was developing a procedure for treatment of breast cancer called super-radical mastectomy. This consisted of removal of the breast and axillary lymph nodes along with the pectoral muscles in the standard Halsted or Handley-type of radical mastectomy. Added to this was a dissection of the cervical and mediastinal lymph nodes. Two of the patients, after undergoing super-radical mastectomy, became comatose. These two patients were reported by Zimmermann and Wangensteen along with 15 other patients who had major operations and developed signs and symptoms of water intoxication during the postoperative period.

This was at a time in the history of surgery when it was generally believed that the postoperative patient was intolerant to salt and that salt solutions should be withheld. The resident staff, therefore, administered fluids to these patients, but withheld use of electrolyte solutions. An intravenous infusion was started the night before operation and 5% glucose was given up until the time that the patient reached the operating theater. The anesthesiologist then continued to give 5% glucose during the operation. After a long operative procedure which involved an extensive operative exposure, including splitting the sternum, the patient was taken to the recovery room where additional intravenous 5% glucose was ordered. The serum antidiuretic hormone levels must have been high during the operative and early postoperative period and probably up until the onset of coma. The relatively large volume of nonelectrolyte solutions given intravenously was retained, diluting body solute.

Water intoxication is not seen very often. Unusual circumstances are likely to precede the condition, circumstances of a long and difficult operative procedure and administration of fluids by a number of different physicians without anyone recognizing the magnitude of the fluid administration. Such patients become confused, act strangely, stare into space, or are unable to talk. They may become sleepy or incoordinated and delirious. There may be periods of violence and noisiness, and muscular weakness supervenes. The patient may have fits or hyperventilate. Nausea and vomiting are not uncommon. Finally the patient becomes comatose. He may develop an extensor, plantar reflex. There are no pathognomonic physical findings for excessive total body water. There is no edema or increase in skin turgor. These latter physical findings are more closely related to abnormalities of extracellular fluid rather than total body water. The most dramatic signs and symptoms of water excess (and of water deficiency as well) are related to the effects upon the central nervous system.

Diagrammatically, the condition should be represented as an expansion in both intracellular and extracellular water, as shown in Figure 2-1. There is no change in total body solute. For this reason the concentration of sodium is decreased, and the concentration of bicarbonate and chloride should be decreased proportionately. There is no change in concentration of hemoglobin or in the hematocrit, since the expansion involves both the plasma as part of the extracellular fluid and the red blood cells as part of the intracellular fluid. The change in the concentration of sodium can be used to calculate the increase in total body water, provided, of course, that there has not been any change in total body solute through the loss or gain of electrolyte-containing fluids. If the concentration of sodium is 10% below normal, this means that total body water is approximately 10% above normal.

The diagrammatic presentation of the abnormality indicates the objective of treatment, namely, a removal of the excess body water. Figure 2-1 also indicates how much water should be removed. If the patient's recent weight is known and his present weight can be determined with a bedside scale, the excess body weight should confirm the calculated excess of total body water as determined from the concentration of sodium. The patient can be given Lasix or a hypertonic solution of mannitol. When the required amount of urine has been excreted, a repeat analysis of the serum electrolytes should show a return to normal concentration of sodium, CO_2 content, and chloride, and this should be exactly equal to the decrease in body weight. For the patient who is comatose and whose cardiovascular system is normal, 300 ml of 3% NaCl can be given as a part of the initial treatment. This will remove some fluid from the intracellular space, increase the extracellular fluid volume, and provide for the replacement of salt which will be lost in the course of the diuretic therapy.

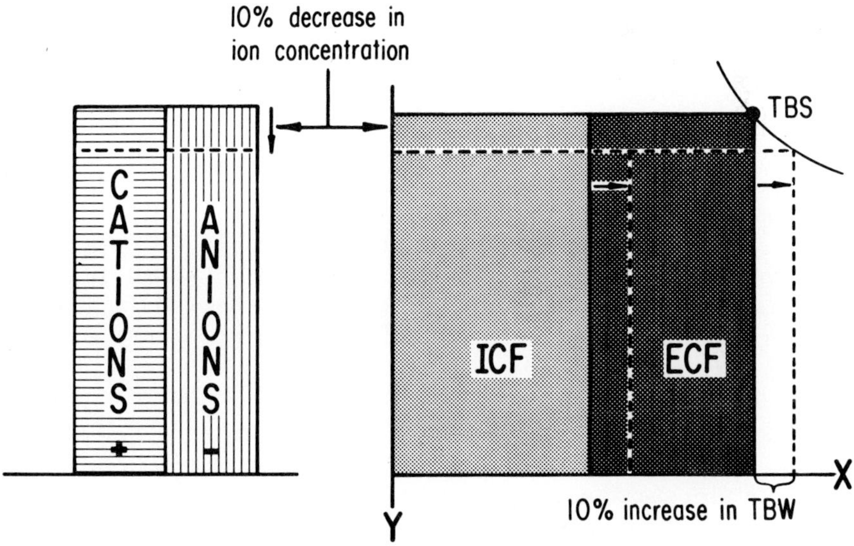

Figure 2-1. Retention of water causes a proportional dilution of both cations and anions in both the extracellular and intracellular spaces. The use of % changes is approximate. Calculation of proportionate changes is more accurate. For example, a decrease in sodium concentration from 143 to 130 mEq/l would suggest an increase in TBW from 25.5 to 28 liters. A pocket slide rule is of great convenience for bedside calculation of such proportions. A 4-inch diameter circular slide rule is easy to carry.

Water intoxication is not always a pure, isolated condition. It frequently occurs in patients who have undergone extensive operative procedures and in patients who have hemorrhaged and have had blood transfusions. There may be an element of inadequate renal blood flow, or there may be mild residual renal injury from the ischemia which resulted from the hemorrhage and the massive endogenous release of vasopressin during the operative procedure which preceded the development of water intoxication. In patients with acute renal failure, where the renal insufficiency is not recognized and infusions of 5% glucose are continued, the same expansion of total body water and dilution of sodium and other electrolytes occur. There is then a retention of creatinine and urea, which helps distinguish renal failure from water intoxication.

Pure salt deficiency causes a low concentration of serum sodium and must therefore be considered in the differential diagnosis of water intoxication. Pure salt deficiency will be discussed in Chapter 3, but is a mixture of extracellular electrolyte deficiency and intracellular water excess, so that a high concentration of hemoglobin or a high hematocrit is helpful in the differential diagnosis of pure salt deficiency.

INAPPROPRIATE ADH

Retention of water with a lowering of concentration of sodium is occasionally observed in patients with bronchogenic carcinoma. Utiger has detected arginine vasopressin in lung cancer tumor extracts by immunoassay and has found as many as half a million micro-units in 4 gm of tissue. This compares with about 7 million micro-units in the average posterior pituitary. Injuries to the hypothalamus, as occur in some instances of hemorrhage from intracranial aneurysms, may interrupt the normal inhibitory relationships so that the supraoptic nucleus increases its firing and causes an inappropriate secretion of antidiuretic hormone. Three such cases were described by Joynt et al. Since the total quantity of body solute is normal and the other homeostatic mechanisms may be working normally, the expansion of extracellular fluid may increase glomerular filtration. There may be a consequent decrease in aldosterone secretion. The expansion of extracellular fluid may also influence a third factor in the kidney which causes a decrease in reabsorption of sodium from the proximal convoluted tubule. Whatever the exact mechanisms, the response to an expansion of body fluids is, according to Bartter and Schwartz, an increased urinary excretion of sodium.

The differential diagnosis of inappropriate antidiuretic hormone secretion (IADHS) should include the possibility of adrenal insufficiency, since sodium is also lost in this latter condition producing a low serum sodium concentration. According to Bartter and Schwartz, the syndrome of inappropriate secretion of antidiuretic hormone is accompanied by adequate urinary 17-hydroxycorticoids and aldosterone secretory rates.

The diagnosis of IADHS should be suspected when, in the presence of hypotonicity, the urine osmolality is persistently higher than that of plasma. In a patient with IADHS and normal renal function, the serum sodium concentration is low, but there is usually sodium in the urine. When fluid intake is restricted, the serum sodium concentration will rise and the urinary sodium concentration decrease.

Lee et al. have recommended the administration of intravenous 5% glucose in a dose of 20 ml per kilogram given over one hour, followed by measurements of urine volume and osmolality as well as serum osmolality for three hours. In a normal person the concentration of solutes in the urine will decrease to between 85 and 184 milliosmoles per liter. In contrast the patient with an inappropriate secretion of antidiuretic hormone concentrates urine to between 255 and 638 milliosmoles per liter in spite of the overhydration. The patient with the syndrome of inappropriate secretion of antidiuretic hormone will excrete only 22 to 69% of the administered water in the course of the three hours, whereas a normal person will excrete between 52 and 98% of the water load in three hours. Calculations of the free water clearance showed a minus 1 to a plus 0.1 ml per minute for the patients with the syndrome as compared with a positive water clearance between 2.1 and 11.2 ml per minute for the control patients. In two patients with IADHS in whom the tests were repeated while 250 mg of diphenylhydantin hydrochloride were injected intravenously, a positive water clearance developed.

Treatment is simply withholding water once the condition is diagnosed. Inappropriate secretion of antidiuretic hormone is infrequent and for this reason alone may go unrecognized. In a real sense water intoxication during the postoperative period may be considered as an inappropriate secretion of antidiuretic hormone. We prevent water intoxication now by not overloading our patients with electrolyte-free intravenous fluids.

POSTCOMMISSUROTOMY SYNDROME

There are two conditions which have been referred to as postcommissurotomy syndrome. One of these is a pneumonitis, pleuritis, and pericarditis with cough, fever, and pain which has been considered as an autoimmune disease and responds to steroids. This condition has nothing to do with water balance except for the effects of edema from the inflammatory reaction. The other postcommissurotomy syndrome is a special case of inappropriate postoperative retention of water from excessive secretion of antidiuretic hormone and is due in part to the pain and other factors which would be present in any major operation. There is, however, in addition a specific increase in antidiuretic hormone due to the decrease in the size of the left atrium.

Wilson et al. studied the body composition of such patients and their fluid and electrolyte balance before and after commissurotomy. These patients are chronically ill and preoperatively many have a below normal total body potassium and an above normal total body sodium with a mild increase in total body water. Following successful operation many months are required in some patients before body composition returns sufficiently to normal to provide a normal concentration of serum sodium. Goodyear and Glenn studied 37 patients before and after mitral commissurotomy and found the postoperative serum sodium concentration below 131 mEq/l in 16. They found the serum chloride concentration to be low as well, but loss of sodium and chloride in the urine was not excessive, and they concluded as had others that the problem was one of water retention from an unusually prolonged antidiuretic stimulus.

Henry et al., in a search for an explanation of the diuresis which occurs during negative pressure breathing, located a stretch-receptor area in the wall of the left atrium. They found that cooling the vagus nerves in the neck abolished the diuresis which was otherwise produced by inflation of a balloon in the left atrium. Actual analyses of antidiuretic hormone in dogs subjected to distention of the atrium carried out by Shauyb et al. indicated a rise in antidiuretic hormone secretion in every instance when atrial distention was released. A bilateral cervical vagotomy abolished any change in antidiuretic hormone secretion resulting from change in atrial pressure. This would seem to provide the final bit of evidence explaining the peculiar predisposition of patients with mitral stenosis to retain water after commissurotomy.

Fluid restriction is an obvious way of preventing the postcommissurotomy syndrome and, according to D'Angelo et al., the administration of alcohol is also effective in treating patients who develop oliguria and the dilutional changes in sodium and chloride concentration. In most instances there are no symptoms. If the patient shows apathy, stupor, disorientation, or delirium, a small amount of hypertonic sodium chloride would be given as part of the initial treatment. Administration of hypertonic saline might be considered also if the patient has been on a sodium-restricted regimen preoperatively, or has been treated with diuretics, so that there is a suspicion of some depletion of total body sodium in addition to retention of water. There is a tendency in some of these patients for a rising concentration of serum and urine potassium, and this should respond to the administration of sodium chloride and glucose. Whenever hypertonic sodium chloride is given, it should be limited to 9 or 10 gm, and the patient should be re-examined before giving additional hypertonic salt. In patients with persistent valvular defects and with cardiac decompensation, the retention of water may be a manifestation of congestive heart failure and indicate a poor prognosis.

CELLULAR DEHYDRATION

Loss of water from the body results in an increase in concentration of solute and, regardless of the etiology, calls for replacement of total body water. Diagrams of body volume and concentration are a great help in understanding the variations which may occur and in analyzing the data from a specific patient. In all situations in which a high osmolarity is found, cellular dehydration is present. Cellular dehydration may be due to simple water loss, as is depicted in A of Figure 2-2, or due to an excess of total body sodium and chloride, as shown in B, or water depletion plus an accumulation of a nonelectrolyte solute such as glucose, as is shown in C of Figure 2-2.

In part A of Figure 2-2, the simplest type of total body water loss is depicted in which there is no change in total body solute. The rise in concentration of sodium is proportional to the fall in total body water. The loss of water is from both the extracellular and intracellular fluid. The diagram demonstrates that with a 10% loss of total body water there is a 10% increase in concentration of sodium and in concentration of measured anions. Treatment for this condition would require expansion of total body water by the 10% that has been lost.

The situation depicted in B of Figure 2-2 is one which might occur if a normal person were given only electrolyte solution for a replacement of his insensible and obligatory urinary water loss until the serum sodium concentration reached 154 mEq/l. This indicates a 10% increase in the concentration of total body solute. The consequence of retention of sodium salt without water is cellular dehydration. One might argue that some of the sodium would go into the cells, but even so, the treatment would require administration of sufficient nonelectrolyte solution to decrease the concentration of the total body electrolytes to a normal of 140 mEq/l with the expectation that as dilution occurred and as total body water volume increased, the excess volume of fluid and sodium chloride would be excreted in the urine.

The diagrams provide a basis for estimating the type and volume of fluid needed. As the patient is being treated, the accuracy of the estimate can be evaluated. For example, if 4 liters of 5% glucose were administered to the patient depicted in B of Figure 2-2, the patient should excrete an equal volume of urine but with a urine NaCl of around 9 gm per liter. Repeat analysis of the serum sodium should show a value of 140 mEq/l provided, of course, the

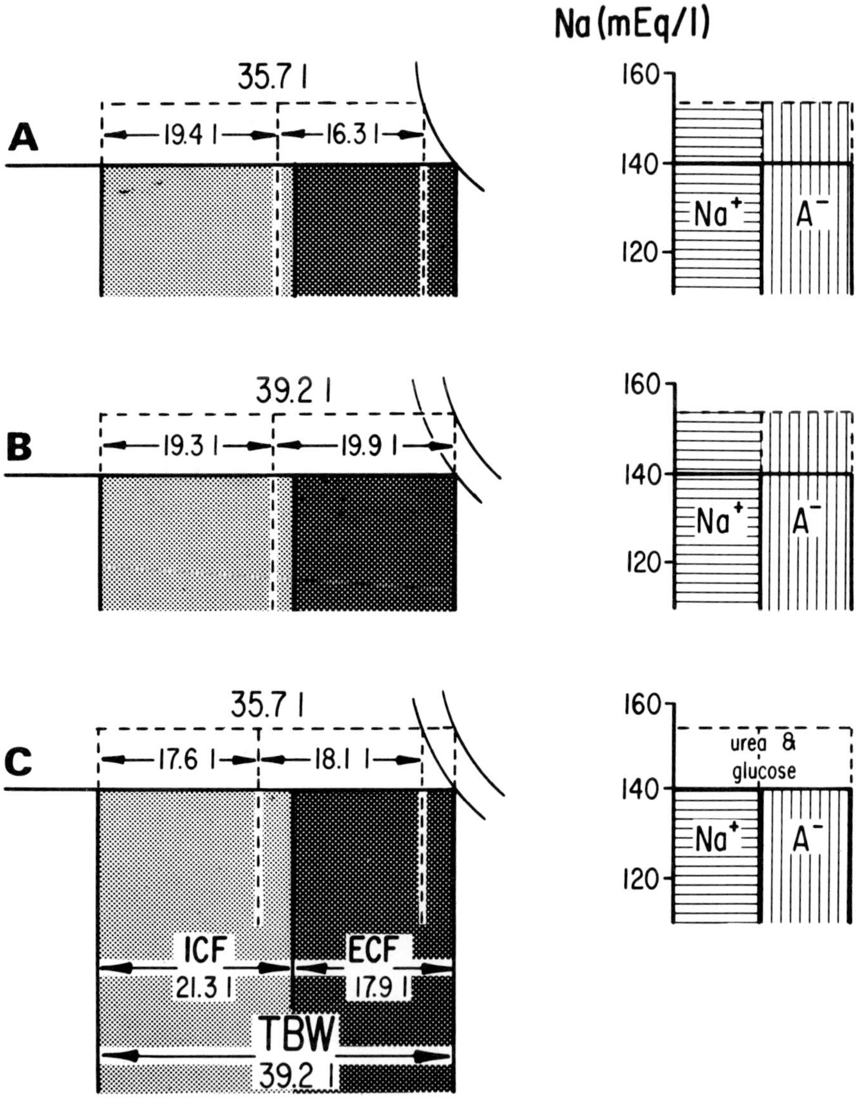

Figure 2-2. Shows three situations in which hypertonicity occurs. A, the simplest of these is a pure decrease in total body water. B, excessive intake and retention of sodium chloride without appropriate water are unusual but a possible cause of hypertonicity. C, retention of nonelectrolyte like urea, mannitol, and glucose may cause hypertonicity and dehydration without a rise in sodium concentration.

patient has been given his complement of metabolic fluids and replacement fluids for ongoing abnormal loss. If the patient is losing gastrointestinal juices, these could be replaced with nonelectrolyte solution, and the excess body salt would not need to be excreted by the kidneys.

A high concentration of sodium indicates cellular dehydration, but it is also possible to have cellular dehydration in the presence of a normal sodium concentration, C of Figure 2-2. To the extent that nonelectrolyte is present and remains in the extracellular fluid, the deficiency in body water comes from the cells, and the extracellular fluid volume may be normal or even above normal. The volume of fluid required to restore the patient's total body water deficit should be calculated upon the per cent increase above normal of total body osmolarity and a normal figure of 310 milliosmoles per liter can be used as an estimate of the desired level.

$$\text{mOsm/l} = 2\ (\text{Na mEq/l}) + \frac{\text{mg\% glucose}}{18} + \frac{\text{mg\% urea}}{2.8}$$

Actually the cellular dehydration will be corrected by movement of water back into the cells as glucose in the extracellular fluid is metabolized. The cellular dehydration in this instance is not entirely due to a total body water deficit but is due also to a solute excess in the extracellular fluid space. As a part of hyperglycemia, glycosuria may cause an osmotic diuresis and total body water deficiency. There may be a combined problem and the needs for water and electrolyte will require further evaluation as the hyperglycemia is corrected through the help of insulin. Cellular dehydration then can be due to a loss of total body water (with an elevated serum sodium concentration) or an internal shift of water due to accumulation of extracellular, nonelectrolyte solute and in both instances the pathophysiology is that of a decrease in cellular volume.

The attraction of cellular water into the extracellular space, illustrated in C of Figure 2-2, is productive of distortion of the brain and disturbance in cerebral function. This occurs during development of the hyperosmotic state. As internal shift of water progresses and water leaves the cells, including the brain, there develops a discrepancy between the size of the rigid cranium and its contents. A negative pressure develops between the brain and the calvarium. Fluid accumulates in the form of hygromata and as cerebral edema. There are tears in small veins with hemorrhages and thromboses and areas of brain destruction. The peripheral manifestations of these changes are increased tendon reflexes, jerky incoordinate movements of the extremities, and disturbed speech. The patient progresses through stages of severe thirst, euphoria, disorientation, stupor, coma, and finally death from respiratory failure. If the patient is properly treated early enough in this sequence he will recover completely, but to the extent that thrombosis, hemorrhage, and brain damage have occurred, there are permanent sequelae which can be so severe as to leave the patient with total and permanent disability. With lesser degrees of damage there may be atrophy of muscles and paralysis, impaired speech, losses in memory, and impairment of intellectual capacity.

In the very exceptional circumstances where a high concentration of sodium is due to retention of salt as in B of Figure 2-2, the urinary electrolyte excretion is above normal. More often a high concentration of sodium indicates a decrease in total body water, including a decrease in extracellular fluid as depicted in A, which activates those homeostatic mechanisms which preserve body salt and preserve extracellular fluid volume and blood volume. As a result the patient with a high concentration of serum sodium has a very low concentration of urine sodium. This is true even though the urine volume may be maintained by a high solute load. Preservation of volume takes preference over correction of tonicity.

The patient who is depleted of total body water is likely to have an increased rate of catabolism and an increased urea excretion. At the same time, his kidneys may be functioning poorly because of a decreased glomerular filtration rate or because of damage to the kidneys from the illness which led to the dehydration. The relatively large volume of urine required to excrete an increased load of solute when the kidneys are unable to concentrate to a maximum degree may mislead the unwary into thinking that the patient is adequately hydrated. Although the urinary sodium and chloride are usually low in patients with high serum sodium concentration, the urinary potassium is usually increased and the serum potassium may also be high. To the extent that there is an extracellular metabolic acidosis, there also is a tendency for potassium to leave the cells.

Treatment is based upon the amount of water required to reduce osmolality of the total body water to normal. This is regardless of any internal shift of fluid. If there is solute excess in the extracellular compartment this solute will require water for excretion. The common mistake in treating patients with a high sodium concentration is to underestimate the requirements of 5% glucose for repair of the total body water deficit. The second most common mistake is to administer saline or other electrolyte-containing solutions as a part of the treatment. The third mistake is to fail to include additional 5% glucose sufficient to supply the current metabolic fluids for urine and insensible loss.

Finally these patients are so ill that the treatment should be planned on a 4- to 8-hour schedule instead of every 24 hours. Usually the physician recognizes that water is needed, orders 2 or 3 liters and then is disappointed after 24 hours or longer to find that the sodium concentration is still as high and the patient is still as ill as before. If a patient has an estimated normal total body water capacity of 40 liters and a sodium concentration 15% above normal, he will need 8 liters of 5% glucose in 24 hours to supply fluid for urine and insensible loss and to reduce tonicity to normal. There are very few physicians who, when first faced with such a problem, are aware of the magnitude of the fluid required or are willing to prescribe such treatment. This is understandable, and the use of an incremental approach is indicated. Instead of 8 liters in 24 hours one should order 3 liters of 5% glucose in 8 hours and then re-evaluate the patient. If the original data and analyses were correct, the patient should be improved and the concentration of sodium, though still 10% high, will be headed in the direction desired. Such diagnosis ex juvantibus (in response to treatment) is reassuring whenever a severe imbalance is under treatment.

The volume concentration diagram of the patient should be modified in a progress note on the basis of response to treatment. Since correction involves adding a known volume of nonelectrolyte fluid to the total body water and measuring the fall in concentration of sodium, one has in essence the information for actually determining the volume of total body water that is being treated. Of course urine and insensible loss of water and salt must be considered as well as any other source of intake and output. These other sources of change in body composition will usually be minimal or subject to measurement. The calculations are simple. The patients and those caring for them will benefit by completion of such calculations and recording them alongside the diagrams used as a basis for the treatment. If an abnormal osmolarity has developed rapidly, it may be corrected within 24 hours. If it has developed over a number of days, then the correction should be prolonged over several days, provided of course the data show a steady improvement. In general, the most vigorous treatment is given when the abnormality is most severe, and treatment is slowed as the target is approached. This obviates overtreatment. It also allows, in the patient with hypertonicity, for a redistribution of fluid and solute so that there is minimal disruption of cells and vessel walls. When tonicity is lowered too rapidly in the extracellular fluid, water will move into cells and into the brain and may cause coma and convulsions at a time when the laboratory data are looking more normal.

The other requirements for complete intravenous fluids must not be overlooked during the treatment of dehydration. The patient may also have lost total body sodium and need, in addition to water, some electrolyte-containing fluid. The replacement should be postponed until tonicity is restored to normal. As acidosis, uremia, and oliguria are corrected, the serum potassium may fall and potassium replacement may be required. If the patient begins to excrete large volumes of urine, this water loss may need to be replaced until such time as a more specific diagnosis is made and some means is found for reducing the urine volume.

As soon as hypertonicity with cellular dehydration is recognized, a search is begun for the sequence of events that led to this observation. The most common cause of total body water deficiency is simple desiccation without replacement (Fig. 2-2A). Evaporation of water is continuous, and all that is required for the production of dehydration is a cessation of intake, or a decrease of water intake below the insensible loss and obligatory loss in urine.

We tend to forget the related and complex mechanisms which are necessary for water balance, namely, thirst and drinking. A patient must be conscious in order to be aware of thirst. He must have normal hypothalamic and related brain function. In addition to being aware of thirst, a patient must be able to reach out and pick up a glass or perhaps to pour water from a pitcher, and the water must be available. An ill or elderly, weakened individual will become dehydrated for a no more complicated reason than that no one helps the patient to drink. If the patient's temperature is elevated or if the air temperature is high, water loss may be increased, and the body composition becomes more and more salt and less and less water (Genesis 19:26).

Once it is recognized that the elaborate homeostatic mechanisms for control of water balance can no longer function because the patient is debilitated or unconscious or has some lesion in his kidneys or head which interferes, then the balance of water for that patient is dependent upon those who are caring for him. Accurate records of intake and output and daily body weights are a necessity. The capacity of the kidneys in diluting, concentrating, and excreting the daily solute load should be known; if the patient has a need for twice the usual volume of fluid in order to excrete his solute load, either this amount of fluids should be provided or the solute load reduced. If the patient is alert, physically active, and has access to water, and still a high concentration of sodium develops then such possibilities as renal insufficiency and diabetes insipidus need to be considered.

Patients receiving tube feedings are predisposed to either dehydration from osmotic diuresis or water overload depending upon the composition of the feeding. When food and fluids are administered by tube and per order of the physician in charge, the normal hunger and thirst mechanisms are bypassed and, not infrequently, the patient who requires tube feedings also has impairment of renal function or of cerebral function or both. In an elderly and debilitated patient who has borderline cardiac failure and who develops oliguria, the administration of excessive water in tube feedings may produce a total body water excess with hyponatremia. To the extent that there is excessive salt in the tube feeding, edema and ascites may develop.

More commonly, the solute load is in excess of the water administered. There is nowadays a myth about the value of high protein feedings. There are not too many variables that can be manipulated in a tube feeding to make it attractive in promoting sales. Many of the tube feedings that are commercially available are made up with an excessive amount of protein. These drinks are promoted as supplements to an inadequate diet, and the objective has been to provide the patient his daily protein requirements in 800 or 1000 ml of formula. It is expected that in addition he will eat what he can and drink enough fluid to provide his needs for the day. Most of these formulas contain a calorie per ml so that a liter of such a solution may supply 90 gm of protein but only 1000 calories. If a physician looks at the caloric content and decides that he would like for his patient to have 2000 or 3000 calories, the patient then receives 180 or 270 gm of protein. The only way that such a formula can be used in the body is to break down much of the protein for energy and excrete the nitrogen as urea. These formulas also contain an excessive amount of sodium and potassium so that the solute load which must be excreted from such a feeding may require an extra liter of urine, and therefore of water intake even though the kidneys are capable of maximum concentration. If the kidneys are functioning poorly, the patient may require 2 or 3 liters of extra water in order to get rid of the excessive solute load. If this water is not provided, the extra solute is still excreted with the production of dehydration and azotemia. These formulas are frequently made from milk protein, which means that they contain lactose, and if the patient has a deficiency of lactase in the intestinal mucosa, he may have diarrhea which further complicates the problem.

Water depletion in patients receiving tube feedings can be prevented by using a formula in which the protein makes up only 15% of the total calories. Then when a high calorie intake is supplied, the protein is proportionate and the amino acids from the protein will be available to build body protein. Energy requirements will be made up from nonprotein sources. It is necessary to make sure that the formula contains sufficient water, so that the intake and output for the day will allow for the obligatory excretion of the solute load in the urine plus the replenishment of that water which is lost from evaporation through the skin and lungs. Frequent urinary specific gravities should be recorded by the nursing staff. This will provide information about the range of osmotic work of which the patient's kidneys are capable and will permit regulation of solute and water intake so that the specific gravity remains in a midrange between a very dilute and highly concentrated urine, Figure 2-3. It is important that urine volume not only be adequate, but that the specific gravity of that urine should be 1.010 to 1.015 in a patient whose kidneys are capable of concentrating and diluting beyond this range.

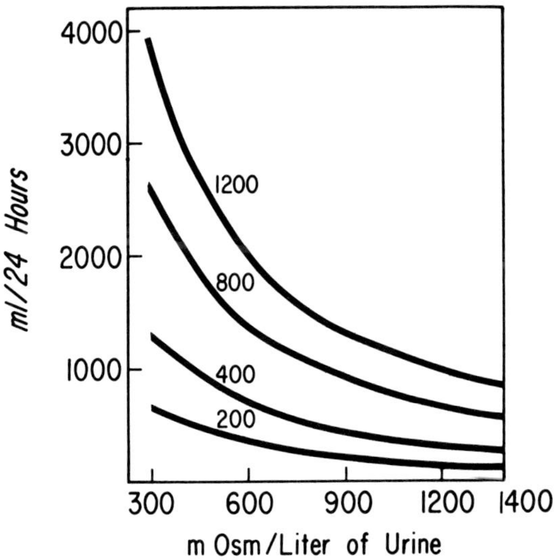

Figure 2-3. Shows the inverse relationship between volume of urine and concentration of urine for four different levels of a day's solute excretion. Urine volume may be high because of a surplus of body water, in which case urine specific gravity will be low. If a high specific gravity is found, it may indicate an osmotic diuresis and need for an increase in water intake. (Modified from Gamble)

Using a formula with only 15% of the calories as protein, 2 liters will provide 74 gm of protein which satisfies the recommended daily requirement for an average adult. If a higher protein intake is indicated, then a higher caloric intake is also needed. Meat-base formulas are tolerated by a greater number of people than milk-base formulas because lactose is not present and there is usually less salt.

There are other situations in which body water may be depleted by an osmotic diuresis. Hypertonic urea is used in treating cerebral edema in order to withdraw water from the brain. It is sometimes overlooked that the use of hypertonic urea for treatment of cerebral edema also takes water out of the body, and if this is repeated and water is not replaced, the patient will become hypertonic due to a total body water deficiency. Hypertonic mannitol will do the same thing, as will hyperglycemia from diabetes mellitus. Hypertonic enemas have been given repeatedly in attempts to remove retained feces from patients with megacolon with a resulting depletion of total body water, just as repeated use of tap water enemas in such patients has led to water intoxication. Patients who have upper gastrointestinal hemorrhage are provided a high protein diet from their own blood. This means an increase in solute load at a time when kidney function is impaired from poor circulation, so that a concentrated urine cannot be formed; as a result the patient is likely to have a total body water depletion and a rising blood urea nitrogen with consequent movement of water out of cells.

Nephrogenic diabetes insipidus should be considered in a patient whose urine volumes are high and whose serum sodium concentration is also elevated. The diagnosis is confirmed when the high volume of urine continues in spite of the administration of Pitressin. The implication is that a lesion in the lower nephron prevents normal response to antidiuretic hormone. The patient with a complete lower urinary tract obstruction, after relief of that obstruction, may demonstrate such a pattern. Patients also have demonstrated this deficiency after prolonged chronic partial obstruction of the lower urinary tract. The lower nephron functions poorly in response to antidiuretic hormone in patients who have a total body potassium depletion and also in patients who have a high concentration of serum calcium.

If the patient with hypertonicity and high volumes of urine does respond to Pitressin, then the diagnosis of hypothalamic posterior pituitary diabetes insipidus should be considered. In the practice of surgery this is most frequently seen in patients with head trauma and in such instances it is usually transient, lasting a week or ten days, but it can be permanent. It may occur from cerebral hemorrhage or from pressure from a tumor in the area of the hypothalamus. The classical sequence of events after injury to the supraoptic, hypophyseal system was described and explained in the work of Fisher et al. There is a transient phase lasting four or five days in which urinary output is increased. Following this there is apparently degeneration of the posterior pituitary and release of antidiuretic hormone so that the urinary volume is again normal. After this more normal phase the urinary output again increases and remains elevated until treatment is instituted. The latent period preceding the permanent phase, including the transient phase of diuresis and the normal interphase, lasted from 6 to 18 days with a mode of 11 days, in the experiments which they carried out on some 85 cats and 2 monkeys. A similar sequence of events is frequently observed in humans. Such patients are usually relatively easy to manage once the condition is recognized and providing the patient is alert and aware of thirst.

If, however, diabetes insipidus is complicated by uncontrolled intake it is not so simple, as was exemplified by an 11-year-old boy who was operated upon in 1959 for a large craniopharyngioma. The difficulties which we had in the management of this patient over the subsequent six months were a revelation as to how much we take for granted regarding the interrelationships of thirst, hunger, and regulation of water excretion by antidiuretic hormone. In this patient all of these mechanisms were deranged. The patient not only did not respond to thirst, but actually refused to drink water, and there were periods of time when it was necessary to place a tube in his stomach in order to supply his water requirement. He did not produce antidiuretic hormone, so pitressin tannate had to be given daily. In addition to this he ate excessive amounts of solid foods so that there were times when his solute load was high. His serum sodium concentration varied between levels which were below normal to levels as high as 170 mEq/l. The usual tendency was for the patient to remain hypertonic because of his adipsia. This was a patient who might have been considered as having "neurogenic hypernatremia," a specific derangement of his "osmostat," or a lesion in some location in the brain which causes the retention of solute. The majority of patients who might be so classified actually represent patients in whom the total body water is allowed to remain deficient over long periods of time. This patient was reported along with a review of the pertinent literature by Skultety and Joynt.

The easiest abnormalities to understand are the simple disturbances of total body water which cause an equal and opposite change in serum sodium concentration. These are abnormalities of hydration and the term "dehydration" is appropriate. Unfortunately, terms have been used loosely, and "dehydration" to some people means a loss of extracellular fluid. Likewise "hypernatremia" to some means a derangement of osmoreceptors rather than simple desiccation. Water balance problems are derangements of total body water. They cause symptoms of abnormal tonicity by changing the size of the central nervous system. They are recognized as abnormalities of osmolarity, tonicity, and sodium concentration.

The next chapters will discuss changes in solute. These changes also involve total body water, but the water is distributed with solute and the signs and symptoms and neurohormonal regulation are related more to changes in volume of the extracellular fluid and circulation and less to cellular volume and the central nervous system and seem to be designed for restoration of a normal relationship between total body water and total body solute.

REFERENCES

Bartter, F. C., and Schwartz, W. B.: The syndrome of inappropriate secretion of antidiuretic hormone. Amer. J. Med. *42*:790, 1967.

D'Angelo, G. J., Murdaugh, H. Y., and Sealy, W. C.: The nature and treatment of post-commissurotomy hyponatremic syndrome. Surg. Gynec. Obstet. *106*:87, 1958.

Edelman, I. S., Leibman, J., O'Meara, M. P., and Birkenfeld, L. W.: Interrelations between serum sodium concentration, serum osmolarity and total exchangeable sodium, total exchangeable potassium and total body water. J. Clin. Invest. *37*: 1236, 1958.

Fisher, C., Ingram, W. R., and Ranson, S. W.: *Diabetes Insipidus and the Neurohormonal Control of Water Balance.* Ann Arbor: Edward Bros., 1938.

Gamble, J. L.: *Chemical Anatomy, Physiology, and Pathology of Extracellular Fluid.* Cambridge: Harvard University Press, 1950.

Goodyear, A. V. N., and Glenn, W. W. L.: Observations on the hyponatremia following mitral valvulotomy. Circulation *11*:584, 1955.

Henry, J. P., Gauer, O. H., and Reeves, J. L.: Evidence for atrial location of receptors influencing urine flow. Circulation Research *4*:85, 1956.

Hickey, R. C., and Hare, K.: The renal excretion of chloride and water in diabetes insipidus. J. Clin. Invest. *23*:768, 1944.

Joynt, R. J., Afifi, A., and Harbison, J.: Hyponatremia in subarachnoid hemorrhage. Arch. Neurol. *13*:633, 1965.

Lee, W. Y., Grumer, H. A., Bronsby, D., and Waldstein, S. S.: Acute water loading as a diagnostic test for the inappropriate ADH syndrome. J. Lab. Clin. Med. *58*: 937, 1961.

Moore, F. D., Olesen, K. D., McMurrey, J. D., Parker, H. V., Ball, M. R., and Boyden, C. M.: *The Body Cell Mass and Its Supporting Environment.* Philadelphia: W. B. Saunders Co., 1963.

Shauyb, W. A., Moran, W. H., Jr., and Zimmermann, B.: Studies of the mechanism of antidiuretic hormone secretion and the post-commissurotomy dilutional syndrome. Ann. Surg. *162*:690, 1965.

Silva, R. E., Jr., and Rosenberg, M.: The release of vasopressin in response to haemorrhage and its role in the mechanism of blood pressure regulation. J. Physiol. *202*:535, 1969.

Skultety, F., and Joynt, R. J.: Clinical implications of adipsia. J. Neurosurg. *20*:793, 1963.

Ukai, M., Moran, W. H., Jr., and Zimmermann, B.: The role of visceral afferent pathways on vasopressin secretion and urinary excretory patterns during surgical stress. Ann. Surg. *168*:16, 1968.

Utiger, R. D.: Inappropriate antidiuresis and carcinoma of the lung: detection of arginine vasopressin in tumor extracts by immunoassay. J. Clin. Endocrinol. *26*:970, 1966.

Wilson, G. M., Edelman, I. S., Brooks, L., Myrden, J. A., Harken, D. E., and Moore, F. D.: Metabolic changes associated with mitral valvuloplasty. Circulation *9*:199, 1954.

Zimmermann, B., and Wangensteen, O. H.: Observations on water intoxication in surgical patients. Surgery *31*:654, 1952.

Chapter 3

Extracellular Solute

The distribution and circulation of body fluids are dependent upon total body solute. This is because of the water-attracting properties of molecules. The smaller the molecule the greater its water-holding properties. Intracellular volume is related to total body potassium which is retained in cells by virtue of the metabolic activity which pumps sodium out of the cells. The body sodium content governs the volume of extracellular fluid, part of which is plasma. While cellular metabolism supplies the energy of life including the energy of maintaining potassium in cells and sodium outside of cells, the extracellular fluid provides the transport of oxygen, substrates, and waste products that allow optimum cellular function.

Sodium-containing fluids, including blood, flow by virtue of the action of heart muscle, skeletal muscle, and vasomotion combined with valves and sphincters in the heart and in the vessels. According to Starling's law of the capillary bed, interstitial fluid is formed on the arterial side where intravascular pressure exceeds colloid osmotic pressure. On the venous side, interstitial fluid returns to the vascular bed because the colloid osmotic pressure exceeds hydrostatic pressure. Albumin by virtue of its size generates most of the colloid osmotic pressure. Albumin is large in comparison with sodium and potassium but is smaller than other plasma proteins. Albumin is large enough to be restrained by the capillary endothelium but small enough to generate osmotic gradients between interstitial fluid and plasma. There is some leakage of albumin from the vascular space, and this is removed from interstitial fluid and returned to the vascular space by the lymphatics which have their own motion and valves.

INTERSTITIAL FLUID

Surgeons have always been concerned about blood volume and are aware of the effect of albumin in maintaining plasma volume. The relationship between interstitial volume and plasma volume has periodically occupied our attention because of recommendations for or against the use of saline or other isotonic sodium-containing solutions in the treatment of patients undergoing major operations or after hemorrhage and trauma. At one time we had the impression that saline might temporarily expand plasma volume but that the saline would soon leak out into the interstitial fluid and become ineffective in sustaining blood volume. Actually, salt-containing solutions expand the entire extracellular fluid and are effective in expanding blood volume to the extent that the plasma portion of extracellular fluid is increased. Three to four times as much isotonic saline is required to expand the blood volume as would be required if blood were the blood volume expander. The regulation of extracellular fluid volume is of importance in the practice of surgery, and surgeons would do well to read the review by Gauer et al., which calls attention to the close relationship between the volume and pressure of the interstitial fluid and the volume and pressure of the intravascular fluid.

Our understanding of the interstitial fluid has been improved by the work of Guyton, who used a sphere of perforated metal which was implanted in the tissues and allowed to remain until it had been encapsulated by connective tissue. A percutaneous puncture of this capsule then allowed recordings of the pressure in the interstitial fluid which is in equilibrium with the capsule. Guyton found that the interstitial fluid pressure was normally around 6 to 7 torr (mm Hg) less than atmospheric. Changes created in the hydrostatic pressure caused appropriate changes in interstitial fluid pressure as would be predicted by Starling's law of the capillaries. Guyton prepared a model of interstitial fluid by using a rubber anesthesiologist's bag and filling it with small rubber balloons to represent cells surrounded by loose cotton to represent the interstitial connective tissue (Fig. 3-1). He inserted a sump drain into this container and by applying negative pressure could evacuate interstitial fluid from the system so that the cell-like balloons were all pulled closely together and the system was relatively small and tight. He then placed increasing amounts of fluid into the interstitial fluid of this model, measuring the changes in volume and the changes in pressure. He found that the relationship was similar to the pressure volume relationships which he observed in isolated limbs and in the intact animal (Fig. 3-2).

The concept of a negative interstitial fluid pressure with connective tissue and cells all in close apposition and with a minimum of free fluid explains tissue turgor and the folds of skin that are so plastic when there is a reduction of extracellular fluid below normal or when a patient has little subcutaneous fat. If interstitial fluid pressure were not negative, why would scrotal skin be so wrinkled and conforming to underlying structure? Guyton measured interstitial pressure by way of the perforated metal spheres chronically implanted in the scrotum and the pressure was -6 torr as in other sites.

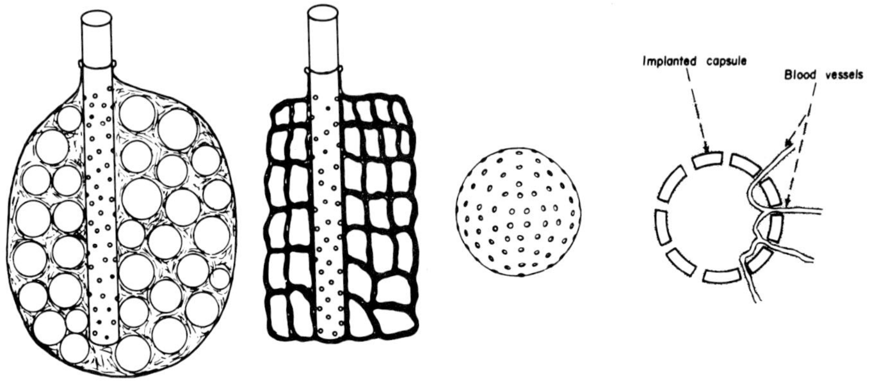

Figure 3-1. Shows the model of tissue fluid made with small balloons for cells, cotton, fluid, and a sump drain, all in an anesthesia bag. This is shown first with an excess of fluid and second with "interstitial fluid" aspirated. On the right is diagrammed the perforated steel ball which, when implanted, becomes impregnated with blood vessels and connective tissue, allowing an in vivo determination of interstitial pressure by insertion of a needle into the lumen. (From Guyton, A. C.; A concept of negative interstitial pressure based on pressures in implanted perforated capsules. Circ. Res. 12:399, 1963, by permission of The American Heart Association, Inc.)

Guyton's model is important in our understanding of patient management as will be indicated below. Part of this concept involves an understanding of compliance. A low-compliance system is one in which very small changes in volume create a considerable change in pressure. This is the situation of the normal extracellular fluid when the interstitial fluid is negative in pressure and when very little fluid is present between cells so that there is stiffness of the tissue and no free movement of interstitial fluid throughout the interstitial space. As fluid accumulates in the interstitial space the cells begin to separate one from another. The pressure rises to atmospheric pressure and with increasing retention of interstitial fluid it becomes evident that the patient has edema. In edema the interstitial fluid moves freely and can be compressed from an area by a thumb print or can accumulate in dependent areas as in the edematous patient who is sitting or standing. When there is an excess volume of interstitial fluid, approaching or actually causing edema, compliance is high and a large change in volume can occur with minimal change in interstitial fluid pressure.

According to the review of the subject by Gauer et al., there is a high correlation between interstitial fluid pressure and intravenous pressure. This means that when interstitial fluid volume is normal or reduced, the administration of isotonic sodium-containing solutions could be expected to have a maximum effect in raising not only interstitial fluid pressure but also central venous pressure. This in turn would increase venous filling pressure of the heart. On the other hand, if the patient is edematous or nearly so from sodium retention and has an expanded interstitial fluid volume, then the administration of isotonic sodium solutions will increase the edema without significantly increasing central venous pressure.

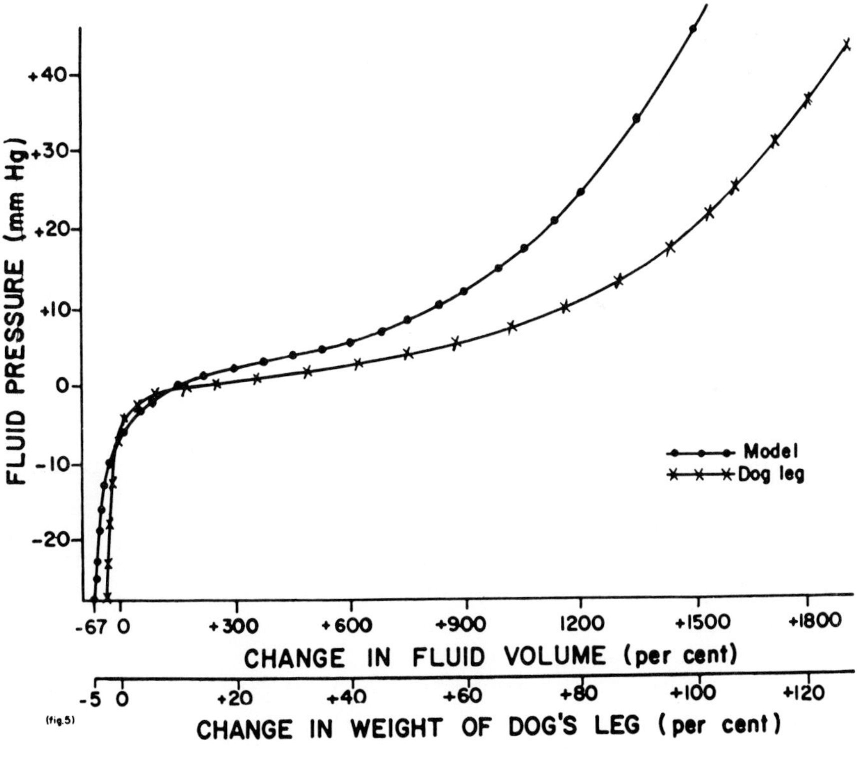

Figure 3-2. Shows the interstitial fluid pressure volume relationships observed in the model shown to the left of Figure 3-1 and in animals. At low tissue fluid volumes, pressure is negative and compliance low. With increasing interstitial fluid, pressure rises but compliance is high. (From Guyton, A. C.; A concept of negative interstitial pressure based on pressures in implanted perforated capsules. Circ. Res. *12*:399, 1963, by permission of The American Heart Association, Inc.)

Patients who are congenitally unable to produce albumin survive by virtue of an expansion of their extracellular fluid volume. The same is true of patients who, because of nutritional deficiencies, develop a depletion of body proteins and a deficit of total body albumin. The hypoproteinemic patient already has an expanded extracellular fluid. His interstitial fluid pressure is closer to atmospheric and the infusion of sodium-containing solutions in such patients could not be expected to have much effect upon interstitial fluid pressure or central venous pressure, unless rather large volumes were used, because of the increased compliance of the system in this part of the pressure volume curve (Fig. 3-2). The normal individual with a negative interstitial fluid pressure can be resuscitated following hemorrhage by the administration of salt-containing solutions because the compliance is low. The chronically ill, hypoproteinemic patient would be less responsive to crystalloid solution in resuscitation because of the high compliance. Such a patient requires colloid such as albumin, plasma, dextran, or whole blood in order to expand blood volume, increase central venous pressure, and restore cardiac filling.

With this brief review of the relationship of interstitial fluid to plasma fluid as a background, several types of body sodium abnormalities will be discussed. These might be classified as (1) internal inactivation, (2) external loss, and (3) pure salt deficiency.

INTERNAL INACTIVATION OF EXTRACELLULAR FLUID

It is intended here to review the effects of acute tissue injury and shock in producing internal inactivation of extracellular fluid. This implies that extracellular fluid has an action in sustaining the circulation and nourishment of cells. Some of the evidence for this has been provided in Guyton's experiments. The concept of inactivation of extracellular fluid implies also that the effectiveness of this fluid in sustaining circulation may be decreased because of changes in distribution and mobility of the fluid within the body rather than because of loss from the body.

Evidence for inactivation of extracellular fluid during shock has been produced by Hopkinson et al., using Guyton's perforated metallic capsules chronically implanted into the tissues of the experimental animal. The animals were subjected to a Wiggers' type of shock in which 35% of the estimated blood volume was removed. If blood was removed and quickly returned there was no change in interstitial fluid pressure, but after a more prolonged period of hemorrhagic shock and subsequent restoration of the blood there was a period of increased negative interstitial fluid pressure. If in addition to return of the removed blood, an amount of Ringer's lactate solution equal to 5% of the body weight was also administered, the interstitial fluid pressure was returned to its normal pre-bleed level. On the other hand, if clinical dextran or low molecular weight dextran was administered along with the return of blood, the interstitial fluid pressure was even lower than normal suggesting that the administration of these colloid-containing solutions extracted fluid from the interstitial space into the plasma volume. In these experiments, the survival rate was equally satisfactory regardless of the solution used for resuscitation and regardless of the postresuscitation interstitial fluid pressure.

These experiments provide evidence that there is inactivation of interstitial fluid in hemorrhagic shock and that the loss causes a decrease in interstitial pressure which can be corrected by the administration of appropriate amounts of salt-containing solutions. Survival, however, is dependent upon reestablishing adequate circulation and does not necessarily require a restoration of a normal 6 or 7 torr of negative interstitial fluid pressure. The normal interstitial fluid is present in low enough volume so that the system is relatively dry and there is low compliance. This implies that restoration of plasma volume from interstitial fluid sources would be relatively slow, but that the replenishment of blood volume and restoration of normal interstitial fluid volume and pressure would be accelerated by the administration of salt-containing solutions. The observations of Hopkinson et al. suggest that the administration of such solutions might be effective in resuscitation following hemorrhage.

Gauer et al., in summarizing the relationships that have been observed between the interstitial space and the vascular bed in a normal animal, called attention to the fact that a 10% change in blood volume would lead to a 3 cm of water change in central venous pressure and that the compliance of the interstitial space is in equilibrium with the compliance of the vascular space. There is considerable logic therefore in the use of saline or Ringer's lactate in resuscitation of hemorrhagic shock even if there were no internal inactivation of extracellular fluid. Ingraham and Wiggers in 1945 observed that well-hydrated animals had a resource for autotransfusion or transcapillary refill of the vascular space when subjected to hemorrhage and that recovery was likely, whereas dehydrated animals failed to reestablish plasma volume after hemorrhage and hemoconcentration, and death was more frequent.

It may be difficult to perceive the internal loss of extracellular fluid in hemorrhagic shock. It is easier to observe loss of extracellular fluid in tourniquet shock which can be produced experimentally by placing a tourniquet around an extremity for a period of time and then allowing blood to flow through the extremity. It is apparent in a patient who has been pinned under a heavy object with compression of blood supply to the extremity but without fractures or significant trauma to the soft tissues. After such compression for a number of hours, when the patient is removed, he initially may appear normal but there is progressive swelling of the extremity due to the ischemic damage. The shock which develops is obviously due to loss or inactivation of extracellular fluid in the damaged tissues.

Ischemia leads to disruption of long chain polymers in tissue so that these become smaller in size and more numerous and there is therefore an increase in osmotic pressure. There is also impairment of vasomotion and function of lymphatics. There is impairment of the endothelial membrane so that albumin is no longer restrained in the vascular space. These changes occur in an extremity during and after tourniquet shock. They also occur throughout the body in those areas which are most ischemic during an episode of hemorrhagic shock.

Rosenthal and Millican in a review of the role of fluids, electrolytes, and plasma proteins in experimental traumatic shock and hemorrhage in 1954 observed that the loss into damaged tissues leads to such a depletion of fluid, electrolytes, and proteins as to be incompatible with life. They remarked that the capacity to swell takes prior claim on administered fluids, most of the fluid accumulating in the injured area. Because of the injury to the capillaries and changes in function of the lymphatics, there does not appear to be any advantage in the use of albumin or other colloid-containing solutions as compared with saline or lactated Ringer's. According to this review, the capacity of injured tissues to swell is limited only by the quantity of fluid administered. This may help to explain the apparent tolerance of some severely injured patients to large volumes of electrolyte solution.

Over 40 years ago Blalock investigated the effects of muscle trauma and handling of the bowel during laparotomy and found sufficient loss of blood volume as a result of leakage of fluids into traumatized tissues to account for the observed reduction in blood pressure. Blalock was cautious in interpretation of these findings. He did mention earlier literature which indicated an impaired potential of the dehydrated individual to replenish an acutely reduced blood volume from tissue fluids.

An increase of fluid around wounds in the course of a few hours has been demonstrated by Rocchio and Randall. There is an increase in water and sodium and a decrease in potassium.

There is probably both an intracellular and an extracellular increase in sodium in this reactive zone which, according to Botelho-Machado and Adamsons, extends for several centimeters into surrounding tissues. With an extensive wound and added trauma from retractors and handling of bowel the inactivation of extracellular fluid could be considerable.

Broido et al. hypothesized that sodium was sequestered in collagen as the result of physical chemical changes occurring during hemorrhagic shock, and they supported this thesis with an experiment in which the collagen of a rat's tail was implanted beneath the skin. In animals subjected to hemorrhagic shock there was an increase in sodium- and water-holding properties whereas in control animals without an episode of hemorrhagic shock there was no increase in weight of the rat's tail implant.

De Palma et al. subjected rats to hemorrhagic shock and by use of electron microscopy showed an increase in hepatocyte water with separation of endoplasmic reticulum. Myocytes showed separation of myofibrillae. Survival was assured in 90% of animals by reinfusion of the shed blood or by administration of either saline or lactated Ringer's in a volume three times that of the shed blood. Use of 5% dextrose in Ringer's solution decreased the survival rate which is difficult to explain.

During the last three or four decades an interesting evolution of thinking has taken place with regard to the effects of trauma on sodium balance. It was recognized early that sodium-containing fluids administered to the postoperative patient were retained. Initially, this was attributed to the increased secretion of mineralocorticoids. These patients were considered to be intolerant to sodium-containing fluids and such fluids were withheld. Randall and Papper in 1958 administered 2000 ml of .9% saline preoperatively and postoperatively and compared the natriuretic responses. Less of the infused sodium was excreted postoperatively despite an increase in glomerular filtration rate suggesting that there was an increase in tubular reabsorption of sodium. If the extracellular fluid was expanded prior to the administration of the 2 liters of saline solution during the postoperative period, a normal natriuresis occurred. This seemed to suggest that the operation had produced a deficiency in effective extracellular fluid volume. In a patient with Addison's disease, who was maintained on a constant dose of cortisone and saline, it was observed that during the postoperative period there was a retention of administered saline similar to that observed in patients with normal adrenal function, indicating that enhanced adrenal function was not necessary for the retention of sodium in the postoperative period. This type of experiment was repeated by Shires and Jackson in 1962, and the observation was again made that if patients received 2000 ml of Ringer's lactate during the operation they would respond by excreting additional administered saline solution during the postoperative period.

Shires et al. in 1961 attempted to demonstrate the postulated postoperative decrease in extracellular fluid volume. They found a reduction of as much as 28% of the control extracellular fluid volume, and they felt that the magnitude of the loss was related directly to the duration of retraction and the extent of trauma produced in the course of operative exposure. This volume of loss is approximately the volume observed by Blalock in his experiments with laparotomy and trauma to the bowel.

Shires et al. in 1964 used the standard Wiggers shock preparation in dogs and found that a mortality rate of 80% without treatment could be reduced to 70% if blood alone was returned but could be reduced to 30% by restoration of the extracellular fluid volume with lactated Ringer's in addition to the return of blood. With their measurements of extracellular fluid volume, they demonstrated a 28% decrease as a result of the hemorrhagic shock and following the return of blood alone. They found that a hemorrhage of 10% of the estimated blood volume did not produce any extracellular fluid loss but that a 25% blood volume hemorrhage with sustained hypotension for 135 minutes led to a deficit of 18 to 26% in extracellular fluid after return of the blood.

Butcher studied the relationship of extracellular fluid volume to sodium excretion by using normal men and gradually depleting them of sodium. He produced a retention of infused Ringer's lactate which was very similar to the retention observed in the postoperative patient. There was no change in the concentration of sodium so that concentration was not an index of the degree of depletion or repletion. There was an increase in both the hematocrit and plasma protein concentration proportional to the degree of sodium depletion. Butcher referred to work reported later by Dillon et al., wherein the efficacy of a modified lactated Ringer's solution in resuscitation of animals subjected to a Wiggers type of hemorrhagic shock was demonstrated. In the Dillon study approximately 70% of the estimated blood volume was removed. A 50% mortality rate resulted when the shed blood was returned and 100% mortality if the blood was not returned. The best results in resuscitation were obtained from the administration of half of the blood removed plus a modified Ringer's lactate solution given in amounts of 2.75 times the blood volume removed. They were able to resuscitate shocked animals with Ringer's lactate solution alone if the solution was given within an hour after the blood loss. The use of 5% dextrose solution without sodium actually increased the mortality rate whether blood was returned or not. The same was true with the use of 10% mannitol.

Physiologically and pathologically the interstitial and vascular fluid volume are in equilibrium. Plasma albumin-induced, intravascular, colloid osmotic pressure balanced against hydrostatic pressure tends to produce refilling of an acutely depleted vascular space. Damaged tissues tend to inactivate extracellular fluid and to interfere with maintenance of an effective flow of blood and may immobilize large volumes of sodium and even colloid-containing fluids if these solutions are given in large volume as part of the resuscitation therapy. There are many variations of this theme, and it is not surprising that there are many seemingly closely related experimental and clinical observations but with marked differences in the results and interpretation of results.

If blood is removed and immediately replaced before any tissue damage occurs there will be no inactivation of sodium-containing fluid. A shock model may be too mild (or too lethal) to demonstrate the efficacy of a proposed treatment. There also is a temporal factor which must be taken into consideration. In situations where there is inactivation of extracellular fluid, the replacement should be provided early as the effective extracellular fluid volume is being lost. In instances where blood is not available or is delayed, hemodilution by expansion of the entire extracellular fluid volume may be required, and the patient may need to be overloaded with saline or lactated Ringer's in order to survive. Only by close observation of the patient can a physician decide how much electrolyte solution must be supplied to take the place of extracellular fluid which is being inactivated in a crushed extremity or in the tissues generally when a patient has been subjected to a sufficiently long episode of shock.

There are two phases to the treatment of shock and injury when treatment with saline or lactated Ringer's is required. First is the resuscitation phase, and the second is the diuretic phase. These phases are well understood in the treatment of thermal injury. In other situations where the degree of tissue injury is obscure there has been and is likely to continue to be confusion, but the principle remains the same. There is an early phase of extracellular fluid inactivation and a later phase of reactivation.

During phase one, in the early hours of resuscitation, saline administration may be required. During the later treatment of phase two saline may be contraindicated, and the patient may in fact need assistance in unloading excessive volumes of salt solution which were required during phase one. Perhaps we are now in a position partially to resolve some of the seeming contradictions between therapy of 30 years ago when saline was considered invidious and more recent reports that saline may be a necessary part of treatment of patients with trauma and blood loss.

TREATMENT WITH SALINE

Fogelman and Wilson clarified our thinking by calling attention to the fact that there are three major types of fluid loss which may lead to shock, namely a major loss of salt solution alone, a combined loss of saline solution and blood, and loss of blood alone. They illustrated these three types of loss as follows: Major salt solution loss is to be expected in patients with burns, peritonitis, multiple contusions, and intestinal obstruction. A combined loss of saline solution and blood is to be expected in patients with multiple fractures, major operations, large gunshot wounds, pancreatic and visceral injury, and in hemorrhage followed by a prolonged period of hypotension. Major blood loss, which is rare, is represented by simple hemorrhage without other injury and without a prolonged period of hypotension.

For those patients whose major and only loss is extracellular fluid, resuscitation with blood alone is likely to lead to pulmonary edema. Blood cannot be substituted for saline solution in the treatment of loss of extracellular fluid although, as has been noted elsewhere in this chapter, extracellular-like fluid can be used as a substitute for blood if the salt solution is given in sufficient volume to expand the entire extracellular fluid space.

The majority of patients in shock have a combined need for blood and saline solution. By saline is meant either isotonic sodium chloride or lactated Ringer's solution. The latter may have some slight advantage, but either solution is effective. The administration of a nonelectrolyte solution containing colloids is worse than no treatment at all as is the use of a nonelectrolyte solution such as 5% glucose. The expansion of effective extracellular fluid should be accomplished early in treatment and before oliguria, hypotension, and other signs of circulatory insufficiency become manifest.

There is no sharp distinction between the use of saline solution as a substitute for blood in the treatment of hemorrhage and the use of saline solution in the treatment of hemorrhagic shock in order to compensate for inactivation of such fluid in the tissues secondary to a prolonged period of hypotension. In the operating room it is common to allow the patient to lose up to a unit of blood without replacing the blood loss provided the patient's vital signs remain stable. The more generous use of saline solution and lactated Ringer's solution in the operating room has decreased the requirement for blood transfusions. There is evidence that, if sufficient bleeding occurs so as to require transfusion, the response to blood transfusion will be improved if the patient has received saline solution as a part of his early treatment.

Rush performed experiments in which dogs were bled rapidly from an artery into a bottle, reducing the mean arterial pressure to 30 mm Hg in 2 to 3 minutes. Pressure was held at this level by adjusting the height of the receptacle until 10 to 25% of the removed blood had spontaneously returned to the body whereupon the remaining blood was returned. This caused death in 37 out of 38 animals within 6 hours. If buffered saline was infused in 4 times the volume of the blood removed, the survival rate was 40%. Rush concluded from these observations and from his clinical experience that the patients who were provided with saline solution were able to refill their vascular space more rapidly, could maintain a lower hematocrit, and were tolerant of a greater volume of blood loss.

Simmons, Anderson, and Heisterkamp measured extracellular fluid volume in combat casualties in Vietnam and found that the deficit was no greater than could be accounted for by transcapillary refilling of the vascular space and dehydration which was present prior to the injury. They felt that shock was often the result of undertransfusion and believe that there has been too much emphasis placed upon the administration of saline solution.

In an earlier report (1969) of some 96 combat deaths, Simmons et al. found pulmonary congestion, edema, and hemorrhage in almost all instances. They again commented that the extracellular fluid requirement should not exceed 3 or 4 liters and that the use of 10 to 12 liters of lactated Ringer's solution did not seem justified on the basis of this study. Such large volumes have been given in the course of resuscitation of many severely injured patients who have survived. It may be that the variation in the amount of saline or lactated Ringer's solution which has been used in some patients demonstrates what Rosenthal and Millican observed in 1954, that administered fluids find their way into the damaged tissues and tend to increase the swelling. Only the clinician who is observing the effects of treatment can decide how much saline solution is required as a part of resuscitation.

When the experience in Vietnam is discussed in conferences in our University Hospitals, the observation is usually made that there is a difference between healthy young soldiers and older patients with arteriosclerosis and varying but significant degrees of pulmonary and heart disease. Patients undergoing operations for abdominal aortic aneurysms are usually given 3 or 4 liters of lactated Ringer's solution in addition to replacement of measured blood loss. This has decreased the incidence of renal failure and has not increased the incidence of pulmonary edema. Such patients would probably not tolerate larger volumes of saline solution and there would be no logic in supplying larger volumes.

Levine et al. produced pulmonary edema in dogs by placing a balloon in the left atrium and increasing the obstruction of movement of blood through this area at the time that saline solution was infused. The normal extravascular lung water is 3.5 ml/kg body weight in dogs, and edema occurred suddenly when the extravascular water exceeded 6 ml/kg body weight. There were no reliable clinical signs warning of the imminence of frank pulmonary edema. The movement of lung water also follows Starling's law of transcapillary exchange. Accumulation of lung water did not occur unless left atrial pressure was raised so as to exceed colloid osmotic pressure. According to Guyton and Lindsey, the normal interstitial pressure in the lung is some 19 torr below atmospheric.

Magilligan et al. found an increase in pulmonary extravascular fluid in dogs resuscitated from hemorrhagic shock by use of lactated Ringer's solution alone but not with reinfusion of blood. They did not study the use of blood combined with lactated Ringer's solution. An increase in pulmonary fluid is the price one pays for the use of salt solutions. Pulmonary edema is the risk of overuse.

One might question how it would be possible to give as much as 12 liters of electrolyte solution along with 8.5 liters of whole blood to patients in the course of 24 hours without observing pulmonary edema or obstructive atelectasis. This was reported by Carey et al. in their study of resuscitation of men injured in Vietnam. One can only conclude that the excessive amount of sodium-containing fluid was either sequestered in areas of injury or caused an elevation of interstitial fluid pressure slowly enough so that the pressure volume relationships were moved into the more compliant zone of Guyton's model (Fig. 3-2). In this zone a relatively large increase in volume can be produced without greatly increasing interstitial fluid pressure or central venous pressure. The severely injured soldiers treated with large volumes of fluid in Vietnam must not have had an excessive elevation of left atrial pressure if they did not develop pulmonary edema. Although "shock lung" and pulmonary edema can probably be exaggerated by overuse of salt solutions, if the resuscitation is carried out early and effectively so that there is minimal damage to the lungs, then the larger amounts of electrolyte solution seem to be tolerated.

There are other limits to the use of noncolloid solutions in the replacement of blood as has been emphasized by Rush and

Eiseman. They were able to remove up to 50% of the blood volume and to replace this by the administration of saline solution in amounts three times the volume of blood removed. As dilution of red blood cells occurred, there was an increase in cardiac output. A critical point is reached, however, wherein the hemoglobin concentration is so low as to provide an inadequate carrying capacity for oxygen. There is an increased oxygen demand from hemodilution because of the required increase in cardiac output. Ideally, the hematocrit should be maintained between 30 and 40%. If the hematocrit is too low there will not be adequate oxygen-carrying capacity, and if the hematocrit is too high the increase in viscosity may be a factor in impairing circulation.

Our main concern in this chapter has been with the use of saline solutions in the treatment of an ineffective extracellular fluid volume or what Fogelman and Wilson referred to as a combined type of fluid loss. Simple blood loss without prolonged hypotension does not require the administration of saline solution although saline solution can be used if blood is not available. Saline solution as a substitute for blood is most effective if given early. Gollub has reported upon the use of 3 to 8 liters of salt solution in patients undergoing open heart surgery while being maintained on an extracorporeal pump oxygenator. These patients did not develop pulmonary edema, and it was felt that the hemodilution might even have certain advantages. The oxygen requirements with extreme hemodilution were increased but were more easily met by the increased blood flow as a result of the reduced viscosity.

REACTIVATION PHASE

Doty, Hufnagel, and Mosley studied the distribution of body fluids following hemorrhage and resuscitation in combat casualties. These patients received an average of 6360 ml of blood and 5390 ml of electrolyte solution. All of the patients survived, and none had renal insufficiency. However, urine output was above 2000 ml/day between the 24th and 72nd hour, suggesting that extracellular fluid had been overexpanded. The term "overexpanded" needs to be qualified. This much fluid may have been necessary for resuscitation, and only became excessive in later hours or during phase two. The important objective in resuscitation is to establish adequate circulation and to end up with a surviving patient.

There may be difficulties in measurement of extracellular fluid or other spaces under such circumstances because of the slow mixing of the trace substance which is used to measure a space. Even if the spaces can be accurately measured and even if there is no demonstrable deficiency in extracellular fluid volume, there may still be justification for the administration of saline or lactated Ringer's solutions as a part of resuscitation. Inactivation of extracellular fluid in collagen, in movement of sodium and water into cells, or in edema in crushed tissue may still allow that fluid to be included in any measurement of the sodium space, but the inactive fluid is not effective in sustaining normal circulation. In this study, the extracellular water was markedly expanded at 72 hours. The plasma volume, blood volume, and total body water volume were fairly close to normal at this time and the red blood cell volume remained contracted.

Fleming and Bowen selected 10 patients who required ventilatory support because of the development of the wet lung syndrome after resuscitation from massive injuries received in Vietnam. These patients received between 6500 and 16,000 ml of electrolyte solution with an average of 11,000. Following resuscitation, most of the patients remained in positive water balance until the wet lung syndrome appeared; it appeared on the average of 4½ days after injury. These patients received more electrolyte solution than was given to the patients studied by Doty, Hufnagel, and Moseley and it can be concluded that if space measurements had been made that the extracellular fluid volume would have been even greater than observed by Doty et al. With such an expansion of extracellular fluid, these patients had reached a place on the pressure volume curve of Guyton's model where the compliance is great, and large increments of extracellular fluid would be required to increase venous filling pressure of the heart. As the lungs accumulate fluid, and fluid moves out of the tissues into the alveolar space, the ventilatory compliance of the lung is greatly reduced. In other words it requires an increased pressure to maintain an adequate ventilation. Fleming and Bowen found the reduced pulmonary ventilation compliance to be one of the more valuable indices of the wet lung syndrome. There was also a reduction in the Po_2 below 80 torr. Interestingly, there was no increase in central venous pressure, which averaged 6.4 cm of saline.

The urinary output in these patients averaged 2165 ml/day, which is approximately the same as that observed by Doty, Hufnagel, and Moseley in individuals who received somewhat less fluid and who did not develop the wet lung syndrome. There was a dramatic improvement in compliance of the lung and in the oxygenation of the blood in all of these patients soon after they were given 40 to 80 mg of furosemide and had developed a vigorous diuresis. One cannot simply conclude that all of these patients received an excessive amount of saline solution during their early phase of resuscitation and at a time when extracellular fluid was becoming inactive as the result of shock and other tissue damage. It can be stated that these patients should have had diuretic assistance sooner in the second phase of fluid activation. Just as the furosemide produced a dramatic improvement after the wet lung syndrome had developed, such treatment given prophylactically should have prevented the development of the wet lung.

It may be that under exceptional circumstances overzealous administration of saline solution may cause pulmonary edema during the first stage of resuscitation. Hardy and Godfrey studied the change in cardiac output by use of a ballistocardiogram in individuals who were normal as compared with individuals who had been dehydrated. They found that the administration of intravenous fluids to the dehydrated person caused a marked increase in cardiac output so that the output was considerably above normal whereas the administration of similar amounts of fluid to a normally hydrated person did not cause any change in cardiac output. In terms of Guyton's model the dehydrated patient has a low compliance so that a small change in volume will have a marked effect on his pressure both in the interstitial fluid and in the central venous space. This is one more argument for keeping patients hydrated when they are to undergo a major operation.

Carey et al. studied 27 patients resuscitated with a combination of balanced salt solution and whole blood compared with 29 patients treated with normal saline solution and blood and 10 treated with protein-containing solutions and blood. They found all of these equally effective. The patients received an average of 12,000 ml of electrolyte solution (5,000 ml in the group receiving protein) and 8,500 ml of whole blood, and none of them developed pulmonary edema or obstructive atelectasis.

As the pendulum of therapy has swung from withholding salt solutions to the administration of saline or lactated Ringer's solution during and immediately after operation, many patients including civilians have received large volumes of salt-containing solutions. Doty, Moseley, and Simmons' recommendation that large volumes of salt solution be avoided is logical, and if the patient can be resuscitated by the administration of lost blood and less than 4 liters of lactated Ringer's or saline solution, this is ideal. The important thing of course is to initiate measures to reestablish normal circulation as soon as possible and to be vigorous in resuscitation so that tissue injury from prolonged shock will not occur. The so-called "shock lung" is likely to result if severe and prolonged shock occurs whether excessive amounts of saline solution are given or not. On the other hand, if the patient is resuscitated even with large volumes of saline and initially little or no blood, providing the circulation can be maintained and the hemodilution corrected, shock lung is unlikely to occur.

There is even some suggestion that shock lung will occur if a patient is resuscitated with blood alone when he actually has sustained a significant loss of extracellular fluid. It may be necessary to somewhat overexpand extracellular fluid volume during resuscitation in order to provide adequate circulating blood volume, especially if blood is not immediately available. Towards the end of the first day, as the patient begins to mobilize these inactivated fluids, it may be necessary to administer furosemide or other diuretics to assist the patient in excreting the excessive sodium and water. There is no question that there have been excesses in the use of saline and that physicians would be well advised to moderate such therapy as suggested by Moore and Shires.

There are situations in which colloids may be useful in resuscitation. It would be preferable to correct protein deficiencies before the patient is subjected to a major operation, but sometimes this is not possible. The malnourished patient or patient with liver disease who has a serum albumin below 3 gm/100 ml prior to trauma may require an excessive amount of salt solution if colloid is not provided. It is probably better to include albumin or plasma early during resuscitation than to use large amounts of saline and then to try to correct the total body albumin deficiency during the later period when pulmonary edema may be more likely to occur.

According to Losowsky et al., the colloid osmotic pressure is around 200 torr when the albumin concentration is in the range of 2 gm/100 ml, and 400 torr with an albumin of 5 gm/100 ml. The osmotic pressure is increased to a greater extent than would be predicted by the mere increase in concentration of protein because of the associated distribution of electrolytes and the Donnan equilibrium. On the basis of plasmaphoresis experiments, Matthews concluded that the intravascular pool of albumin is maintained at the expense of the extravascular pool, and reduction in the latter is probably the stimulus for albumin synthesis. In a patient who is depleted of albumin, all of the albumin is restricted to the vascular pool, and when some of this is also lost there is no extravascular albumin to help in reestablishing the plasma volume. Colloid osmotic pressure is generated by virtue of the effect of molecules that are large and are confined to the vascular space by the endothelial membrane. Part of the effect of hypotension and trauma is to increase the permeability of the endothelium. Patients who have a normal concentration of serum protein preoperatively are likely to demonstrate a drop of as much as 1 gm/100 ml in the plasma albumin concentration after an operation of the magnitude of a gastric resection.

Beattie et al. observed a sustained hypovolemia and extracellular fluid volume expansion following cardiopulmonary bypass which they attributed to a decrease in oncotic pressure as a result of a decrease in concentration of plasma albumin. There is a delay in the mobilization of extravascular albumin in these patients probably because of a persistent increase in capillary permeability. They theorize that there may be release of a factor from white blood cells and platelets in the course of damage from the pump oxygenator which increases the capillary permeability. This explanation would not seem to account for a persistence of the increase in extracellular fluid and a decrease in circulating blood volume for as long as 6 days. Such a finding is similar to the situation in the nephrotic syndrome where there is an increase in capillary permeability. A practical point is made by Beattie that such patients may require the increase in total body water and extracellular fluid volume in order to sustain an adequate circulation. The use of diuretic agents to reduce the extracellular fluid load could reduce the blood volume sufficiently so as to interfere with circulation.

Dieter et al. observed that patients who had been depleted of sodium by preoperative diuresis tended to retain more sodium and fluid during the early postoperative period because of the increase in secretion of aldosterone and the exchange of sodium for potassium in the distal convoluted tubule. Patients who have undergone diuresis preoperatively have an increased loss of potassium in the urine postoperatively. If they are digitalized and the digitalis is near a toxic level, a sudden decrease in concentration of serum potassium may induce digitalis intoxication. There are, therefore, patients in whom the phase two excess of extracellular fluid should not be treated vigorously. In most patients in whom the intraoperative and immediate posthemorrhage resuscitation fluids are limited to 3.5 liters of saline it is not necessary to use diuretics, and pulmonary edema is unlikely as long as additional electrolyte-containing solutions are not administered during the first postoperative week. This does not mean that fluids that are lost from the gastrointestinal tract should not be replaced, but additional electrolyte solutions are not required.

Prevention is always better than treatment. Trudnowski reviewed a three-year experience involving the intraoperative use of Ringer's lactate solution containing 5% glucose. This is fairly widely used and is consistent with the guidelines laid down in the *Manual for Preoperative and Postoperative Care* of 1971 in a section written by Shires. During a major operation 700 ml/hour of electrolyte solution should be given up to a limit of 3500 ml and all blood loss should be replaced as it is lost provided the volume lost is in excess of 500 ml.

In the treatment of hemorrhagic shock for an average-sized

adult, several liters of lactated Ringer's can be given fairly rapidly while the blood is being cross-matched and, if needed, additional electrolyte solution can be given along with the blood up to a total of 3.5 liters of lactated Ringer's plus whatever amount of blood is necessary to restore normal circulation. Five per cent glucose in the lactated Ringer's solution is probably advantageous since the glucose will be used for energy and will help to suppress fatty acids and to prevent fatty acid toxicity. During an operation and during resuscitation in hemorrhagic shock, or following accidental trauma, nonelectrolyte solution should not be given. Mannitol should probably not be used except in those instances wherein the physician has given as much blood and electrolyte solution as he feels is required, and the patient remains oliguric. In most instances, oliguria is an index of inadequate resuscitation, and the treatment should be an increase in blood transfusion or administration of electrolyte solution or both.

Following the day of resuscitation no further electrolyte solution should be given beyond replacement of abnormal fluid losses such as from the stomach or other parts of the gastrointestinal tract. Careful monitoring of body weight and intake and output will assist the physician in deciding whether diuretics are indicated to help unload the electrolyte solution that was administered during resuscitation.

DIGESTIVE TRACT FLUID LOSS

The digestive juices are secretions which are derived primarily from extracellular fluid, but there is alteration in the electrolyte composition in the course of secretion. Acute loss of digestive juices does not alter the tonicity of the fluid remaining in the body (Fig. 3-3). Of course, associated with the fluid loss there may be an inability of the patient to eat and drink, and over a period of time there would be a total body water deficiency and an increase in concentration of sodium and other body solutes. In other situations where the patient is able to ingest water, there might develop a pure salt deficiency which will be discussed later in this chapter. With severe acute vomiting and diarrhea, the patient may lose a large volume of extracellular fluid to the extent of being hypotensive and still have a normal sodium concentration in the fluids remaining.

If the fluid loss is neutral, the anion composition of the blood may also remain normal. If the fluid is lost from an acid-secreting stomach, the blood chloride will be low and CO_2 high, as discussed in Chapter 6. If bile and pancreatic juice are the predominant fluid lost, the result is a hyperchloremic acidosis, as is illustrated in Figure 3-3.

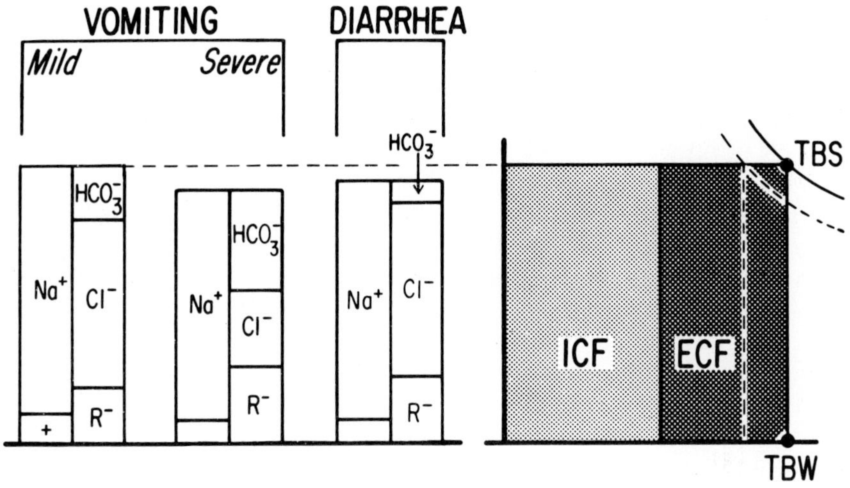

Figure 3-3. Loss of digestive tract fluid decreases extracellular fluid volume but does not alter tonicity. There is likely to be a change in chemical composition and acid-base balance.

In contrast to the sequestration or inactivation of fluids discussed earlier in this chapter, loss of gastrointestinal fluid is more likely to be measured. Replacement can be designed on the basis of the volume and approximate composition of the fluids lost. Since all of the fluids in the body and in the gastrointestinal secretions are of approximately the same tonicity and since isotonic saline and 1/6 molar sodium lactate can be combined in varying proportions to simulate the type of fluid lost, the treatment is simple and can be based upon information obtained at the bedside. For example, while making morning ward rounds, if the bottles are emptied at midnight, there will be approximately one-third of the day's loss of digestive juices in the gastric suction bottle. Determination of the pH with pH paper indicates the ratio of necessary replacement fluids. If the gastric aspirate is below pH 3, saline is used (Fig. 3-4). If the pH is around 7.4, a ratio of saline to 1/6 molar sodium lactate of 4:1 is approximately the composition of the fluid loss. If the pH is above 7.4, a ratio of 2 parts isotonic saline and 1 part 1/6 molar sodium lactate is indicated. Following the recommendation of Lans et al., 40 mEq of potassium chloride are added to each liter of replacement solution, provided, of course, that the urinary output is adequate.

All of these replacement fluids should include 5% glucose in order to provide additional calories. Obviously patients receiving treatment for loss of gastrointestinal juices are not eating, and the caloric intake from intravenous fluids is seldom adequate. In addition to the replacement of loss of abnormal fluid, as with loss from the gastrointestinal tract, the prescription must include fluids for metabolic needs such as insensible loss and urine as well as the fluid and electrolytes necessary for correction of the patient's past deficit. When the total requirements for the day have been estimated, an order should be written for the nurse so that she can provide standard units of intravenous fluids that are available in the hospital with a minimum of mixing and adding of substances to the intravenous fluids. For example, the following order might be written for a patient who is losing alkaline digestive juices at a rate of 1500 ml per day on the first day after operation. It is assumed that this patient has no existing abnormalities of volume, tonicity, and chemical composition and no acid-base imbalance; therefore no fluids are required for correction of past abnormalities.

1) 1000 ml isotonic saline in 5% glucose, 40 mEq KCl
2) 500 ml 1/6 molar sodium lactate in 5% glucose, 20 mEq KCl
3) 1000 ml 5% glucose, 40 mEq KCl, 1 ampule vitamin B complex
4) 500 ml 5% glucose

Run at 33 drops/min (16 drops equal 1 ml) or 3000 ml/24 hours

TABLE 3-1. TOTAL VOLUME OF DIGESTIVE SECRETIONS PRODUCED IN 24 HOURS BY ADULT OF AVERAGE SIZE

Saliva	1500 ml
Gastric secretions	2500 ml
Bile	500 ml
Pancreatic juice	700 ml
Secretions of intestinal mucosa	3000 ml
Total	8200 ml

GASTRIC JUICE

Gastric juice usually has around 60 mEq/l sodium and 100 mEq/l of chloride. Isotonic saline has 155 mEq/l of sodium and 155 mEq/l of chloride. If the gastric juice volume is in the range of 500 to 1500 ml per day, then isotonic saline will provide some excess of both sodium and chloride, but the kidneys will be able to excrete the surplus of these ions. Empirically, following the experience of Lans et al., mentioned in Chapter 1, 40 mEq of potassium chloride should be added to each liter of saline used for replacement of gastric juice loss. This also may require ex-

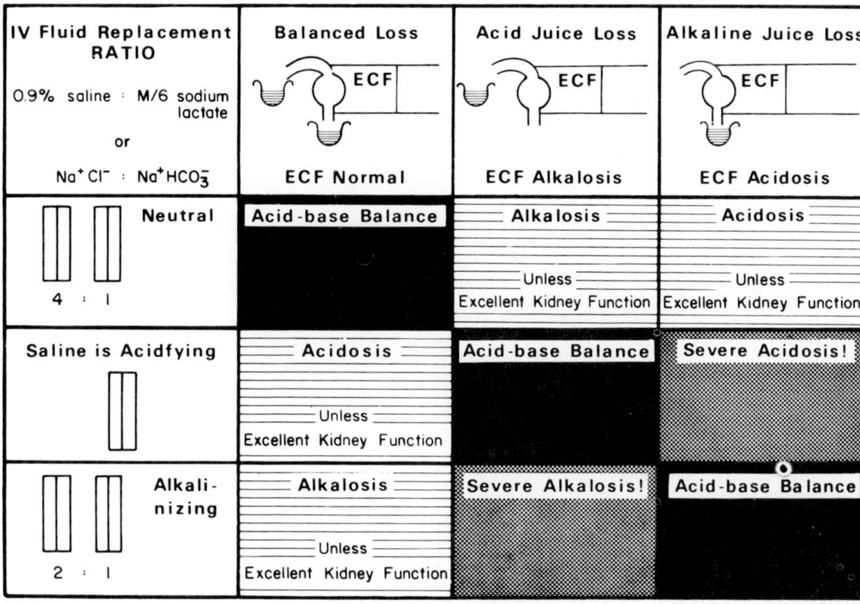

Figure 3-4. Summarizes the types of digestive juice loss and resulting acid-base balance across a contingency table and the three major types of fluid treatment in the first column at the left. Appropriate treatment corrects and inappropriate treatment exaggerates the abnormal acid-base balance resulting from loss of digestive tract contents. Testing with pH paper provides a bedside means of monitoring the fluid lost and urine so as to maintain acid-base balance.

cretion of some of the excess potassium since gastric juice normally has approximately 8 to 10 mEq/l potassium. If a patient loses 2 or more liters of gastric juice having a pH less than 1, it may be necessary to make up a solution with 0.5% saline containing 78 mEq each of sodium and chloride plus 60 mEq of chloride as ammonium chloride and 20 mEq as potassium chloride.

Repeated examination of the pH of the urine is an inexpensive way to determine the appropriateness of the replacement solution. A patient who loses acid gastric juice is likely to develop an alkaline urine unless, of course, a potassium deficiency exists. Under the latter circumstances the urine will be acid even when the patient has a metabolic alkalosis because of the intracellular acidosis which results from replacement of intracellular potassium with 1 part hydrogen and 2 parts sodium. During the course of management, the occasional determination of serum chloride, CO_2, potassium, and sodium concentrations will assist one in determining the need for some change in the composition of replacement solutions.

A patient requiring liters of replacement for very acid gastric juice may have a gastrin-secreting adenoma or carcinoma of the pancreas or duodenum, and such a patient may require a total gastric resection. Early attention to the patient's nutrition will improve the chances of success of such operative treatment. Since the total daily intravenous fluid therapy may require 5 or 6 liters of fluid, it is possible to incorporate amino acids and hypertonic glucose in a day's fluids and still to use a replacement solution which is less concentrated than would be required to nourish most patients. If prolonged parenteral fluid therapy is a possibility and central venous nutrient is to be used, the latter should be ordered to be given at a constant rate throughout the 24 hours so as to maintain a uniform blood glucose level and a relatively uniform stimulation of insulin secretion. The other fluids can then be given in a side arm proximal to the millipore bacterial filter.

PURE SALT DEFICIENCY

Patients who lose digestive tract juices acutely have a decrease in volume of the extracellular fluid but no change in the concentration of serum sodium (Fig. 3-3). If, however, a patient loses extracellular fluid by wound drainage, vomiting, diarrhea, or intestinal fistula and is allowed to drink water or is given intravenous glucose solution without replacement of any of the electrolytes that are lost, the result is a pure salt deficiency. This condition was produced experimentally in animals by Darrow and Yannet in 1935, and by Elkington et al. in 1947, and in man by Butcher in 1965. If the pure salt deficiency is sufficiently severe, the patient will develop circulatory insufficiency, oliguria, and anuria, and as observed by Darrow and Yannet, such animals do not respond to blood transfusion but require replacement of the electrolytes that have been lost.

Although the fluid lost from the body comes from the extracellular space, as the patient drinks water, the water distributes throughout all of the body water. If enough water is taken to replace that which has been lost the result is a normal total body water, but an internal shift produces a deficit of extracellular fluid including plasma volume and an expansion of intracellular fluid (Fig. 3-5). Total body solute is decreased and the concentration of all of the body electrolytes is decreased, which is evidenced by the low concentration of serum sodium. The sequence of events leading up to the observation of a low sodium concentration should, in most cases, allow the physician to decide whether the patient has a pure water excess, a pure sodium chloride deficiency, a total body potassium deficiency, or possibly the retention of glucose and/or urea, all of which produce a low concentration of sodium in serum.

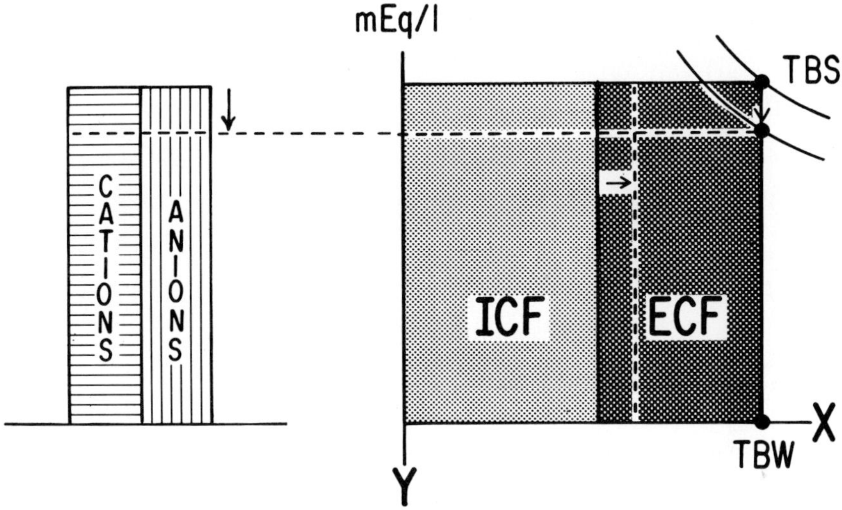

Figure 3-5. A pure salt deficiency causes an increase in intracellular fluid volume and a decrease in extracellular fluid volume as well as a decrease in tonicity (decrease in concentration of major cations and anions).

The contraction of extracellular fluids in pure salt deficiency includes plasma, and the expansion of the cellular fluids includes the red blood cells. The result is that the hemoglobin and hematocrit are markedly increased in pure salt deficiency, whereas they would be normal or lowered in the other conditions mentioned. The white blood count is usually elevated more than the hematocrit or hemoglobin. For example, in a patient who was admitted with a sodium of 112 mEq/l, the hemoglobin was observed to be 19 gm% and the white blood count 53,000/mm.[3] Such a high white blood count leads one to suspect a severe infection, but the temperature in such patients is subnormal. In the course of the next 4 days as the serum sodium rose to 130 mEq/l, the hemoglobin fell to 12.9 gm% and the white blood count decreased to 10,900/mm^3.

The treatment of pure salt deficiency involves simply the replacement of extracellular electrolytes. In the above-mentioned patient, peritoneal dialysis was used because the patient was anuric, elderly, and of normal body weight, and we were concerned that in the course of the administration of large amounts of sodium chloride solution, that we might precipitate cardiac decompensation. The use of peritoneal dialysis allowed us to restore extracellular fluid electrolytes without changing total body water. Of course the water moved from the cellular space into the extracellular fluid as sodium and chloride moved from the dialysate into extracellular fluid.

In most instances, the patient is not as depleted as the patient mentioned, and there is still adequate renal function so that it is safe to start out with hypertonic saline solution and then subsequently to complete the replenishment by the use of isotonic saline or lactated Ringer's solution. The patient is allowed to excrete the water which moves from the cellular space into extracellular fluid and to retain the electrolytes. Moyer recommended that not more than 9 gm of salt be given at any one time as a hypertonic salt solution. This amounts to 300 cc of 3% saline or approximately 200 cc of 5% saline. Before repeating such a dose, the patient should be reexamined and the serum electrolytes reanalyzed.

The total amount of salt which will be required can be predicted on the basis of the percentage decrease in concentration of sodium observed when the diagnosis is first made. If the concentration of sodium is 15% below normal, it will require enough salt to raise the total body solute by 15%. In other words, it will require that amount of salt which would normally be present in 15% of the total body water. This amount of salt should not be given in one fluid order. Often patients have a combination of salt depletion and total body water excess, and some of the correction of the low serum sodium concentration requires hypertonic and isotonic saline solution but some of the increase in sodium concentration results from a diuresis of excess total body water. Serial sodium determinations, body weights, and careful records of intake and loss during treatment should resolve any question about the original diagnosis.

PANCREATITIS

Replacement of extracellular fluid and plasma is a prominent part of the successful early care of patients with pancreatitis, and the choice of fluids depends upon one's estimate of the nature and severity of the disease. Without going into the etiology of pancreatitis, the sequence of events can be described as an increase in permeability of the pancreatic ducts with pancreatic enzymes leaking out into the interstitial fluid where they become active and cause inflammatory reactions and further disruption of membranes. There results an outpouring of protein-rich fluid from the plasma and the production of a glary, gelatinous edema. What happens next depends on the relative amounts of pancreatic enzymes and the antiproteolytic activity of plasma proteins as well as the amount of vasoactive and toxic material that is developed in the edematous gland. It depends as well on how rapidly the edema fluid can be carried away by the lymphatics draining into the thoracic duct and the movement of fluid away from the pancreas through the lymphatics in the diaphragm and through the retroperitoneal tissues and peritoneal cavity.

The loss of red blood cells into the area and particularly the appearance of *Esch. coli* will convert the process into a hemorrhagic pancreatitis with necrosis. It is not necessary to have a diffuse hemorrhagic pancreatitis for bleeding to occur. In some instances, the erosion into a larger vessel may cause severe hemorrhage, and if the bleeding point is secured the prognosis may still be satisfactory. There may be infarction and necrosis of the entire pancreatic gland. The destruction of tissue may be more localized with formation of a pseudocyst which is well circumscribed. Occasionally the pancreatic juice and edema fluid leak out into the peritoneal cavity and cause a massive ascites which interferes with breathing. The enzyme-rich fluid may diffuse toward the diaphragm and be carried through into the pleural cavity by the diaphragmatic lymphatics. This may cause a pleural effusion with compression of the lung.

It is evident that the local effects will cause severe pain and interference with breathing from compression of the diaphragm and lung, as well as interference with the function of the digestive tract, especially the stomach and duodenum. In addition to the loss of fluid into the area and into the peritoneal cavity, there may be loss of fluid from vomiting. If the patient is obese, as is often the case in patients with pancreatitis secondary to biliary tract disease, there may be little evidence of extracellular fluid loss insofar as there is any change in skin turgor, but the loss of extracellular fluid and plasma proteins may amount to 2 or 3 liters. The process often does not come and go with the rapidity of a traumatic or thermal injury. Comparisons of various treatments of experimentally produced pancreatitis in the laboratory have given misleading results when the experimenter has administered different types of fluid in conjunction with the initial production of pancreatitis but failed to continue therapy with that regimen over a longer time span.

The progressive nature of the changes in the pancreas and surrounding tissue was illustrated by the observation made by Edmondson and Berne that the average serum calcium for a group of these patients reached its lowest point on the sixth day, at which time it was 8.4 mg%. From patients who had died from severe pancreatitis, they removed the pancreas and surrounding tissues at the time of autopsy and found, after one day of disease, as much as 200 mg of calcium and, on the seventeenth day, as much as 1732 mg of calcium in these tissues. Calcium is removed from the body fluids by the formation of soaps with the released fatty acids, as pancreatic lipase hydrolyzes triglycerides. They observed a slow return to normal in the more severe episodes of pancreatitis and observed that in those patients whose serum calcium dropped below 7 mg/100 ml, that a fatality was likely. The relationship between the development of tetany and the serum calcium level was poor, giving rise to the suggestion that perhaps magnesium was also precipitated in the soaps and that a low serum magnesium level might account for tetany observed in those patients in whom the serum calcium was only mildly depressed.

Hernandez et al. administered calcium repeatedly in the intravenous fluids to a patient with pancreatitis, without correcting hypocalcemic tetany, and finally administered parathyroid hormone, with a marked improvement in the serum calcium level, and with relief of symptoms. They subsequently concluded that this particular patient had adrenal insufficiency and also parathyroid insufficiency. This led to a series of experiments in animals subjected to parathyroidectomy and premedicated with Dihydrotachysterol and calcium before being subjected to experimental pancreatitis. The lowering of serum calcium and magnesium was greater in parathyroidectomized than in normal animals subjected to pancreatitis. Injections of parathyroid hormone in animals made hypocalcemic by pancreatitis and hypoparathyroidism resulted in an elevation of the serum calcium and serum magnesium and an increase in phosphate excretion in the urine. It appeared, therefore, that the parathyroid glands permitted compensation for loss of calcium and magnesium into areas of fat necrosis. These data also add incentive to analyze serum magnesium in patients who have become hypocalcemic and especially those with tetany, which does not seem to be explained by a mild hypocalcemia.

Another manifestation of the progressive and evolutionary nature of this complicated disease is the development of pulmonary insufficiency. It has been said that there are stages of acute pancreatitis running through shock, pulmonary insufficiency, and sepsis. Respiratory complications have been observed in 20 to 70% of patients, according to a review by Finley. Whenever pulmonary complications develop in a disease requiring vigorous treatment of shock and administration of fluids, the question will arise as to whether pulmonary complications have resulted from overtransfusion or overinfusion of electrolyte solutions. In some instances this may well be a factor.

I remember a child in whom the distention of the abdomen was the prominent manifestation of pancreatitis, and elevation of the diaphragm was so marked as to interfere with ventilation. We could have made the diagnosis by determining the amylase concentration of peritoneal fluid. We should have been highly suspicious of the diagnosis since a sister had been operated upon as an infant for what was thought to be a retroperitoneal fibrosarcoma and had subsequently developed a pseudocyst of the pancreas and diabetes. The diagnosis in my patient was actually made during a laparotomy which was performed in part to relieve the patient of respiratory distress. Postoperatively it was necessary to give large amounts of saline in order to replace the fluid which was lost into the peritoneal cavity as ascites reformed. When the child became distressed again by distention of the abdomen and elevation of the diaphragm, the fluid was aspirated for a few days as needed to allow adequate respiration. There was no evidence of toxicity in this patient, but respiratory distress was created by the mechanical effect on the diaphragm.

Usually respiratory distress is not so obviously due to mechanical factors and is not so easily relieved. Atelectasis, pneumonitis, pulmonary emboli and thrombosis, added to the mechanical difficulties, create a problem which is as intractable as the chemical stage of massive fat embolism or the post-traumatic wet lung syndrome which is discussed in Chapter 9.

Vogel and Zieve have demonstrated a lecithinase in the duodenal contents in man. Surfactant contains lecithins that are excellent substrates for this pancreatic enzyme, and it has been postulated that the atelectasis observed in patients with severe pancreatitis may result from the inactivation of surfactant by lecithinase, which is released from the pancreas and carried through the blood stream to the lung. That such an enzyme could remain active in the blood stream was demonstrated when Morgan et al. injected phospholipase obtained from cobra venom into peripheral veins of dogs. Surface tension in the lungs increased following the injection.

PANCREATITIS AND RENAL FAILURE

Renal failure does not occur as frequently as pulmonary failure in patients with pancreatitis, but the factors causing renal failure may be both as obvious in some patients and as obscure in others. The obvious cause of renal failure is massive loss of fluid with obvious signs of shock. In a review of 60 patients with pancreatitis observed at the University of Iowa between 1940 and 1960, Foster and Ziffren found 23 who had developed circulatory collapse; 20 of these died. Nine of the 23 became anuric or had oliguria or azotemia. Only 2 patients developed azotemia in the absence of vascular collapse.

In most instances, renal failure is probably due to circulatory insufficiency. Many surgeons have observed patients, however, who developed renal insufficiency without any obvious circulatory collapse. Beisel et al. reviewed some 32 patients with pancreatitis and 63 patients with acute renal failure observed over a 4-year period. There were 5 patients who had a combination of pancreatitis and renal failure. One of these patients had no documented evidence of shock. Appropriate observations could have been overlooked, but it may be that active enzymes, vasoactive substances, and other substances released from the pancreas made sufficient contribution to the renal failure so that an obvious change in vital signs really did not occur. Lee and Hills reported no cases of renal failure in some 30 patients observed at Kings College Hospital over a period of 10 years. In their recent experience, however, they observed 4 patients and in 2 instances there was no recognizable cause for the renal failure. In one patient the pancreatitis was not even diagnosed until autopsy. It has been suggested that perhaps the local inflammation causes an extreme discharge from the celiac plexus which adds to renal ischemia in these patients.

In most instances where renal failure occurs it is probably primarily the result of unrecognized and inadequately treated deficiencies in extracellular fluid and blood volume. Elliott found blood volume deficits averaging 1500 ml in patients with severe pancreatitis who had been treated with what clinically seemed to be an appropriate volume of fluid. He recommended 50 to 75 gm of albumin in addition to electrolyte solution. Hoxworth, who discussed the paper, suggested that stored plasma could be used in preference to albumin and at much lower cost.

EARLY MANAGEMENT OF PANCREATITIS

The severely ill patient who is seen early after the onset of pancreatitis will have a nasogastric tube in place in order to remove the acid gastric juice and prevent stimulation of secretin. This juice should be checked for pH and, if the gastric juice is acid, it should be replaced with 0.9% saline in 5% glucose. The deficit from local loss of fluid may be difficult to estimate but should be replaced with a liter of stored plasma (or 50 gm of albumin) and 2 liters of lactated Ringer's (or 1500 ml of 0.9% saline and 500 ml of M/6 sodium lactate). The rate at which this fluid is given and the addition of more of the replacement solution will depend upon the patient's response in terms of his blood pressure, pulse, urinary output, alertness, warmth of skin, and capillary refill. As soon as it is established that normal circulation is assured, serious consideration should be given to the infusion of high-calorie nutrient solution with amino acids and vitamins. The details of this are given in Chapter 4. Provision of a high normal blood sugar is one of the more effective ways of suppressing secretion of the pancreatic digestive enzymes. Nakajima and Magee used secretin-stimulated dogs with chronic pancreatitic fistulas and found a linear inverse relationship between pancreatic enzyme output and blood glucose levels following infusion of D-glucose. The inhibition was greatest for amylase and least for protease with lipase in between. The blood glucose levels were in a range which is frequently achieved in the course of providing patients with central venous nutrient. Dudrick observed a decrease in pancreatic fistula drainage in a patient treated with central venous nutrient. From these observations it would appear that the use of central venous nutrient in patients with pancreatitis not only should sustain a more healthy state of nutrition but may have a specific and beneficial effect in reducing secretion of pancreatic enzymes and thereby reduce the autodigestion which sustains the disease.

Kenwall and Wels reported 11 consecutive patients with severe pancreatitis who were treated with serum albumin. They were under the impression that the postoperative course was much less stormy and that the patients were able to leave the hospital sooner. The effectiveness of albumin has been explained as due to its plasma volume expansion, but it has also been suggested that it may provide a more specific antiproteolytic effect. Dextran has been used in place of plasma or albumin. The higher molecular weight or so-called clinical dextran has been used as a plasma expander without any significant improvement in the mortality rate in experimental pancreatitis. Schiller et al. administered clinical dextran, 75,000 average molecular weight, to a group of animals and compared the results with the administration of 40,000 molecular weight dextran and felt that the latter actually decreased the survival rate. They did observe, however, that the combination of low molecular weight dextran and steroids reduced the fluid loss and lowered the mortality.

In many of the experiments the fluid or agent tested has been given once and for a brief period of time. In view of the progressive and prolonged nature of pancreatitis the experimental treatment should probably be given over a longer period of time. Wright and Goodhead injected a mixture of blood and trypsin into the pancreatic duct and then ligated the duct in dogs and proceeded to treat different groups with infusions of the specific fluid every 8 hours for 3 days. In this study they produced 100% death in the control group. When plasma was used the mortality rate was reduced to 36%. The higher molecular weight dextran produced a mortality rate of only 20%, and the low molecular weight dextran group of animals had no deaths and no hemorrhagic pancreatitis. In a small group of dogs with treatment delayed for 12 hours, the low molecular weight dextran still was effective in preventing death and minimizing the severity of pancreatitis as observed at autopsy after sacrifice of the animals on the third day. These results were interpreted as showing that the higher molecular weight dextran and plasma were effective in expanding plasma volume and the clinical dextran was thought to have an antithrombotic action. The low molecular weight dextran was felt to produce an improvement in capillary blood flow preventing thrombosis and assisting in dissemination of the highly concentrated enzymes and other vasotoxic materials from the region of the pancreas.

The requirement for replacement of extracellular fluid and proteins and even blood will be reduced and the prognosis improved if fluids exuding from the pancreas can be drained away before their local irritating actions and toxic products give rise to further edema and fluid loss. If, in spite of nasogastric suction, maintenance of an adequate blood glucose level, the use of anticholinergics and antibiotics, there is not a rapid improvement, or if there is evidence of hemorrhagic pancreatitis, then an operation should be considered to assess the degree of damage and to establish drainage of the pancreatic area. The treatment was recently outlined by Jordan and Spjut. Gillesby, in discussion of this paper, recommended that if the pancreas were necrotic and black in appearance that, in addition to external drainage, a Roux-en-Y loop of small bowel be sutured over the area so that the necrotic material could drain into the lumen of the bowel.

In addition to establishing adequate drainage of the area, the surgeon will simplify further management of fluids and nutrition if he will place a suction gastrostomy and feeding enterostomy. This makes it possible to remove the nasogastric tube, keep the upper digestive tract at rest, administer nourishing fluids, and replace the aspirated juices removed from the stomach.

During the earlier stages of the disease it might be possible to drain away tissue fluids with their high concentration of noxious enzymes by cannulation of the thoracic duct. There is resistance to flow at the lymphatic-venous junction in the neck, and Dumont and Martelli have been able to minimize the edema in the pancreas in the experimental animal by this technique. Dreiling has used this in a few patients for the relief of massive pancreatic ascites which he feels is due to blockade of pancreatic lymphatics. In order for this to be effective, the block would need to be greatest above the site of cannulation. Much of the improvement in these few patients may have been due to the diversion of this toxic fluid away from the blood stream. In one of their patients the fluid removed from the thoracic duct was inadvisedly given intravenously and precipitated pulmonary edema. If thoracic duct drainage were attempted too late in the course of the disease—after the lymphatics were so obstructed as to prevent flow through the thoracic duct, after there already had been necrosis of the pancreas, and after appearance of red blood cells in the lymph—it is less likely that this would be of benefit. Schiller et al. drained the thoracic duct in dogs subjected to pancreatitis and observed initially a high flow rate but a precipitous reduction in lymph flow coincident with the appearance of red cells in chyle. Duprez, who participated in the study, had observed earlier that if the sanguineous lymph from such animals was injected into the pancreatic ducts of normal dogs this induced severe pancreatitis. Schiller commented about the difficulties of maintaining flow from a cannulated thoracic duct because of plugging with fibrin and cellular debris. If the thoracic duct drainage could be instituted early enough in the course of the disease and was maintained, this would be an ideal way to drain the toxic fluids away from the gland.

Schiller found that the use of low molecular weight dextran increased the loss of peritoneal fluid and increased the mortality rate when only 1 dose was given during the time of the initial insult, but if steroids were combined with low molecular weight dextran the fluid loss was reduced and mortality rate lowered. Perhaps some combination of steroids to reduce the permeability of endothelial and cellular membranes, drainage of the thoracic duct, and the use of low molecular weight dextran for maintaining lymph flow should be given further study in the laboratory.

Another approach to removing toxic fluids is the use of peritoneal dialysis. Wall observed that hemodialysis has not been effective in improving the prognosis of pancreatitis, probably because the chief area of damage is in the region of the pancreas and in some instances throughout the peritoneal cavity. The extent of this type of reaction is evident to the surgeon who finds masses of omental fat necrosis at the time of exploration. The time that it takes to develop the effects of this local action of the pancreatic juice is indicated by the fact that the lowest serum calcium is usually observed on about the sixth day of illness. Peritoneal dialysis would be likely to remove much of the enzyme-rich fluid from the peritoneal cavity and from the area of the pancreas and to so dilute the pancreatic enzymes as to minimize fat necrosis and the production of other toxic materials. Wall used Trasylol in the dialysate but it was probably the dilution and removal of the pancreatic enzymes rather than their inactivation in situ which was of benefit. He thought that three severely ill patients treated in this way demonstrated an improvement in their course coincident with the initiation of peritoneal dialysis.

Bolloki and Gliedman began peritoneal dialysis late in the course of the disease when all other treatments seemed to have failed and in a seemingly preterminal stage of the disease and observed dramatic improvement. One theoretical advantage of peritoneal dialysis is that it should remove toxic fluids coming from the pancreas even late in the disease when lymphatics and small vessels are thrombosed and when parts of the gland might be inaccessible to agents given via the intravenous route. One of the objections to the use of thoracic duct drainage has been that the drainage might be difficult to maintain in the later stages of the disease either because of occlusion of lymphatics in the region of the pancreas or because of plugging of the thoracic duct at a higher level. Peritoneal dialysis, in the experience of Bolloki, is effective even in late stages of the disease.

Rosato et al. injected taurocholate in the pancreas of guinea pigs and were then able to reduce the mortality from 77% to 32% by the use of peritoneal irrigation. The irrigations were given 90 min after the taurocholate and again in 150 min. During the first series of irrigations the amylase in the dialysate was observed to be markedly reduced between the first and the last exchange of fluid. Only a small rise in amylase concentration was observed in the peritoneal effluent at the beginning of the second set of irrigations indicating that this particular model of pancreatitis did not produce a progressive destruction. The treatment which was limited to 150 min was therefore effective.

ABDOMINAL FLUID ACCUMULATION

Accumulation of extracellular fluid in gastric dilatation, bowel obstruction, pancreatitis, peritonitis, and rapidly formed or re-formed ascites results in loss of effective extracellular fluid and requires replacement just as if a neutral extracellular-like fluid was being lost to the environment or was inactivated in damaged tissues. The volume may be difficult to estimate and depends upon the same type of clinical experience that serves in estimating the volume of fluid required for the traumatized patient. The fluid usually is lost rather than being temporarily inactivated so that a later period of reabsorption and potential pulmonary edema may be of less concern.

With massive and rapid increase in intra-abdominal fluid there is an increase in intra-abdominal pressure which may cause compression of the inferior vena cava and interference with venous return. Treatment requires replacement of lost fluid but of even greater urgency is evacuation of the fluid. Passi et al. have reviewed this mechanism in the pathophysiology of acute gastric dilatation. In the early postoperative period, in any patient who is developing signs of impaired circulation and in whom there is no functioning nasogastric tube, stomach contents should be aspirated.

Classically and in the late stages of gastric dilatation the venous circulation becomes obstructed before arterial flow is completely blocked. There is bleeding into the lumen along with an even more rapid expansion of the stomach. Some of this blocked fluid will run out the patient's mouth or be seen on the pillow, cheek, and bed clothes. Such a patient may have over a gallon of fluid in the stomach. Evacuation leads to a dramatic improvement as a result of increased venous return. The measured volume of lost fluid should be replaced with isotonic saline or Ringer's lactate and the infusion rate should be rapid at first and then slowed as urinary output, pulse, blood pressure, and other signs show a return to normal circulation.

REFERENCES

Beattie, H. W., Evans, G., Garnett, E. S., and Webber, C. E.: Sustained hypovolemia and extracellular fluid volume expansion following cardiopulmonary bypass. Surgery *71*:891, 1972.

Beisel, W. R., Herndon, E. G., Myers, J. E., and Stones, L.: Acute renal failure as a complication of acute pancreatitis. Arch. Intern Med. (Chicago) *104*:539, 1959.

Blalock, A.: Trauma to the intestines: the importance of the local loss of fluid in the production of low blood pressure. Arch. Surg. (Chicago) *22*:314, 1931.

Blalock, A.: Experimental shock: the cause of the low blood pressure produced by muscle injury. Arch. Surg. (Chicago) *20*:959, 1930.

Bolloki, H., and Gliedman, M. L.: Peritoneal dialysis in treatment of acute pancreatitis. Surgery *64*:466, 1968.

Botelho-Machado, J., and Adamsons, R. J.: Dimensions of the reactive zone of wound delineated by shifts of water between major fluid compartments. Surg. Gynec. Obstet. *134*:942, 1972.

Broido, P. W., Butcher, H. R., and Moyer, C. A.: A bioassay of treatment of hemorrhagic shock. II. The expansion of extracellular ions during hemorrhagic hypotension and possible relation to alterations in extravascular-extracellular tissue. Arch. Surg. (Chicago) *93*:556, 1966.

Butcher, H. R.: The pathophysiology of sodium depletion in man. Surg. Clin. N. Amer. *45*:345, 1965.

Carey, L. C., Cloutier, C. T., and Lowery, B. D.: The use of balanced electrolyte solution for resuscitation. In *Body Fluid Replacement in the Surgical Patient.* Fox, C. L., Jr., and Nahas, G. G., eds. New York: Grune & Stratton, 1970.

Darrow, D. C., and Yannet, H.: The changes in the distribution of body water accompanying increase and decrease in extracellular electrolyte. J. Clin. Invest. *14*:266, 1935.

DePalma, R. G., Holden, W. D., and Robinson, A. V.: Fluid therapy in experimental hemorrhagic shock: ultrastructure effects in liver and muscle. Ann. Surg. *175*: 539, 1972.

Dieter, R. A., Jr., Neville, W. E., and Pifarre, R.: Serum electrolyte changes after cardiopulmonary bypass with Ringer's lactate solution used for hemodilution. J. Thorac. Cardiov. Surg. *59*:168, 1970.

Dillon, J., Lynch, L. J., Jr., Myers, R., Butcher, H. R., Jr., and Moyer, C. A.: A bioassay of treatment of hemorrhagic shock. I. Blood, Ringer's solution with lactate, and macromolecules in experimental hemorrhagic shock. Arch. Surg. (Chicago) *93*:537, 1966.

Doty, D. B., Hufnagel, H. V., and Moseley, R. V.: The distribution of body fluids following hemorrhage and resuscitation in combat casualties. Surg. Gynec. Obstet. *130*:453, 1970.

Doty, D. B., Moseley, R. V., and Simmons, R. L.: Sequential changes in blood volume following injury and transfusion. Surg. Gynec. Obstet. *130*:801, 1970.

Dreiling, D. A.: Inhibitory effect of new anticholinergics on the basal and secretin stimulated pancreatic secretion in patients with and without pancreatic disease. Amer. J. Dig. Dis. *5*:639, 1960.

Dreiling, D. A.: The lymphatics, pancreatic ascites, and pancreatic inflammatory disease. Amer. J. Gastroent. *53*:119, 1970.

Dudrick, S. J., Wilmore, D. W., Steiger, E., Mackie, J. A., and Fitts, W. T., Jr.: Spontaneous closure of traumatic pancreaticoduodenal fistulas with total intravenous nutrition. J. Trauma *10*:542, 1970.

Dumont, A. E., and Martelli, A. B.: Pathogenesis of pancreatic edema following exocrine duct obstruction. Ann. Surg. *168*:302, 1968.

Edmondson, H. A., and Berne, C. J.: Calcium changes in acute pancreatic necrosis. Surg. Gynec. Obstet. *79*:240, 1944.

Elkinton, J. R., Winkler, A. W., and Danowski, T. S.: The importance of volume and tonicity of the body fluids in salt depletion shock. J. Clin. Invest. *26*:1002, 1947.

Elliott, D. W.: Treatment of acute pancreatitis with albumin and whole blood. Arch. Surg. (Chicago) *75*:573, 1957.

Finley, J. W.: Respiratory complications of acute pancreatitis. Amer. Surg. *35*:591, 1969.

Fleming, W. H., and Bowen, J. C.: The use of diuretics in the treatment of early wet lung syndrome. Ann. Surg. *175*:505, 1972.

Fogelman, M. J., and Wilson, B. J.: A different concept of volume replacement in traumatic hypovolemia: observations on injured man and animal. Amer. J. Surg. *99*:694, 1960.

Foster, P. D., and Ziffren, S. E.: Severe acute pancreatitis. Arch Surg. (Chicago) *85*:252, 1962.

Gauer, O. H., Henry, J. P., and Behn, C.: The regulation of extracellular fluid volume. Ann. Rev. Physiol. *32*:547, 1970.

Gollub, S.: Extreme hemodilution in man. In *Body Fluid Replacement in the Surgical Patient.* Fox, C. L., Jr., and Nahas, G. G., eds. New York: Grune & Stratton, 1970.

Guyton, A. C.: A concept of negative interstitial pressure based on pressures in implanted perforated capsules. Circ. Res. *12*:399, 1963.

Guyton, A. C.: Interstitial fluid pressure. II. Pressure volume curves of interstitial space. Circ. Res. *16*:452, 1965.

Guyton, A. C., and Lindsey, A. W.: Effect of elevated left atrial pressure and decreased plasma protein concentration on the development of pulmonary edema. Circ. Res. *7*:649, 1959.

Hardy, J. D., and Godfrey, L., Jr.: Effect of intravenous fluids on dehydrated patients and on normal subjects, cardiac output, stroke volume, pulse rate and blood pressure. J.A.M.A. *126*:23, 1944.

Hernandez, I. A., Powers, S. R., and Frawley, T. F.: The role of the parathyroid glands in calcium and magnesium metabolism in acute hemorrhagic pancreatitis. Surgery *50*:143, 1961.

Hopkinson, B. R., Border, J. R., Heyden, W. C., and Schenk, W. G., Jr.: Interstitial fluid pressure changes during hemorrhage and blood replacement with and without hypotension. Surgery *64*:68, 1968.

Ingraham, R. C., and Wiggers, H. C.: Alkalizing agents and fluids priming in hemorrhagic shock. Amer. J. Physiol. *144*:505, 1945.

Jordan, G. L., and Spjut, H. J.: Hemorrhagic pancreatitis. Arch. Surg. (Chicago) *104*:489, 1972.

Kenwall, H. N. and Wels, P. B.: Acute hemorrhagic pancreatitis. Surg. Gynec. Obstet. *96*:169, 1953.

Lee, H. A., and Hills, E. A.: Acute pancreatitis and renal failure. Postgrad. Med. J. *41*:471, 1965.

Levine, O. R., Mellins, R. B., and Fishman, A. P.: Quantitative assessment of pulmonary edema. Circ. Res. *17*:414, 1965.
Losowsky, M. S., Alltree, E. M., and Atkinson, M.: Plasma colloid osmotic and its relation to protein fractions. Clin. Sci. *22*:249, 1962.
Magilligan, D. J., Oleksyn, T. W., Schwartz, S. I., and Yu, P. N.: Pulmonary intravascular and extravascular volumes in hemorrhagic shock and fluid replacement. Surgery *72*:780, 1972.
Matthews, C. M. E.: Effects of plasmaphoresis on albumin pools in rabbits. J. Clin. Invest. *40*:603, 1961.
Moore, F. D., and Shires, G. T.: Moderation (Editorial). Ann. Surg. *166*:300, 1967.
Morgan, A. P., Jenny, M. E., and Haessler, H.: Phospholipids, acute pancreatitis and the lungs. Ann. Surg. *167*:329, 1968.
Moyer, C. A.: *Fluid Balance: A Clinical Manual.* Chicago: Year Book Medical Publishers, 1952.
Nakajima, S., and Magee, D. F.: Inhibition of exocrine pancreatic secretion by glucagon and D-glucose given intravenously. Canad. J. Physiol. Pharmacol. *48*:299, 1970.
Passi, R. B., Kraft, A. R., and Vasko, J. S.: Pathophysiologic mechanisms of shock in acute gastric dilatation. Surgery *65*:298, 1969.
Randall, R. E., Jr., and Papper, S.: Mechanism of postoperative limitation in sodium excretion: the role of extracellular fluid volume and of adrenal cortical activity. J. Clin. Invest. *37*:1628, 1958.
Rocchio, M., and Randall, H. T.: Wound kinetics. Amer. J. Surg. *121*:460, 1971.
Rosato, E. F., Chu, W. H., Mullen, J. L., and Rosato, F. E.: Peritoneal lavage treatment of experimental pancreatitis. J. Surg. Res. *12*:138, 1972.
Rosenthal, S. M., and Millican, R. C.: The role of fluids, electrolytes and plasma proteins in experimental traumatic shock and hemorrhage. Pharm. Rev. *6*:489, 1954.
Rush, B. F.: Treatment of experimental shock: comparison of the effects of norepinephrine, dibenzyline, dextran, whole blood and balanced salt solutions. Surgery *61*:938, 1967.
Rush, B. F., and Eiseman, B.: Limits of non-colloid solution replacement in experimental hemorrhagic shock. Ann. Surg. *165*:977, 1967.
Scott, V. B., Collignon, U. J., Bugel, H. J., and Johnson, G. C.: The relation of external pancreatic secretion to variations in blood sugar. Amer. J. Physiol. *134*:208, 1941.
Schiller, W. R., Duprez, A., Iams, W. B., Suwa, M., and Anderson, M. C.: Experimental pancreatitis. Arch. Surg. (Chicago) *98*:698, 1969.
Shires, G. T.: Fluid and electrolyte therapy. In *Manual of Preoperative and Postoperative Care.* Kinney, J. M., Egdahl, R. H., and Zuidema, G. D. eds. Philadelphia: W. B. Saunders Co., 1971.
Shires, G. T., Carrico, J., and Cohn, D.: The role of the extracellular fluids associated with major surgical procedures. Ann. Surg. *154*:803, 1961.
Shires, G. T., Cohn, D., Carrico, J., and Lightfoot, S.: Fluid therapy in hemorrhagic shock. Arch. Surg. (Chicago) *88*:688, 1964.
Shires, G. T., and Jackson, D. E.: Postoperative salt tolerance. Arch. Surg. (Chicago) *84*:703, 1962.
Simmons, R. L., Anderson, R. W., and Heisterkamp, C. A.: Blood and crystalloid requirements of combat casualties in Vietnam. In *Body Fluid Replacement in the Surgical Patient.* Fox, C. L., Jr., and Nahas, G. H., eds. New York: Grune & Stratton, 1970.
Simmons, R. L., Heisterkamp, C. A., Collins, J. A., Bredenburg, C. E., and Martin, A. M.: Acute pulmonary edema in battle casualties. J. Trauma *9*:760, 1969.
Trudnowski, R. J.: Ringer's lactate in operative hydration. J.A.M.A. *195*:545, 1966.
Vogel, W. C., and Zieve, L.: A lecithinase A in duodenal contents in man. J. Clin. Invest. *39*:1295, 1960.
Wall, A. J.: Peritoneal dialysis in treatment of severe acute pancreatitis. Med. J. Aust. *2*:281, 1965.
Wright, P. W., and Goodhead, B.: The value of dextrans in the treatment of experimental pancreatitis. Surgery *67*:807, 1970.

Chapter

4

Intracellular Solute

The healthy body has a cellular mass of sufficient size to accommodate the physical activity to which that body is accustomed. The same activity produces motion in the lymphatics so that albumin which leaks out of the vascular space is moved along in lymph and returned to the vascular space. There is thus a minimal amount of interstitial fluid and a negative interstitial fluid pressure with the skin held in tight approximation to the underlying tissues. The cells pump sodium out and maintain the potassium within. The young healthy body is full of potassium and vigor.

POTASSIUM AS CELLULAR CATION

As the years go by there is a steady decrease in muscle mass and total body potassium. The absolute volume of extracellular fluid remains fairly constant; but expressed as a percentage of body weight, the extracellular fluid tends to increase provided there is no accumulation of fat. If the older individual becomes ill and is confined to bed or has further decrease in his physical activity, there is further decrease in cellular mass. Interstitial fluid increases in volume during an illness, perhaps because of less physical activity. There is more albumin outside the vascular space and in compensation the kidneys retain enough sodium to maintain plasma volume. Antidiuretic hormone increases water retention enough to cause a mild lowering in concentration of sodium in the extracellular fluid and a lowering in concentration of potassium in cells. The cellular metabolic machinery is less well nourished, less efficient and less active in extruding sodium so that more sodium accumulates within cells. Potassium which leaks out of cells is excreted. Superimposed upon the changes of age and decreasing activity, there may be a specific additional change in body composition due to some disease process, with a further decrease in total body potassium and increase in total body sodium.

Serum potassium concentration is influenced by the total body potassium but also by current intake and loss, hydrogen ion concentration, and varying rates of potassium entrance into and exit from various organs so that plasma potassium concentration bears a poor relationship to total body potassium. Whereas sodium concentration can vary considerably within the cells, the variability of potassium in the extracellular fluid is limited to a ±4 mEq per liter. In a 70-kg man, there are around 3300 mEq of potassium in the body but only 70 mEq in the extracellular fluid. The intracellular potassium is inaccessible not only to diagnosis but also for treatment. Diagnosis must be by indirect observation. Treatment of even the most severe depletion must be with caution so as not to overload the extracellular fluid.

There are really two problems that may require management, total intracellular potassium and the serum potassium concentration. A nearly lethal high level of serum potassium may coexist with a total body potassium deficit, as in severe acidosis or renal failure. Obviously measures to reduce such a high serum potassium concentration must take precedence over measures to restore total body potassium. Such a patient requires close monitoring in order to begin the administration of potassium as soon as the acidosis or anuria is improving and before the serum potassium level drops to a dangerously low level. In other circumstances a treatment which restores a total body potassium deficit may cause a lowering of serum potassium to the extent of causing cardiac arrhythmia. For example, the administration of potassium in glucose to a patient with a marked total body potassium deficiency may cause a more rapid deposition of potassium in the cells than is balanced by the rate of administration of potassium in the infusion, with a resulting decrease in serum potassium to dangerously low levels. This is particularly hazardous if the patient is receiving digitalis, because the myocardium is rendered especially sensitive to a lowering of plasma potassium concentration.

The magnitude of potassium depletion may be as much as 300 mEq in a 70-kg man without causing any decrease in plasma potassium concentration and without causing signs or symptoms of potassium deficiency. As the total body potassium depletion reaches 10%, there usually does develop a lowering of plasma potassium concentration. The patient may lose as much as 1000 mEq of total body potassium and still survive. According to Schloerb and Grantham, as the percentage of body potassium deficit rises above 10%, there is a steady decrease in concentration of plasma potassium. A serum potassium of 3 mEq/liter is suggestive of approximately a 16% total body potassium deficiency. A serum potassium level of 2.5 mEq/liter is consistent with a 25% total body potassium deficiency. Such estimates are extremely crude and may be unreliable in a specific situation.

Potassium deficiency causes a patient to develop muscular weakness, lethargy, apathy, confusion, delirium, muscle twitching, abdominal distention, intractable edema, arrhythmias, tetany, and postural hypotension. These signs and symptoms are produced by other deficiencies which may well be present in a patient who has a marked depletion of potassium. Acid-base imbalance, magnesium deficiency, hypocalcemia, phosphate depletion, vitamin deficiencies, abnormal concentrations of fatty acids and amino acids could also be present in a seriously ill patient and could contribute to the signs and symptoms observed.

A potassium deficiency is likely to be present in a patient who has required intravenous fluids for a considerable period of time because of inability to take food and fluid by mouth. If in addition to intake failure there has been a loss of fluid from the gastrointestinal tract, potassium deficiency should be a consideration. Even without any abnormal loss from gastric suction, vomiting, diarrhea, purging, or a villous adenoma, there may well be sufficient loss from the kidneys to account for a total body potassium deficiency.

It is possible for a total body potassium deficiency to be the cause of a low concentration of serum sodium. Fichman et al. demonstrated this in patients with diuretic-induced hyponatremia. These patients had a 17.5% decrease in total body sodium plus total body potassium and a 25% decrease in concentration of serum sodium (Fig. 4-1). Total body water remained normal probably because of an increase in antidiuretic hormone secretion. Extracellular fluid was expanded and intracellular fluid contracted by 1.5 liters. There was a shift of sodium into the cells. Normally about 16% of the body sodium is in the cells, but in these patients 26% of the sodium was within the cellular fluid.

Plasma bicarbonate concentrations are a better index of total body potassium than potassium concentrations, provided the patient does not at the same time have some other basis for an abnormality in acid-base balance. The reason for this is that when total body potassium is decreased, the kidney is unable to excrete bicarbonate and excretes chloride in its place. This will be covered in more detail later on in this chapter when the interaction of steroids and diuretics is discussed in relation to the function of the nephron. It is also discussed in Chapter 6 since metabolic alkalosis, which will not respond to the administration of chloride, requires potassium for its correction.

The electrical activity of the heart is influenced by changes in extracellular fluid potassium to the extent that the electrocardiogram is used in diagnosis and in monitoring serum potas-

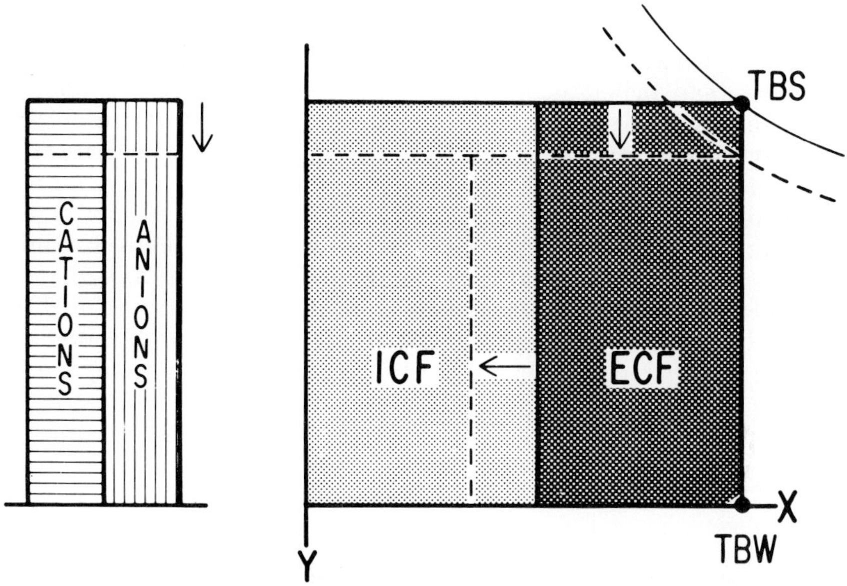

Figure 4-1. Illustrates the decrease in concentration of serum sodium which results from a body potassium deficit. Fichman described a patient with a decrease in potassium of 9 mEq/kg body weight. Twenty-six per cent of the body sodium was intracellular (16% is normal). There was a decrease in cellular volume by 1.5 l, and total body water was normal. The concentration of serum sodium was decreased by 25%.

sium levels. If the serum potassium rises or falls more than 4 mEq/liter from normal, the patient will die from cardiac arrhythmia. The chest lead used in monitoring variations in potassium concentrations during treatment should be securely taped to the chest since slight movement of this lead will cause variations in the height of the T-waves. In hypokalemia, the T-wave is depressed, and there is prolongation of the QT interval. As serum potassium levels rise above 7 mEq/l, the T-waves become high and peaked and there is prolongation of the PR interval. Atrial arrest may occur. The QRS widens and fuses with the enlarged T-wave and such a bizarre pattern is soon followed by asystole or ventricular fibrillation.

KIDNEY AND POTASSIUM

The kidney was designed to conserve body fluid and electrolytes and to excrete waste. Twenty per cent of the cardiac output passes through the kidney, and a large portion of this is filtered through the glomerulus. Eighty-five per cent of the filtrate is reabsorbed in the proximal tubule and all of the potassium is reabsorbed (Fig. 4-2). As the remaining fluid passes through the loop of Henle, sodium is pumped out of the lumen leaving a hypotonic fluid for the distal tubule. In the distal convoluted tubule, cation exchange occurs under the stimulus of aldosterone. Sodium is reabsorbed in exchange for potassium. This exchange occurs only slightly if aldosterone levels are low but can result in a marked saving of sodium at the expense of potassium if aldosterone levels are high.

Potassium retention or excretion by the kidney is closely related to ongoing sodium homeostasis. There are three factors which influence sodium conservation. The first of these is a reduction in glomerular filtration rate. The second is aldosterone. The third factor, which is not otherwise identified, is thought to cause an increased rate of sodium reabsorption in the proximal tubule. If reabsorption in the proximal tubule is sufficiently complete so that there is no sodium left for the loop of Henle, then the countercurrent concentrating process does not take place. The medulla does not become hypertonic, and there is no possibility for action

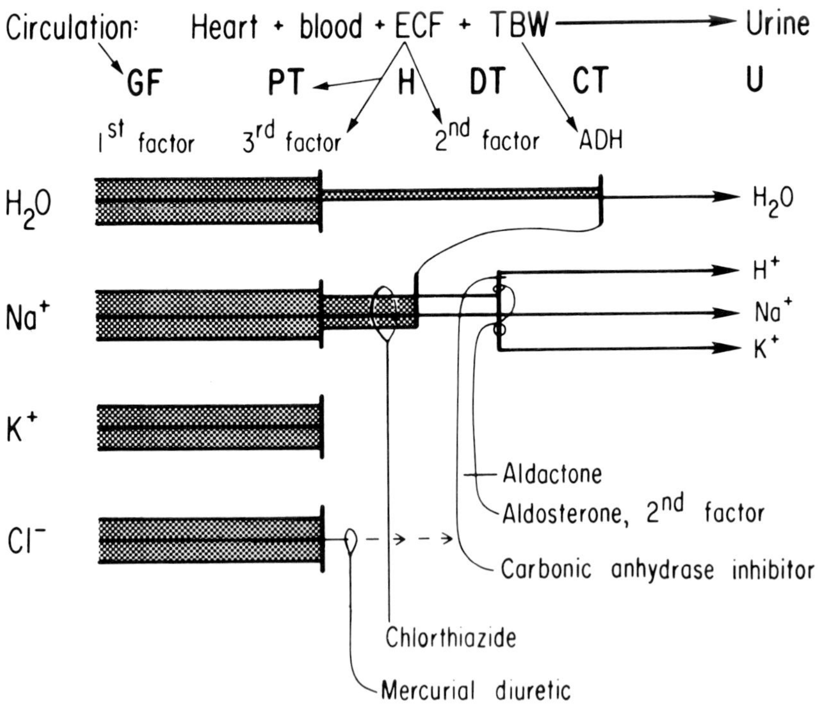

Figure 4-2. This is a suggestion as to how you might doodle your way through the text regarding the renal excretion of potassium under the influence of variations in sodium excretion, diuretics, and aldosterone. Urine is formed as a consequence of various circulatory variables and by action of successive parts of the nephron. There are three *factors* which regulate total body sodium. Diuretics also influence sodium and potassium loss. Conservation of sodium in the kidney causes an increase in potassium loss. See text.

of antidiuretic hormone. Also there is no action of aldosterone in the distal tubule since no sodium is present to be exchanged with potassium.

Diuretics have the potentiality of increasing potassium loss through two mechanisms, by causing more sodium to reach the distal convoluted tubule and by stimulating the production of renin, angiotensin, and aldosterone through a reduction in effective blood volume. Under such circumstances, spironolactone, an inhibitor of aldosterone, acts as a diuretic in that it blocks the cation exchange and promotes further secretion of sodium and preservation of potassium. Mercurial diuretics prevent the reabsorption of chloride in the proximal convoluted tubule, and sodium and water move along with the chloride into the distal tubule. The chlorothiazide diuretics act predominantly to prevent reabsorption of sodium in the proximal convoluted tubule, but also function as carbonic anhydrase inhibitors and prevent the formation of hydrogen ion which is otherwise exchanged for sodium in the distal convoluted tubule. Excretion of hydrogen normally permits reabsorption of sodium and to the extent that there is inhibition of hydrogen secretion, the exchange in the distal convoluted tubule is shifted in the direction of potassium loss (Fig. 4-2).

Patients who have received diuretics should be carefully evaluated for a possible potassium depletion, especially if there is a basis for suspecting increased aldosterone secretion or if the patient has been given steroids along with the diuretic. Spironolactone is not a diuretic but produces an increase in sodium and water excretion in those patients who have an increased secretion of aldosterone. It can therefore be used as a diuretic in selected patients without the risk of increasing potassium loss. Spironolactone can also be used as a functional test for aldosterone secretion. If a good diuresis can be induced with spironolactone, this indicates that the patient does have an increased secretion of aldosterone.

In view of the above-described relationship between aldosterone and renal potassium loss, you may wish to probe more deeply into the control of aldosterone secretion. Coghlan and Blair-West as well as Boyd and Peart have reviewed these relationships. In brief, a reduction in arterial pressure in the kidney may be the stimulus for the secretion of renin by the juxtaglomerular apparatus in the kidney. An alternative theory is that a reduction in the concentration of sodium in the distal convoluted tubule stimulates the secretion of renin. Renin functions as an enzyme with a substrate which is carried by α-2 globulin, producing angiotensin I, a decapeptide. A converting enzyme which is located primarily in the lungs converts angiotensin I to angiotensin II, an octapeptide, which is in turn degraded in the tissues by specific enzymes. Angiotensin II has a vasopressor effect but also stimulates the glomerulosa or outer portion of the adrenal cortex to secrete aldosterone. Aldosterone, acting upon the distal convoluted tubule, promotes potassium excretion and sodium retention. Patients with renal artery stenosis are likely to have a high plasma renin level and a high level of aldosterone with elevation of blood pressure.

In 1955 Conn described a syndrome, due to excessive aldosterone secreted by an adrenal cortical adenoma, in patients with hypertension, low serum potassium concentrations, elevation of serum sodium, metabolic alkalosis, polyuria, polydipsia, paresthesias, intermittent tetany, and periodic muscular weakness. Conn subsequently found that some of these patients did not have a low serum potassium. The diagnosis is made on the basis of a high aldosterone secretion rate with a low plasma renin level and a failure of elevation of plasma renin when the patient assumes an upright position after several days of a low sodium intake. According to a review by Boyd and Peart, Conn now feels that at least 7% of unselected patients with a diagnosis of essential hypertension harbor adrenal adenomata.

There are many causes for secondary hyperaldosteronism, including chronic heart failure and cirrhosis with ascites. Prolonged and major operations, particularly if they are accompanied by periods of hypotension or excessive blood loss or depletion of effective extracellular fluid, lead to increased secretion of aldosterone through the renin-angiotensin mechanism and in some instances through the stimulation of ACTH. In Chapter 3 some of the evidence was presented for internal inactivation of sodium and a decrease in effective extracellular fluid in patients following hemorrhage or trauma. Retention of sodium and an increased loss of potassium in urine in these patients are a sign of increased production of aldosterone.

POTASSIUM AND THE HEART

Surgeons operate upon the heart. They take care of patients who have cardiac disease, and they produce changes in electrolyte concentrations which influence the heart. The most frequent alteration of electrolytes influencing cardiac function is in potassium. Renal failure causes an elevation of serum potassium concentration and acidosis. Stimulated diuresis causes a loss of potassium and an alkalosis. Changes in hydrogen ion concentration in the extracellular fluid influence the concentration of potassium in extracellular fluid by virtue of exchange of hydrogen for cellular potassium. Acidosis causes a rise in plasma potassium concentrations, and alkalosis causes a fall in plasma potassium concentration. The dangers of abnormal serum potassium concentrations are related to the molecular biology of heart muscle. A brief review follows, but additional information may be obtained from the writings of Hoffman and Cranefield, Harris and Opie, and Laks and Elek.

Heart muscle has properties of excitation, conduction, and contraction. Excitation involves two types of fibers. There are automatic fibers in the atrium which, during diastole, slowly leak potassium and gradually depolarize until the electromotive force reaches a threshold, whereupon an action potential begins. Figure 4-3A depicts how a recording might appear from a single automatic fiber. Zero on the ordinate is the base line recording of an electrode placed in the fluid outside of the fiber. The negative potential of approximately 80 millivolts is the recording within the fiber at rest. There is a high concentration of potassium within the fiber and a low concentration outside, with a relatively impermeable membrane between, and a movement of potassium along this concentration gradient maintains the negative electromotive force within the fiber. There is a gradual depolarization of the automatic fiber due to a decreasing rate of potassium egress and when the threshold level is reached as indicated by the dashed line, there is a sudden influx of sodium which causes a shift of potential in a positive direction. Other fibers which are not automatic and which make up the majority of fibers in the heart maintain their resting potential until a wave of depolarization is propagated in the area. Rapid depolarization corresponds with the QRS complex in an electrocardiogram, which is the average effect of the changing potential of many fibers in the heart. Repolarization gradually occurs as the membrane becomes less permeable, as sodium is extruded, as potassium moves into the cytoplasm, and as the high potassium gradient again governs the resting potential by promoting movement of potassium out of the fiber. The resting potential is never quite as negative for automatic fibers as it is for the majority of myocardial cells and slowly decays towards the threshold potential and another excitation. The rate of decay of resting potential is increased by epinephrine, threshold potential is reached more quickly, cardiac rate is increased. Acetylcholine and vagal stimulation have an opposite effect. Calcium moves into the fiber immediately after depolarization and delays the redevelopment of a negative potential. The T-wave in the electrocardiogram marks the repolarization.

When the concentration of potassium in the plasma is lower than normal, the resting potential is even more negative. With increasing concentrations of potassium, the resting potential is raised and the slope of the resting potential in the automatic fibers is increased. The concentrations of calcium and magnesium have little effect upon the resting potential. The threshold potential is, however, governed by the concentration of calcium in the bathing fluid. An increase in calcium concentration shifts the threshold potential away from the resting potential, and a decrease in calcium concentration causes the threshold potential to move towards the maximum diastolic potential.

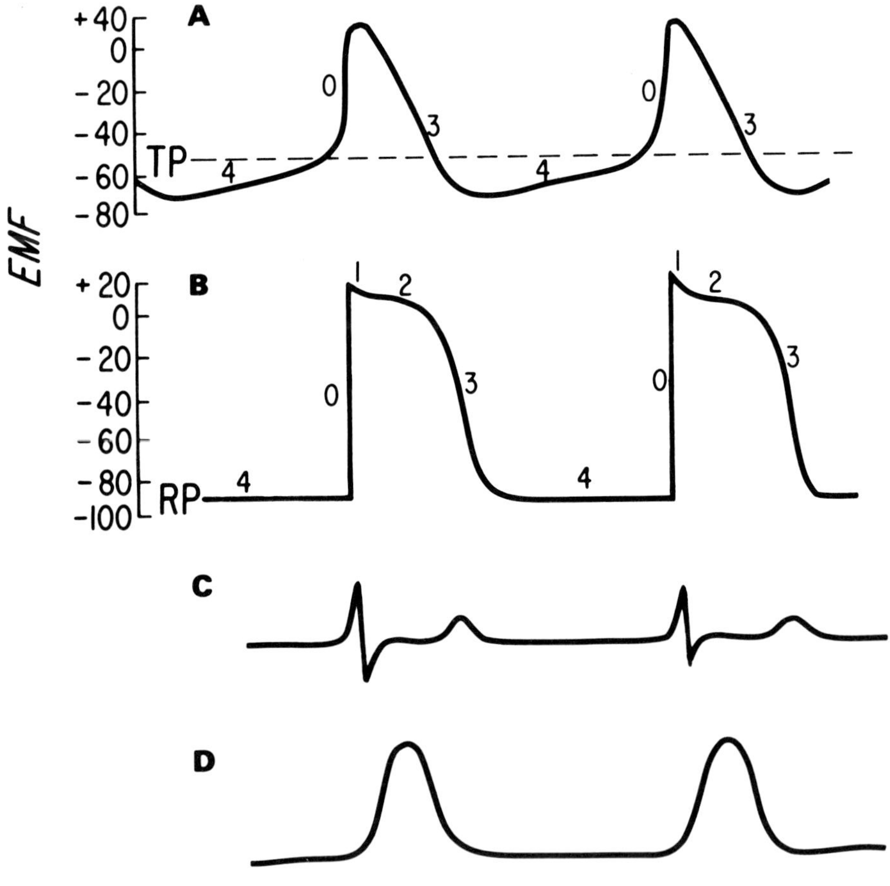

Figure 4-3. Shows the approximate temporal relationships between unipolar potentials in (A) an automatic fiber and, in a (B) Purkinje or other non-automatic type fiber. (C) shows how the rate of change in EMF appears on an ECG and (D) shows the rise and fall in muscle contractile force. TP = threshold potential towards which the automatic fibers resting potential drifts and marking the point at which an action potential "O" is initiated. RP = resting potential which is governed by the ratio of internal/external concentration of potassium. Phase "3" is the period of repolarization. (Modified from Hoffman and Cranefield.)

What was reviewed above had to do only with excitation. Calcium is also important in initiating contraction and in governing the strength of contraction of cardiac muscle. Contraction begins as rapid depolarization occurs and is thought to be due to a sudden increase in free calcium within the muscle fiber. Calcium probably moves into the fiber through a tubular system and is in addition released from the sarcoplasmic reticulum when rapid depolarization occurs. The increased internal concentration of free calcium activates an ATPase, and high phosphate bond energy is made available for muscle contraction. Anything which will increase the concentration of free calcium within the fiber will increase the tension of the contraction. Since additional calcium moves in during each contraction, an increase in rate tends to increase the amount of calcium within the fiber and to increase the tension of the contractions. An increase in concentration of calcium in the bathing fluid will promote the movement of more calcium into the fiber and increase the tension. Isoproterenol is one of the most potent agents for increasing calcium concentration within myocardial fibers. According to Fleckenstein, who participated in the symposium edited by Harris and Opie, an increase in concentration of potassium or magnesium will inhibit excessive isoproterenol-induced calcium incorporation. Cardiac glycosides facilitate calcium release from the sarcoplasmic or mitochondrial stores within the fiber during excitation so that more free calcium is available to activate ATPase and increase the strength of the contraction.

From what has been reviewed it is evident that extreme levels and rapid changes in levels of potassium and calcium in the plasma are to be avoided. A patient who is fully digitalized is near the toxic effect of that drug, and a slight lowering of potassium may precipitate digitalis toxicity. A patient treated with thiazide diuretics who has some depletion of his total body potassium and who is also digitalized is in a particularly vulnerable position. If he receives a number of blood transfusions during a major operation and from the sodium citrate is left with a metabolic alkalosis and if, in addition, he is overzealously ventilated so as to superimpose a respiratory alkalosis, the movement of potassium into his cells may lower the serum potassium concentration enough to cause cardiac arrhythmia or even death.

Davis and Fisch have reviewed the antiarrhythmic action of potassium which they feel is due to suppression of the slow diastolic depolarization of automatic fibers. Increasing the concentration of potassium also enhances conduction which serves to synchronize depolarization throughout the myocardium. Potassium should not be used for blocking abnormal rhythms in a situation where the serum potassium level is already high, where there is impaired renal function or where there is any significant degree of A-V block. Potassium must be given slowly in an intravenous drip and never pushed with a syringe.

Kunin et al. studied the effects of varying concentrations of glucose and varying concentrations of potassium in intravenous fluids and found little effect upon the electrical activity of the heart in normal individuals, but in patients depleted of potassium the stimulated deposition of potassium in the tissues as a result of glucose administration could exceed the rate of potassium infusion with resultant decrease in the plasma concentration of potassium. He therefore suggested that potassium might more safely be given in saline without added glucose in the early stages of repletion. Electrocardiographic monitoring was recommended if glucose solutions of potassium were to be used. Wright and Digiovanni reported a patient who had bursts of ventricular arrhythmias and ventricular fibrillation which were repeatedly corrected with direct current counter-shock conversion. Lidocaine and quinidine helped at first, but toxic levels of these drugs were soon reached. This was a patient who was being ventilated mechanically and there was variation in the P_{CO_2}. The patient finally became stable, with a normal rhythm, when the serum potassium was returned to normal, after a continuous intravenous infusion of potassium.

Hyperkalemia is a common cause of death in renal failure. We have learned to manage these patients with chronic dialysis, which has prolonged the life of individual patients, but this has also increased the number of opportunities for a patient to become involved in a potentially dangerous situation of potassium imbalance. Goggin and Joekes discussed the management of anesthesia during operations in patients with renal failure. These patients are often acidotic and have a total body potassium depletion at the same time that they have a normal or high concentration of serum potassium. When a patient is anesthetized, his P_{CO_2} becomes the responsibility of the anesthesiologist. A rapid change in ventilation rate may be sufficient to precipitate arrhythmia and death. This is because of the effect of extracellular hydrogen ion concentration upon movement of potassium into cells and the reciprocal relationship between the concentrations of extracellular potassium and extracellular hydrogen. Before induction of anesthesia an arterial blood gas and pH analysis should be performed, and then the P_{CO_2} should be maintained throughout the period of anesthesia and recovery at the same level as existed prior to induction. Frequently these patients are hyperventilating before operation; if this is true, the hyperventilation should be maintained at the same rate.

SMALL BOWEL FLUID LOSS

Potassium deficiency was recognized as a clinical problem first in infants with diarrhea and later in adults with prolonged gastric drainage, poor intake, and continued potassium loss in urine. Adults with diarrhea also lose large amounts of potassium. Surgeons have become sensitized to the problem through caring for patients with pseudomembranous enterocolitis, WDHA syndrome, ulcerative colitis, and occasional instances of villous adenoma. Cholera is not a surgical disease, but it causes a clinical pattern somewhat analogous to pseudomembranous enterocolitis and may help us to understand other severe diarrheal disease where potassium loss is a prominent part of the potential imbalance. Stimulated secretion of intestinal mucosa, rather than impaired absorption, is now considered as the mechanism of fluid and electrolyte loss in cholera and in some other diarrheal diseases.

PSEUDOMEMBRANOUS ENTEROCOLITIS

Pseudomembranous enterocolitis is an uncommon disease which is frequently unrecognized, but requires massive fluid replacement if the patient is to recover. In this respect it is very much like cholera. My first experience with this disease was a 78-year-old man weighing 70 kg, who was operated upon late one evening for a bowel obstruction secondary to a Richter's hernia. He had been given penicillin and streptomycin prior to being sent to our hospital. Twelve hours after the operation he began to have diarrhea; by the 36th hour after operation he appeared to be extremely ill with a pulse of 120/minute. His blood pressure, which had been 150/96 torr, was found to be 70 torr. He was having profuse rectal drainage, which was cultured. The rate of infusion of intravenous electrolyte solution was increased. This was a solution made up of isotonic saline and 1/6 molar sodium lactate in a ratio of 2:1 and with 40 mEq/l of potassium chloride added. He was given paregoric to try to decrease the diarrhea, but this only resulted in abdominal distention. In the course of the next 13 days the patient received 126 liters of intravenous fluid. On the fifth day of the illness, the patient received 17 liters of fluid. One morning the intravenous fluids infiltrated, and the nurse decided to wait until the physicians made rounds. This led to a 2-hour accumulation of fluid deficit which caused the patient to become hypotensive again. The patient was gradually depleted of serum proteins and reached the stage of having pulmonary edema when his blood pressure was satisfactory. If the intravenous infusion was slowed enough to relieve him of his pulmonary edema, he became hypotensive. He died shortly thereafter.

The cause of this patient's difficulty was never documented, but it is likely that he had an overgrowth of staphylococci in the intestine and that the diarrhea was due to excessive secretion of the intestinal mucosa stimulated by enterotoxin. Such patients may come to the attention of a physician because of the onset of shock, and only in retrospect is the magnitude of fluid loss recognized. Some patients do not pass a large amount of fluid from the rectum but simply develop distention of the abdomen. They may lose fluid both from the rectum and from the stomach. The fluid may have a light yellow color and appear very much like normal urine. It is not uncommon for a physician first seeing this fluid to raise the question of a rectovesical fistula with urine passing from the rectum.

This disease has always been present but perhaps at times has been unrecognized. In the early days of use of broad-spectrum antibiotics there may have been an increase in the incidence of the disease. An overgrowth of staphylococci may follow the suppression of normal colonic bacteria by antibiotics. The diagnosis should be made from smear or culture of the stool or of scrapings from the rectal mucosa. Isolation of the organism requires a culture medium treated with phenylethyl alcohol to inhibit the growth of coliform organisms. The disease has been produced in the chinchilla by Prohaska.

Successful treatment requires early recognition and vigorous replacement of fluid and electrolytes using isotonic saline and 1/6 molar sodium lactate solutions in the ratio of 2:1 with 40 mEq/l of potassium chloride added. This solution can be run at whatever rate is necessary to reestablish and maintain a normal pulse and blood pressure and normal skin turgor. This is the same sort of treatment which is effective in cholera. The difference is that cholera is self-limiting, and the first day of the disease is the worst, whereas pseudomembranous enterocolitis may go on for several weeks and lead to death, if the cause is not found and treated. A specific organism should be isolated and its bacterial sensitivities determined. As soon as the bacteriologic investigation is under way, all antibiotics that have been in use should be discontinued. Specific antibiotics are needed but while waiting for cultures and sensitivities, an educated guess should be made as to the antibiotic which would most probably be effective in the treatment of a staphylococcal infection. Prohaska et al. found that the effect of staphylococcal enterotoxin was blocked by ACTH. Blood and albumin may be required in the prolonged treatment of these patients, and as with other conditions in which the gastrointestinal tract cannot be used, nutrients should be added to the intravenous route.

The infrequency of occurrence of staphylococcal enterocolitis is both an advantage and a disadvantage. We seldom observe the condition, and it is likely not to be recognized until the patient is so depleted that he may not recover. The mortality rate has been reported as between 60 and 100%. If recognized early and treated appropriately, it should be no more lethal than properly managed cholera. Even better than early recognition is prevention. This is one argument for the use of mechanical bowel preparation and preservation of the normal flora which in turn suppresses overgrowth with hemolytic staphylococci.

WATERY DIARRHEA, HYPOKALEMIA AND ACHLORHYDRIA (WDHA) SYNDROME

Some of the patients with gastrin-secreting tumors of the pancreas and duodenum have diarrhea and may have large volume fluid loss. There is a related group of patients with non-beta islet cell tumors of the pancreas who have a syndrome of **watery diarrhea, hypokalemia,** and **achlorhydria,** the WDHA syndrome. Kraft et al. summarized the reports and the literature of 27 patients with this condition. These patients lose large volumes of fluid, which is more alkaline than pH 7.4, and is appropriately replaced with isotonic saline and 1/6 molar sodium lactate in the ratio of 2:1 with addition of 40 mEq of potassium chloride to each liter. According to Kraft, the average potassium loss is 350 mEq per day and the patients develop a hypokalemic metabolic alkalosis which is difficult to correct. The serum potassium level averages 2.2 mEq/liter and remains low until the tumor has been located and removed. Serum calcium levels are usually above normal. The reason for this is not known although it was suggested by Kraft that it might be secondary to magnesium depletion. Glucose tolerance curves are commonly diabetic in the WDHA syndrome.

Secretin may be the hormone in excess in this syndrome. Secretin stimulates secretion of water and bicarbonate by both the liver and pancreas and also inhibits acid secretion by the stomach. Many of these patients do not secrete acid until after the tumor has been removed, whereupon the stomach resumes a normal response to acid secretory stimulation. Dilated gallbladders have been observed in four of the patients reviewed by Kraft, which is also consistent with the thesis that secretin is the hormone in excess. Intestinal secretions may also be increased. The majority of the patients have had adenomata or carcinomas of pancreatic islet tissue, but in other patients there was found to be diffuse hyperplasia or so-called nesidioblastosis.

Such a patient at the University of Iowa Hospitals was a 28-year-old woman whose gallbladder had been removed in another hospital because it was very large, but no stones were found. She was unable to eat and passed 4 to 6 yellow to green liquid stools each day. She had continuous abdominal pain suggestive of chronic pancreatitis. She had lost 14 kg of body weight. Attempts to eat increased the diarrhea, particularly if fatty foods were ingested. Because of this and because of the upper abdominal pain, pancreatitis was suspected, so an exploratory laparotomy and a pancreatic biopsy were performed. The pancreas had a relatively normal gross appearance and an operative pancreatogram, obtained through the amputated tail, showed normal pancreatic ducts emptying into the duodenum. The exocrine pancreas had been replaced by fibrous tissue, and there was marked hyperplasia of the islet tissue with junctional areas between the ductal epithelium and the hyperplastic islet tissue, nesidioblastosis.

Prior to this exploration and biopsy of the pancreas, the patient had been given feedings through a central venous catheter as described in Chapter 7. These feedings were resumed for an additional 12 days after the exploration and prior to a 95% pancreatectomy. The use of central venous nutrient solution, along with replacement of gastrointestinal fluids, improved the nutritional status and permitted a third and major operation despite a prolonged and debilitating illness. Healing was normal and the patient was soon able to take fluid and foods by mouth and, with the help of pancreatic extract to assist in the digestion of her food, she made a satisfactory recovery and has remained well now for over 4 years.

Too often in the past, when such problems presented, attention has been limited to replacement of fluids and electrolytes, nutritional needs have been overlooked until malnutrition became obvious. This is discussed in detail in Chapter 7, but requires continual emphasis. Even the management of the fluid and electrolyte balance is simplified if the patient's nutrition is maintained.

DIARRHEA

Loss of 16 liters of fluid from the gastrointestinal tract in a day cannot be explained on the basis of impaired absorption of normal secretions. Studies of the action of various hormones and toxins involved in the production of voluminous watery stools have shown that a stimulated mucosal secretion, in addition to impaired absorption, is probably the explanation for such large volume fluid loss as is observed in cholera, pseudomembranous enterocolitis, and other conditions in which diarrhea is a prominent symptom. Zollinger et al. have identified the diarrheagenic hormone associated with non-beta islet cell tumors of the pancreas as secretin, which would seem to explain stimulation of bile and pancreatic juice and possibly stimulation of intestinal secretions, as well as inhibition of gastric acid secretion. Medullary carcinomas of the thyroid have been observed to cause diarrhea, and Williams et al. found that medullary carcinoma produces appreciable amounts of prostaglandins which are capable of stimulating intéstinal secretion. Kimberg et al. studied the toxin produced by *Vibrio cholerae* which stimulates intestinal secretion through an increase in the activity of cyclic AMP. Toxins produced by *Escherichia coli* and some strains of staphylococcus may stimulate intestinal secretion in a manner similar to the endotoxin of *Vibrio cholerae.*

The diarrhea which occurs in gastrin-secreting tumors of the pancreas and duodenum is probably related to the large amounts of very acid juice which, in the duodenum, interferes with the function of pancreatic enzymes.

The cause of diarrhea must be found and treated, by use of an appropriate antibiotic or by removal of the tumor which is producing a diarrheagenic hormone. As we learn more about stimulation of intestinal secretion it may be possible to counteract such stimulation either by a blocking action or by stimulating increased absorption of the secreted intestinal fluids. Fromm et al. have found that glucose in the intestinal lumen serves to increase absorption by small bowel mucosa, and may in addition inhibit mucosal secretion stimulated by cyclic AMP. Until specific measures can be found for decreasing the fluid and electrolyte loss, the patients must be kept alive by replenishing the fluids lost.

The large volume of loss from the gastrointestinal tract should not be looked upon as some new kind of regulatory organ like a third kidney, although as mentioned before, the color of the fluid may suggest urine. The fluid loss calls for accurate replacement in volume and composition rather than attempts to slow the loss by withholding intravenous fluids. Circulatory collapse may occur within a few hours if infusions are stopped. The loss of alkaline intestinal juices will produce a hyperchloremic acidosis especially if isotonic saline is used to replace the loss. Saline with its excess of chloride will exaggerate the hyperchloremic acidosis. Replacement should be with a ratio of 2:1, saline to 1/6 molar sodium lactate, with 40 mEq of potassium chloride added to each liter. Magnesium may be required if the diarrhea persists for more than a few days. The larger the volume of fluids required, the greater the opportunity for supplying nutrients and also the greater the importance of maintaining nutrition, since there is loss of protein in the fluids draining from the bowel.

MAGNESIUM

Magnesium is a divalent cation similar to calcium. Out of a total of around 1000 mEq of magnesium in an average-sized adult, 540 mEq are located in bone. Magnesium, like potassium, is also an important intracellular cation, and 450 mEq are located in cellular fluid. Total body magnesium is even less accessible to measurement than total body potassium because magnesium is concentrated in mitochrondria where it is important as a cofactor for many enzymatic reactions. The smallest portion of total body magnesium is located in extracellular fluid. Normal plasma magnesium levels range between 1.6 and 2.3 mEq/liter. Like calcium, about 1/3 of magnesium is loosely bound to albumin. An average diet supplies 30 mEq of magnesium per day. Ten mEq of this are absorbed, and 20 mEq excreted in the feces. One mEq of magnesium is excreted into the intestines and reabsorbed. The kidneys excrete 10 mEq of magnesium a day, maintaining the patient in balance. In contrast to potassium, magnesium, like sodium, can be conserved by the kidneys; there may be as little as 1 mEq of magnesium excreted per day if the kidneys are functioning normally and if the patient has a total body magnesium deficit.

Magnesium deficiency is likely to cause confusion of the patient, which in turn often confuses those caring for the patient. Such a patient is likely to have a serious illness with a number of possible causes for disturbed function of the central nervous system. Abnormalities in concentration of potassium, calcium, and hydrogen ion are especially likely. The physician's initial reaction to the patient's tremor, plucking at the bed clothes, twitches, hyperreactive reflexes, and positive Babinski may well be to suspect liver or central nervous system disease. The patient is initially disoriented in one or another spheres, but then becomes intensely confused. There are visual and even auditory hallucinations. Often the patient becomes combative and requires restraints to protect him from himself and to prevent the dislodgement of dressings or any tubes or catheters that are in place.

The diagnostic difficulties of magnesium deficiency are reminiscent of the problems in the diagnosis of potassium deficiency some 30 years ago. Perhaps there will come a time when serum magnesium concentrations will be part of the routine electrolyte analysis, and the correct diagnosis will be thrust before us. Even so physicians will need to know something about the patient's course and the signs and symptoms of magnesium depletion, because the manifestations of this depletion, and the serum concentrations, do not always correlate.

You may recall that neuromuscular irritability is related to the ratio: $\frac{(K^+) + (Na^+)}{(Ca^{++}) + (Mg^{++}) + H^+)}$ and usually more than one of these ions is abnormal. Whenever the serum potassium concentration is abnormal, an abnormal magnesium level should also be considered as a possibility. Patients with hypercalcemia from any cause are likely to develop a magnesium deficiency since there is competition between magnesium and calcium for reabsorption by the renal tubule. Malnutrition of sufficient severity to depress serum potassium levels is also likely to deplete magnesium stores. It takes somewhat longer for the patient to develop a magnesium deficiency which is symptomatic. When it does develop, the hypokalemia may be perpetuated by the magnesium deficit, and it will be necessary to correct both. Prolonged loss of gastrointestinal juices from intestinal fistulas, chronic diarrhea, or ulcerative colitis will, in time, produce a magnesium depletion unless adequate replacement is provided.

The patient with diabetic ketosis illustrates similarities between the management of potassium and magnesium depletion. During the early stages of oliguria the serum magnesium and potassium may both be high and then, as the patient is treated and his acidosis is corrected, both serum magnesium and potassium drop to dangerously low levels unless replacement is provided.

It is not necessary to provide magnesium in the intravenous fluid of a patient who is only receiving parenteral fluids for a few days and whose fluid and electrolyte balance has been normal up until that time. If the patient's illness is of a more serious nature or of longer duration and especially if there are abnormal losses of body fluids, then magnesium should be provided on a maintenance basis. Abnormal loss of magnesium should be replaced, and past deficits should be estimated and restored. Magnesium is present in some of the more complex intravenous solutions. The maintenance requirements may be supplied by these. A patient needs about 10 mEq of magnesium per day. This is the amount that he would normally absorb from his diet. If an actual symptomatic inadequacy of total body magnesium is suspected, because of the typical signs and symptoms noted above, and because of an illness which might produce this picture, the extent of the depletion may still be obscure because only 1% of the magnesium is normally present in the plasma and there are a number of factors which may influence the plasma concentration.

The serum concentration in magnesium deficiency is likely to be below 1.6 mEq/l. A cell biopsy can be easily obtained by use of the red blood cells which normally contain 5 mEq/l of magnesium. If the kidneys are functioning normally in other respects, they will conserve magnesium to the extent of reducing urinary magnesium concentrations to as little as 1 mEq/l, in contrast to 10 mEq/l in a healthy person. Even when the suspicion of magnesium depletion has been documented by these laboratory analyses, the treatment must be one of filling up the cells until plasma levels remain normal. There have been occasions when as much as 150 mEq of magnesium was given in a day's fluids and with a progressive decrease in the amounts on subsequent days until the serum magnesium level was normal and maintained by a daily dose of 10 to 20 mEq.

The signs and symptoms of magnesium deficiency are likely to show up a few days after a major operation in patients who are severely ill and in whom the possibility of magnesium deficiency has not been considered. As with potassium, there is an increased loss of magnesium which results from the starvation and trauma associated with a major operation. If the patient has previously been normal there would be no problem; but the patient who is on the verge of being symptomatic from magnesium depletion may lose just enough additional magnesium to cause the onset of a most disturbing clinical picture. In an emergency situation this sequence may be unavoidable. In patients undergoing elective operations for chronic and debilitating disease, total body magnesium deficiencies, like other manifestations of malnutrition, should be corrected before any operation is undertaken. Symptomatic depletion of magnesium can be avoided by adding magnesium to the daily fluids for patients whose parenteral fluids and nutrition are likely to be prolonged and for patients with chronic debilitating disease known to predispose to magnesium deficiency. Henzel et al. have reviewed the significance of magnesium metabolism in the surgical patient.

REFERENCES

Boyd, G. W., and Peart, W. S.: The relationship between angiotensin and aldosterone. Advances Metab. Disord. 5:77, 1971.

Coghlan, J. P., and Blair-West, J. R.: Aldosterone. In *Hormones in Blood*. Vol. 2. Gray, C. H., and Bacharach, A. L., eds. New York: Academic Press, 1967.

Conn, J. W.: Presidential Address. Part I. Painting background. Park II. Primary aldosteronism, a new clinical syndrome. J. Lab. Clin. Med. 45:3, 1955.

Davis, R. H., and Fisch, C.: Potassium and arrhythmias. Geriatrics 25:108, 1970.

Fichman, M. P., Vorherr, H., Kleeman, C. R., and Telfer, N.: Diuretic-induced hyponatremia. Ann. Intern. Med. 75:853, 1971.

Fromm, D., Field, M., and Silen, W.: Effects of insulin on sugar, amino acid and ion transport across isolated small intestine. Surgery 66:145, 1969.

Goggin, M. J., and Joekes, A. M.: Gas exchange in renal failure. I. Dangers of hyperkalemia during anesthesia. Brit. Med. J. 2:244, 1971.

Harris, P., and Opie, L.: *Calcium and the Heart*. London: Academic Press, 1971.
Henzel, J. H., DeWeese, M. S., and Ridenhour, G.: Significance of magnesium and zinc metabolism in the surgical patient. Arch. Surg. (Chicago) *95*:974, 1967.
Hoffman, B. F., and Cranefield, P. F.: The physiological basis of cardiac arrhythmias. Amer. J. Med. *37*:670, 1964.
Kimberg, D. V., Field, M., Johnson, J., Henderson, A., and Gershon, E.: Stimulation of intestinal mucosal adenyl cyclos by cholera enterotoxin and prostaglandins. J. Clin. Invest. *50*:1218, 1971.
Kraft, A. R., Tompkins, R. K., and Zollinger, R. M.: Recognition and management of the diarrheal syndrome caused by non-beta islet cell tumors of the pancreas. Amer. J. Surg. *119*:163, 1970.
Kunin, A. S., Surawicz, B., and Sims, E. A. H.: Decrease in serum potassium concentrations and appearance of cardiac arrhythmias during infusion of potassium with glucose in potassium depleted patients. New Eng. J. Med. *266*:228, 1962.
Laks, M. M., and Elek, S. R.: The effect of potassium on the electrocardiogram. Dis. Chest *51*:573, 1967.
Prohaska, J. Y.: Pseudomembranous enterocolitis. Arch. Surg. (Chicago) *79*:197, 1959.
Prohaska, J. Y., Govostis, M. C., and Taubenhaus, M.: Postoperative pseudomembranous entercolitis: successful treatment with corticotropin (ACTH). J.A.M.A. *154*:320, 1954.
Schloerb, P. R., and Grantham, J. J.: Body composition and plasma concentrations in gastric alkalosis. Ann. N. Y. Acad. Sci. *110*:984, 1963.
Williams, E. D., Karim, J. M., and Sandler, M.: Prostaglandin secretion by medullary carcinoma of the thyroid: a possible case of the associated diarrhea. Lancet *1*:22, 1968.
Wright, B. D., and Digiovanni, A. J.: Respiratory alkalosis, hypokalemia, and repeated ventricular fibrillation associated with mechanical ventilation. Anesth. Analg. *48*:467, 1969.
Zollinger, R. M., Tompkins, R. K., Amerson, J. R., Endahl, G. L., Kraft, A. R., and Moore, F. T.: Identification of the diarrheagenic hormone associated with non-beta islet cell tumors of the pancreas. Ann. Surg. *168*:502, 1968.

Chapter

5

Carbon Dioxide

Henderson in 1908 presented a theory of *neutrality regulation,* which Nuttall has suggested might be a better term for what is commonly called "acid-base balance." This is only the first example of many variations of terminology used in discussion of patients with disturbances of their hydrogen ion concentration. The subject is commonly divided into two parts, namely, respiratory and nonrespiratory (metabolic). The present chapter will concentrate on the respiratory regulation and abnormalities, whereas Chapter 6 is concerned with nonrespiratory or metabolic abnormalities. Repetition is inevitable and provides perspective, so do read on if parts are foggy the first time through these two chapters.

Physicians are usually thinking about mechanisms when they discuss acid-base disturbances. For example, a surgeon may say that a patient has a respiratory acidosis and a nonrespiratory alkalosis. This means that there are two mechanisms at work which cause opposite changes in hydrogen ion concentration. The statement does not indicate anything about the pH, which could be high, low, or normal. *Acidosis* and *alkalosis* are also used to designate a pH below or above 7.4. *Acidemia* and *alkalemia* have been suggested as clinical terms for actual increase or decrease in blood hydrogen ion concentration, but these terms have not been accepted by physicians in everyday use.

When physicians write and talk about these problems, they know by the context of use what is meant. Whenever a patient has both an alkalosis and an acidosis, the terms obviously imply mechanisms. When these terms are used to indicate an actual deviation from pH 7.4, only the one appropriate term is selected. Another source of confusion arises from the clinical definition of 7.4 as a neutral pH, whereas the chemist would consider 7.4 as alkaline and defines 7.0 as neutral. For the clinician acidosis means a blood that is less alkaline than normal.

According to the definition of Bronsted and Lowry, H_2CO_3 is an acid because it is capable of donating H^+. Bicarbonate is a base because it will accept H^+. Carbonic acid is a weak acid because it is in equilibrium with only a relatively low concentration of hydrogen ion and because it is in equilibrium with a relatively high concentration of dissolved CO_2. According to Winters et al., the proportions of dissolved CO_2, carbonic acid, and hydrogen ion are as indicated for the following reactions:

$$\underset{(800)}{CO_2\ (d) + H_2O} \rightleftharpoons \underset{(1)}{H_2CO_3} \rightleftharpoons \underset{(0.03)(0.03)}{H^+ + HCO_3}$$

There are many buffers in blood, extracellular fluid, and cellular fluid, so that some 900 mEq of hydrogen ion can be buffered in the body before death occurs. Since all of these buffers are in equilibrium with the concentration of hydrogen ion (isohydric), it is possible to determine the status of the body buffers by observation of changes in the bicarbonate buffer. The bicarbonate buffer is composed of carbonic acid and its conjugate base, bicarbonate. The dissociation of carbonic acid into hydrogen ion and bicarbonate is a constant, giving rise to the Henderson-Hasselbalch equation, which is used as a means of defining abnormalities of acid-base balance (Table 5-1). The numerator of this equation is related to the total body buffer capacity. The denominator is related to the P_{CO_2} in the blood which in turn is governed by the CO_2 in alveolar air. Normally, approximately 5% of alveolar air is CO_2, which gives a P_{CO_2} of 40 torr.* The solubility coefficient of CO_2 is 0.03, which gives a normal carbonic acid concentration of 1.2 mEq/l and a normal ratio of numerator to denominator of 20 to 1.

Figure 5-1 illustrates the relationship of carbonic acid to cellular metabolism and pulmonary ventilation. Carbon dioxide is produced continuously, dependent upon the rate of metabolic activity, and excreted continuously through the lungs. Any impairment of the excretion of CO_2 causes an increase in the P_{CO_2} in the alveolar air and in the body fluids and in a lowering of pH, as is shown in Figure 5-2. The slope of the line shown is related to the buffering characteristics of the body. If the increase in P_{CO_2} occurs for the entire organism, the slope is different than if the blood is removed and equilibrated with a higher concentration of CO_2 in vitro, as will be explained in relation to Figure 5-8. Increasing the P_{CO_2} not only increases the denominator but causes some increase in the amount of bicarbonate in the numerator of the Henderson-Hasselbalch equation. Increase in the numerator, however, is limited by the buffer capacity of the body

*Torr in newtons per cubit meter is approximately equal to millimeters of mercury. See Smith.

in vivo or the blood when P_{CO_2} is changed in vitro. The ratio falls with increased P_{CO_2} and the pH therefore falls, and since this is brought about by retention of CO_2 this is referred to as a respiratory acidosis.

TABLE 5-1. DERIVATION OF THE HENDERSON-HASSELBALCH EQUATION

$$H_2CO_3 = H^+ + HCO_3^- \qquad (1)$$

$$K = \frac{H^+\ HCO_3^-}{H_2CO_3} \qquad (2)$$

$$H^+ = K\ \frac{H_2CO_3}{HCO_3^-} \qquad (3)$$

$$\text{Log } H^+ = \text{Log } K + \text{Log}\left(\frac{H_2CO_3}{HCO_3^-}\right) \qquad (4)$$

$$\frac{1}{\text{Log } H^+} = \frac{1}{\text{Log } K} + \frac{1}{\text{Log}\left(\frac{H_2CO_3}{HCO_3^-}\right)} \qquad (5)$$

$$\text{pH} = \text{pK} + \text{Log}\left(\frac{HCO_3^-}{H_2CO_3}\right) \qquad (6)$$

$$\text{pH} = 6.1 + \text{Log}\left(\frac{HCO_3^-}{S \cdot P_{CO_2}}\right) \qquad (7)$$

$$7.4 = 6.1 + \text{Log}\left(\frac{24 \text{ mEq/l}}{(0.03)\ (40 \text{ torr})}\right) \qquad (8)$$

The questions most commonly asked in the interpretation of P_{CO_2} and pH or HCO_3^- and pH are: (1) is there a deviation from neutrality and, if there is, (2) is the deviation due to (a) abnormal ventilation or (b) a change in body buffer or (c) a mixture of both, and (3) if there is an abnormality in buffer capacity, how many mEq of acid or base might be needed to restore total body buffer to normal? Over the years efforts have been made to increase the accuracy of answers to these questions by various in vitro manipulations of the blood sample and various graphs and nomograms for manipulation of the data. Carbon dioxide combining power, the Astrup method, and in vitro titration of CO_2 are examples of these efforts; each has limitations and advantages, enthusiasts and critics, a waxing and waning. All are abstractions of the same subject and therefore they focus attention upon what we need to know and seek to grasp.

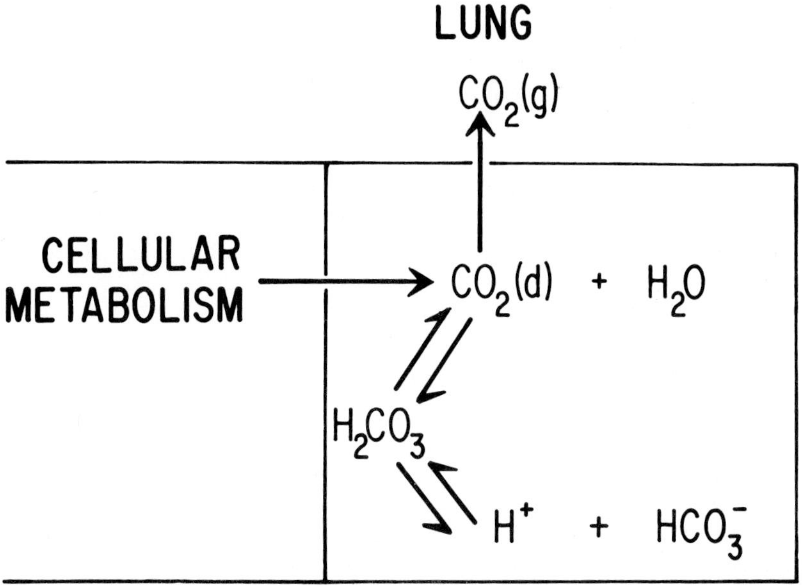

Figure 5-1. Carbon dioxide is produced by cells as a byproduct of energy metabolism and is released into the alveolar air where the P_{CO_2} is normally maintained at 40 mm Hg by control of ventilation through the respiratory center. (d = dissolved; g = gaseous) (Modified from Winters et al.)

CO_2 combining power was an estimate of the buffer capacity when the blood sample was equilibrated in vitro with a normal alveolar P_{CO_2}. The Astrup method provided sets of P_{CO_2} and pH for the blood as obtained from the patient and after in vitro equilibration with two different known concentrations of carbon dioxide. This has been used as a buffer curve for the blood sample which would mirror the buffer capacity of the entire body. Neither method reveals total body buffer capacity. Serial sets of data from arterial blood samples obtained during treatment will provide the most accurate information about total body buffer and total body carbonic acid.

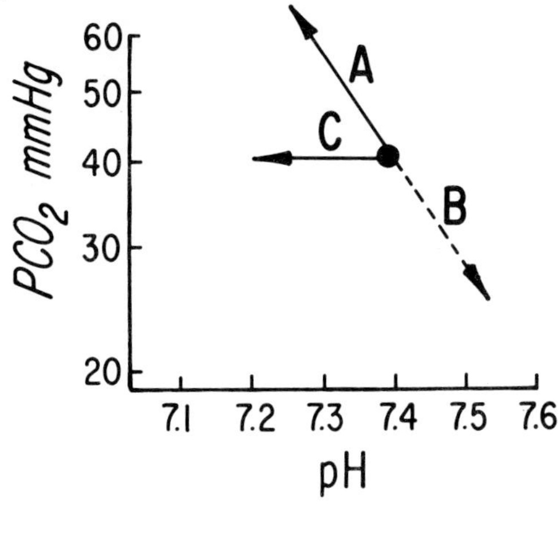

Figure 5-2. Represents P_{CO_2} and pH in a coordinate system with an arrow along the course of an acute respiratory acidosis (line A). The arrow extending down and to the right represents the area of uncompensated hypocapnia as would result from hyperventilation (line B). Pure nonrespiratory acidosis is associated with change in pH without any change in P_{CO_2} (line C).

Interpretation is facilitated by graphic representation of single or sequential sets of data in the plot of pH and plasma HCO_3 introduced by Van Slyke and Simmons, popularized by Davenport, and shown in Figure 5-3, or in the pH-P_{CO_2} plot shown in Figure 5-2. The most recent innovation has been the incorporation of 95% confidence limits, as shown in Figure 5-4. The graph of choice is one of personal preference. Each has advantages, and the value of each is greatly enhanced by knowledge of the patient's history, pertinent physical findings, recent treatment, and other laboratory data.

Huckabee has criticized the use of P_{CO_2} and pH because these are not expressed in moles and has suggested the use of Arrhenius' mass action law (equation 3 in Table 5-1) rather than the Henderson-Hasselbalch equation (equation 6 in Table 5-1). This would allow the use of millimicroequivalents (also called nanoequivalents) to indicate the concentration of hydrogen ion. The normal would be 37 to 42 nanoequivalents per liter, and the maximum range compatible with life for arterial blood hydrogen ion concentration would be 20 to 120. The use of nanoequivalents was discussed by Campbell, who suggested the use of the graph shown in Figure 5-5.

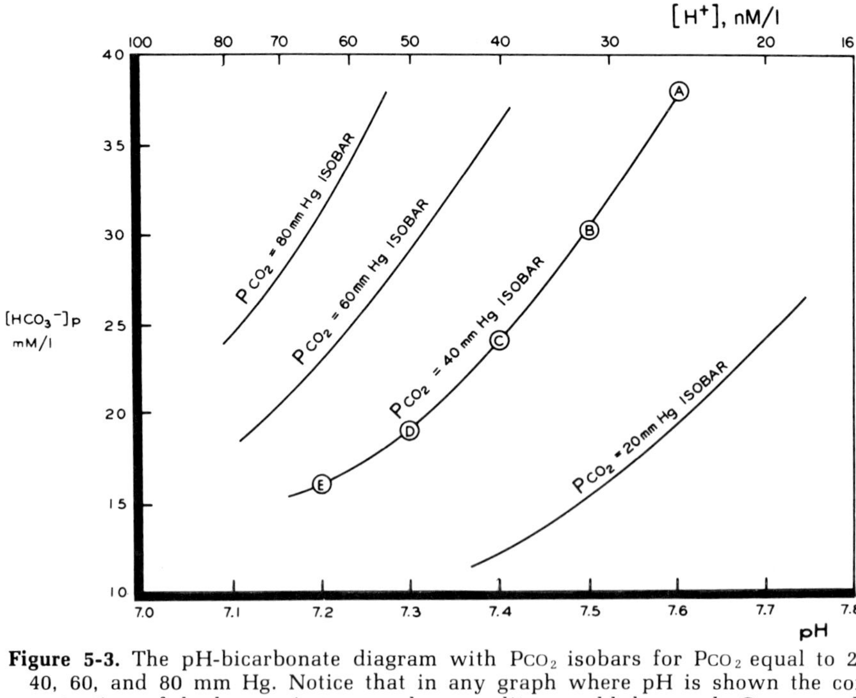

Figure 5-3. The pH-bicarbonate diagram with P_{CO_2} isobars for P_{CO_2} equal to 20, 40, 60, and 80 mm Hg. Notice that in any graph where pH is shown the concentration of hydrogen in nanomoles per liter could be used. Compare the graph with Figure 5-5 recommended by Campbell. Is there any advantage of one over the other? (From Davenport, H. W.: *The ABC of Acid-Base Chemistry*, 5th ed., 1969. By permission of the University of Chicago Press.)

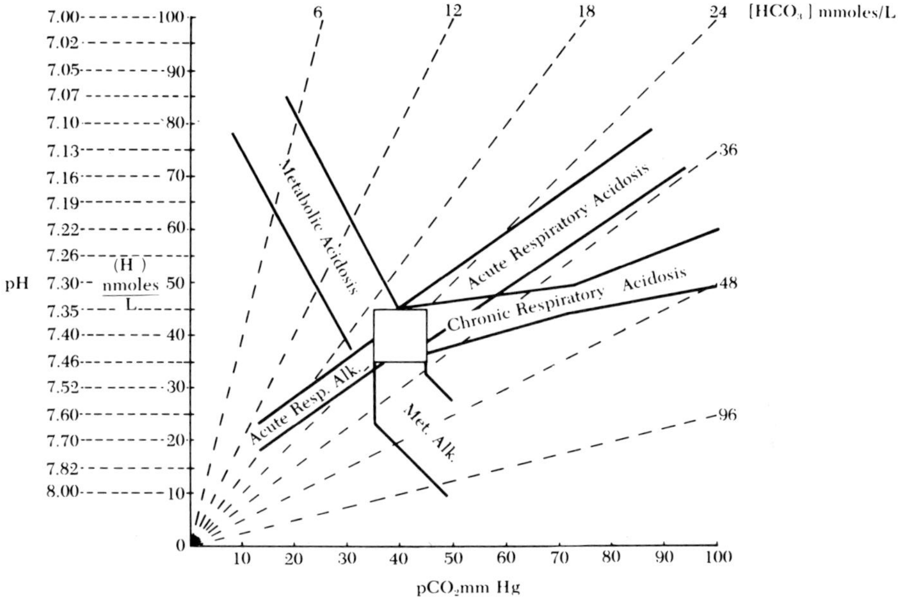

Figure 5-4. Composite acid-base diagram showing the 95% confidence limits for patients with five different and well-defined disturbances. Any patient whose data fall outside of these areas probably has a more complicated mixture of conditions. (From Masoro, E. J., and Siegel, P. D.: *Acid-Base Regulation: Its Physiology and Pathophysiology*. Philadelphia, W. B. Saunders, 1971.)

Schwartz and Relman have criticized the use of the Singer and Hastings buffer base and the Astrup standard bicarbonate and base excess as being superfluous since, without accompanying knowledge of the sequence of events in a particular patient, these calculations can be misleading. Arbus and others, including Schwartz, subsequently proposed the use of significance bands for groups of patients with pure respiratory or nonrespiratory acidosis or alkalosis which was acute or chronic (Fig. 5-4). These significance bands may be of some help but do not obviate the need for a physician who is informed of both acid-base physiology and the sequence of events for his patient.

ACUTE RESPIRATORY ALKALOSIS

Acute respiratory alkalosis represents an excessive removal of CO_2 and therefore of carbonic acid. This is common in patients during recovery from anesthesia following a major operation at which time they tend to breathe in a rapid shallow pattern which is more efficient in the removal of CO_2 than it is in the provision of oxygen. Mild hypoxia may be the stimulus to rapid breathing. Pain is probably also a factor in causing both the shallowness and increased rate of breathing. Anxiety alone is a common cause of overbreathing, even in patients who are otherwise well, and can, on occasion, be so severe as to cause tetany, dizziness, and fainting: *the hyperventilation syndrome.*

Acute hypocapnia accompanied by low oxygen tension is an indication of atelectasis and requires an increase in pressure against which the patient breathes, plus prolongation of full inspiration. Administration of oxygen without correcting the alveolar collapse will not improve the patient and is on occasion

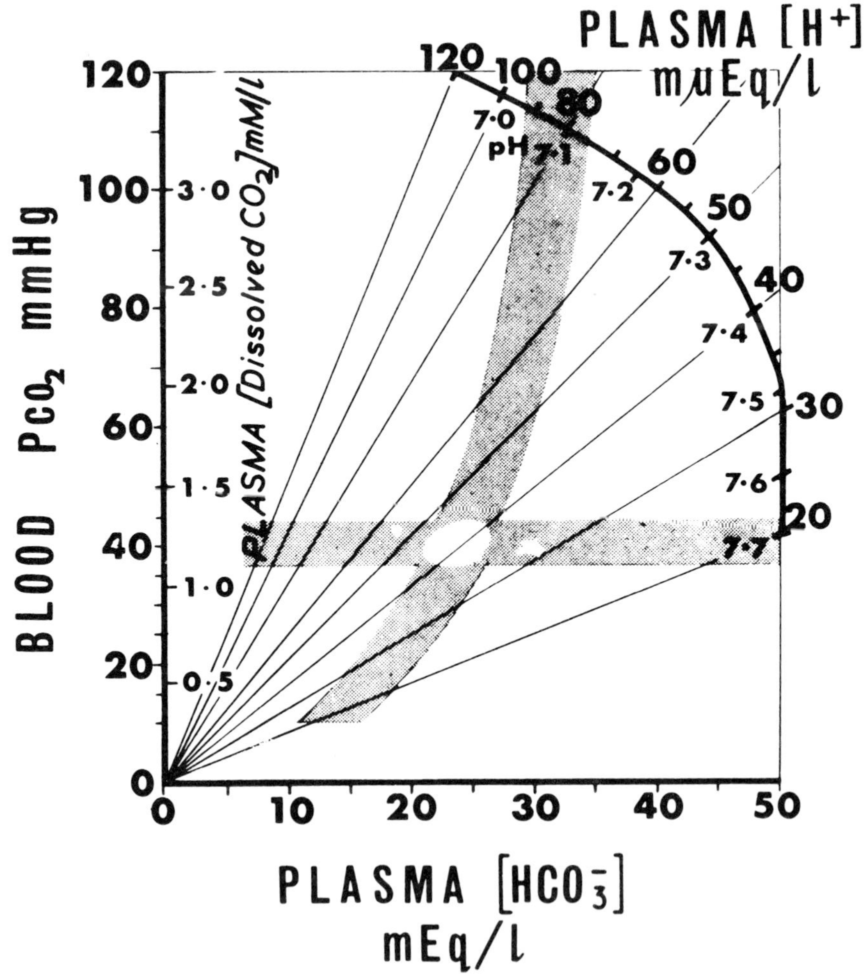

Figure 5-5. For those who prefer working with hydrogen ion concentration in millimicroequivalents per liter instead of its negative log (pH), this graph is recommended by E. J. M. Campbell. The shaded upward curving band covers the normal range of plasma bicarbonate. The transverse shaded band covers the normal range of arterial P_{CO_2}. Concentration of hydrogen (or pH) can be read from the point at which radians intersect the curving dark line in the right upper corner of the diagram. (From Campbell, E., J. M.: R I pH, Lancet 1:681, 1962.)

an unintended coup de grace. An associated hazard relates to the confusion and physical activity of asphyxia. Sedation should be used to relieve anxiety only when it can be determined with assurance that the patient's anxiety is not secondary to hypoxia.

Hypocapnia is occasionally due to overactivity of the respiratory center. Increased blood ammonia levels in patients with liver disease cause stimulation of increased respiration and hypocapnia. The alkalosis converts more of the ammonium (NH_4^+) to ammonia (NH_3), and the latter diffuses more readily across the blood-brain barrier, as reviewed by Child.

ACUTE RESPIRATORY ACIDOSIS (HYPERCAPNIA)

In acute and severe hypercapnia the formation of bicarbonate occurs most rapidly in the blood and less rapidly in interstitial fluid. As a consequence, a concentration gradient for bicarbonate is formed, and bicarbonate moves out of blood into interstitial fluid, as was demonstrated by Shaw and Messer in 1932. This actually decreases the buffer capacity of the blood and if a sample of blood is withdrawn from the patient and equilibrated in vitro with a lower P_{CO_2}, it may appear that the patient has a reduced buffer capacity. In fact, if the P_{CO_2} is returned to normal for the whole patient and a sample of blood removed from the patient, this blood will have a normal bicarbonate. This was demonstrated by Brown and Clancy, who also showed that blood equilibrated with an increased P_{CO_2} in vitro had a higher concentration of bicarbonate than if the entire body was allowed to equilibrate with the same elevated P_{CO_2}. When blood in a test tube is equilibrated with an elevated P_{CO_2}, the bicarbonate which is formed cannot move out of the blood. This illustrates how determinations requiring a change in P_{CO_2} for blood in a test tube may be misleading insofar as total body buffer estimation is concerned.

Acute hypercapnia occurs in the heavily sedated or anesthetized patient and may occur without an associated hypoxia especially if the gas mixture is enriched with oxygen. A progressive elevation of blood pressure should suggest hypercapnia in such patients. Sudden lowering of the P_{CO_2} after several hours of hypercapnia produces hypotension, arrhythmia, and, on occasion, ventricular fibrillation. Miller et al. used a portable mass spectrometer built by the physicist Nier at the University of Minnesota and recorded the alveolar carbon dioxide levels during and after operation. They were able to confirm the suspicion that "cyclopropane shock" was the posthypercapnic phenomenon which they had studied in dogs. There is no direct myocardial toxicity of carbon dioxide, but the sudden lowering of P_{CO_2} after prolonged elevation caused death in 79% of their dogs; review of sudden deaths on the surgical service suggested that this probably had been the mechanism of death in some patients. There is neither time nor adequate renal function during an operation for hypercapnia to produce a compensatory metabolic alkalosis, but there is time enough for other changes which may make the patient unable to readjust to the sudden removal of the increased carbon dioxide stimulus. Miller suggested the analogy of sudden removal of a pheochromocytoma or the sudden stopping of a norepinephrine infusion. Later in this chapter the hazard of alkalosis in patients with chronic hypercapnia will be discussed. In Chapter 4 the relationship of changes in serum potassium to changes in CO_2 were mentioned.

CHRONIC RESPIRATORY ACIDOSIS

In contrast to acute hypercapnia, there is in chronic hypercapnia a gradual increase in total body buffer which is brought about by the increased excretion of chloride and a retention of bicarbonate by the kidney, producing a hypochloremic alkalosis of the type which will be described in Chapter 6 as resulting from loss of acid gastric juice. The retention of CO_2 results in a rise in the concentration of carbonic acid in both extracellular and intracellular fluid, but there is better buffering in the cells than outside of the cells, so that the concentration of hydrogen ion is higher in the extracellular fluid than it is in the intracellular fluid. Whenever there is a concentration gradient across the cellular membrane for hydrogen, an exchange occurs between hydrogen outside of the cell and potassium within the cell. As a result, patients with hypercapnia tend to lose cellular potassium. Such patients are also commonly treated with diuretics which may further deplete the body potassium. The nonrespiratory alkalosis which is found in chronic hypercapnia may therefore represent a hypokalemic as well as a hypochloremic alkalosis. These terms, as mentioned earlier, describe mechanisms and not the actual pH. In chronic respiratory acidosis or hypercapnia the pH is usually below but may be above 7.4, depending upon the current relationship between bicarbonate and carbonic acid, as is shown in the Henderson-Hasselbalch equation.

Emphysema and duodenal ulcer are commonly associated in the same patient. It may be of interest to determine whether a patient with an obstructing duodenal ulcer has developed a low concentration of chloride and potassium because of vomiting or whether this is the result of renal compensation for a chronic hypercapnia. Whatever the sequence of events, the objective of treatment is to provide a normal pH. This may require both improvement in ventilation and restoration of chloride and potassium.

The presentation of a rather complex example may assist in the transfer of theory to practice. A 47-year-old man was in the hospital for ten days because of an empyema secondary to a bronchopleural fistula in the right upper pleural cavity. He had been treated for tuberculosis five years earlier, and his sputum was negative for acid-fast bacilli. When he was admitted his sputum cultured beta-hemolytic streptococcus and *Hemophilus parainfluenzae*. The empyema cavity was drained, and from the drainage *Diplococcus pneumoniae* was also cultured. The chest x-ray at the time of admission showed a large hydropneumothorax in the upper half of the right pleural space and an infiltrate in the lower lobe of the right lung.

Physicians were called to see the patient because he was confused and had twitching of muscles. There were no breath sounds heard over the right lung field. The blood pressure was 240/120 mm Hg. An endonasal-endotracheal tube was inserted and after suctioning and hyperinflation the tube was attached to a humidifier with 70% oxygen running at 8 liters/minute. Several hours later the patient was observed to be sweating profusely, was hypotensive, unresponsive, and breathing poorly. Physicians were again called and assisted ventilation by hand, causing a rapid return of responsiveness and cessation of sweating. A sample of arterial blood was drawn during the institution of assisted ventilation so that we do not know the values when the patient was most acidotic, but the first data are shown in Table 5-2 and as point 1 in Figure 5-6. He had a pulse of 100/minute. He became hypotensive and appeared to be in a terminal state. Not only was he vigorously hyperventilated by hand, but because of his shock-like state and the supposition that he would have produced excess lactic acid, it was elected to give him 150 ml of molar sodium bicarbonate. After he seemed to be somewhat improved, a positive pressure respirator was attached to the endonasal-endotracheal tube. The blood pressure at this time was 80/50 torr and the central venous pressure 11 cm of water.

The diagnosis was still in question, and blood was drawn for culture on the possibility that this was septic shock. Five hundred ml of blood were started as a transfusion. Antibiotics and steroids were ordered, isoproterenol was given as an intravenous drip. The patient improved during the next twelve hours. His urinary output remained at 30 ml/hour and his central venous pressure at 14 cm of water. Isoproterenol was used to maintain the blood pressure, but according to notes on the patient's record, the cause of the hypotension remained an enigma. No growth occurred from two blood cultures. The physicians in their notes in the chart also speculated that respiratory acidosis might have caused myocardial insufficiency. By the second day the arterial pH was 7.62 (Fig. 5-6, point 2). The laboratory reported the serum sodium

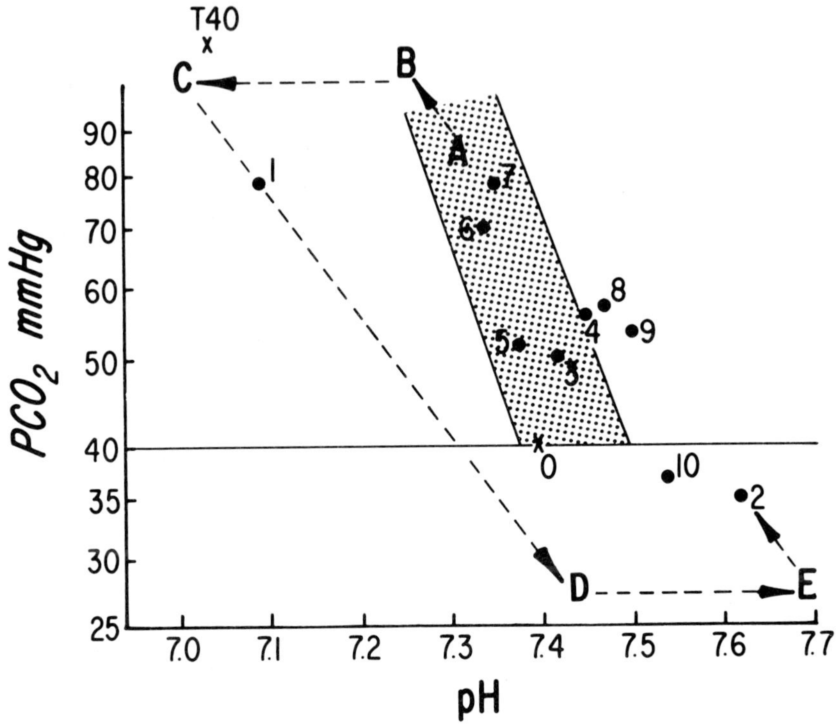

Figure 5-6. Shows a plot of a patient with chronic respiratory acidosis whose data were probably at A when he developed an acute increase in CO_2 at B and then circulatory failure which probably placed his data at C. The numbered points indicate blood samples drawn in sequence during treatment as discussed in the text. This patient was subjected to both extremes of abnormal hydrogen ion concentration within a period of a few minutes.

was 135 mEq/l with a CO_2* of 36, chloride 80, and potassium 5.8 mEq/l, all of which was consistent with a diagnosis of hypochloremic metabolic alkalosis as is usually found in patients with chronic respiratory insufficiency.

By the end of the second day the blood pressure was sustained without isoproterenol. Positive pressure had been reduced, but arterial ventilation was still required. Notes on the chart indicated that septicemia was considered as the cause of shock, but most of the therapeutic effort was now directed toward sustaining the improved pulmonary function. A tracheostomy was substituted for the endonasal-endotracheal tube. The patient gained strength

*CO_2 content of blood sent to the laboratory in a tube exposed to room air. The CO_2 + Cl = 116 or 14 mEq below an average normal of 130 whereas the concentration of Na is 135 or 8 less than 143, the usual normal. There must be some unmeasured anions accumulated to 6 mEq/l or a laboratory error. Otherwise, the difference between observed and expected concentration of anions should be the same as for cations. Work this out with Gamble bar graphs as you would in a progress note.

and remained alert. Frequent suctioning and stimulated coughing were effective in removing secretions. Repeated trials with humidified oxygen and without the respirator were tolerated for increasingly long intervals but led on days 6 and 7 to a high P_{CO_2} (Table 5-2).

TABLE 5-2.

Day of Observation	P_{O_2}	pH	P_{CO_2}	COMMENTS
1	100	7.09	79	
2	170	7.62	35	Respirator
3	144	7.42	50	Humidifier 40% O_2
4	114	7.45	56	Respirator
5	152	7.38	52	Respirator
6	160	7.34	70	Humidifier 40% O_2
7	97	7.35	78	Humidifier 40% O_2
8	112	7.47	57	Respirator
9	43	7.50	53	Room Air
10	49	7.54	37	Room Air

Finally, the patient was able to breathe room air without assistance, but his breathing was labored and P_{O_2} low. By the tenth day, P_{CO_2} was 37 torr, P_{O_2} 49 torr, and pH 7.54. The empyema cavity which had been treated with closed drainage was converted to open drainage after a month, and the patient was transferred back to the state tuberculosis sanitarium. The discharge summary stated that the period of confusion and hypotension was still not fully explained but was probably due to CO_2 narcosis. The slow response of the hypotension to emergency measures seemed to remain a puzzling part of the picture. The patient's breathing gradually improved, and he did not require further respiratory assistance.

A detailed trip around Figure 5-6 will help to explain the sequence of events in this patient's illness. The shaded area represents the 95% confidence limits for chronic respiratory acidosis as observed in man by Brackett, Wingo, et al. This area contains data from patients whose chronic respiratory insufficiency had been partially compensated by excretion of titratable acid, ammonia and chloride in the urine.

When patients develop acute respiratory acidosis, starting with a normal acid-base balance, the P_{CO_2} rises and the pH falls. Their data would fall along the buffer line running approximately through point 0 and the point marked T40. As the kidneys compensate by excreting organic acids and ammonium ion, the shaded area is entered; it is highly probable that the upper part of this shaded area is the site of our patient's data at the time that he entered the hospital and for most of the ten-day period up to the time when he was first seen with muscle twitching and coma.

At this time it is likely that he had an acute increase in PCO_2 and a decrease in pH and that his data moved from A to B along a buffer line which ran through the area of chronic metabolic alkalosis. For a time his drive to breathe was hypoxia. When he was given oxygen to breathe without any assistance in ventilation, the hypoxia was relieved, but he then had an increasing PCO_2 and CO_2 narcosis with depression of his respiratory center. Originally, during this period he had a high blood pressure secondary to the high PCO_2 but when CO_2 narcosis increased, circulatory failure developed and his cells began to produce lactic acid. This addition of a metabolic acidosis moved his data to C and his buffer line to the left. At this time after two minutes of artificial ventilation an arterial blood sample was drawn which is shown as point 1. With continued ventilation the PCO_2 decreased and the patient's data, if frequently obtained, would have shown movement along the buffer line to a point below a PCO_2 of 40 and an increasingly severe alkalosis, possibly in the area designated as D.

This degree of rapid change from a high to a low PCO_2 is likely to result in cardiac arrhythmias. It is not always possible to distinguish the symptoms of severe acidosis and severe alkalosis. Monitoring of arterial pH and PCO_2, as was done here, is essential to understanding the cause and the best means of treatment. Extremes of pH and a rapid fall in pH are all disturbing to cardiac and central nervous system function. Kilburn has listed a pH of 7.54 as a level above which mental and neurological dysfunction is likely to occur and mentioned the observations of Ketz and Smith that a decrease of PCO_2 from a normal 45 to 26 mm Hg causes a decrease in cerebral blood flow from a normal 52 ml to a level of 34 ml/100 gm of brain/minute and causes an increase in cerebrovascular resistance to almost twice the normal value. Hypoxia and hypocapnia are additive.

Not only was there a shift to a respiratory alkalosis from overzealous ventilation but because 150 mEq of sodium bicarbonate were given, the buffer curve was shifted to the right, giving him in addition a metabolic alkalosis. A blood sample was not obtained at D or E, but was sampled the following morning, approximately 12 hours after point 1, and this second sample is shown at the area marked 2 in Figure 5-6.

It is probable that the pH was lower than 7.1 at the beginning of treatment and higher than 7.6 during the early period after establishment of assisted ventilation and after administration of sodium bicarbonate. Even with the data as actually recorded, this is a change of pH from 7.1 to 7.6, and such a change of pH in a short period of time, extending over almost the full length of the tolerable pH scale, might be expected to cause disturbances in cardiovascular and cerebral function.

Rotheram et al. found that weaning patients from a mechanical ventilator after restoration of a normal P_{CO_2} was often a major undertaking and could pose as many problems as have been reviewed in the course of instituting mechanical ventilation. They observed marked respiratory depression and return to hypercapnia and stupor. Intracerebral alkalosis may persist longer than in other cells. Prevention of serious central nervous system injury and consequent tremor, coma, and convulsions requires that these changes in treatment be carried out gradually and with close monitoring of blood gas and pH levels and appropriate correction of electrolyte balance if hypochloremia, hypokalemia, or other abnormalities are contributing to the problem.

During the subsequent days, our patient's data moved back into the shaded area of the 95% confidence limits for chronic respiratory acidosis with compensatory metabolic alkalosis. The last sample shown on the tenth day left the patient with a near normal P_{CO_2}, but with a metabolic alkalosis. He was at this time hypochloremic and needed salt in order to be able to correct the hypochloremia and alkalosis. Points numbered 7 through 10 show how the patient moved from hypercapnia to a normal P_{CO_2} and was left with a hypochloremic alkalosis. This was accomplished through improved ventilation and a lowering of P_{CO_2} and almost represents another in vivo titration of CO_2 and a total body buffer curve. Such an in vivo carbonic acid titration line, to be uncontaminated by changes in relative concentrations of cations and nonrespirable anions, should be derived over a shorter span of time. It does require time, however, for readjustment between the cellular and extracellular buffers. Such a line would theoretically allow determination of the total body bicarbonate or so-called T40 bicarbonate. From knowledge of the abnormality of the body bicarbonate when the whole body is equilibrated with a P_{CO_2} of 40 torr, it would be possible to estimate how much ammonium chloride or excess chloride would be required to restore the pH to normal and to restore the chloride and bicarbonate concentrations to normal.

WHOLE BODY BUFFER ESTIMATION

Brown and Clancy have illustrated experimentally how bicarbonate, after generation from CO_2 in the red blood cells, moves out into plasma and interstitial fluid. They made repeated and frequent measurements of the plasma bicarbonate in samples of arterial and venous blood starting at the time of institution of breathing 30% CO_2 (Fig. 5-7). The red blood cells passing through the lungs took up the high concentration of CO_2 and the bicarbonate generated appeared in high concentration as the blood passed initially through the arteries, but then diffusion into interstitial fluid occurred. The plasma bicarbonate of venous blood rose more slowly. Within a few minutes the bicarbonate concentration in the arterial blood decreased enough so that the venous bicarbonate again exceeded the arterial bicarbonate and both arterial and venous levels were then elevated but with the venous higher than the arterial. The initial peak in the arterial bicarbonate is the important part of this graph and is due to the generation of bicarbonate and its subsequent diffusion into the interstitial and cellular fluid. Figure 5-8 shows the plasma bicarbonate when the blood is equilibrated with a high P_{CO_2}, using the total animal. The rise in plasma bicarbonate is not as great as when a blood sample is equilibrated with a high P_{CO_2} in vitro.

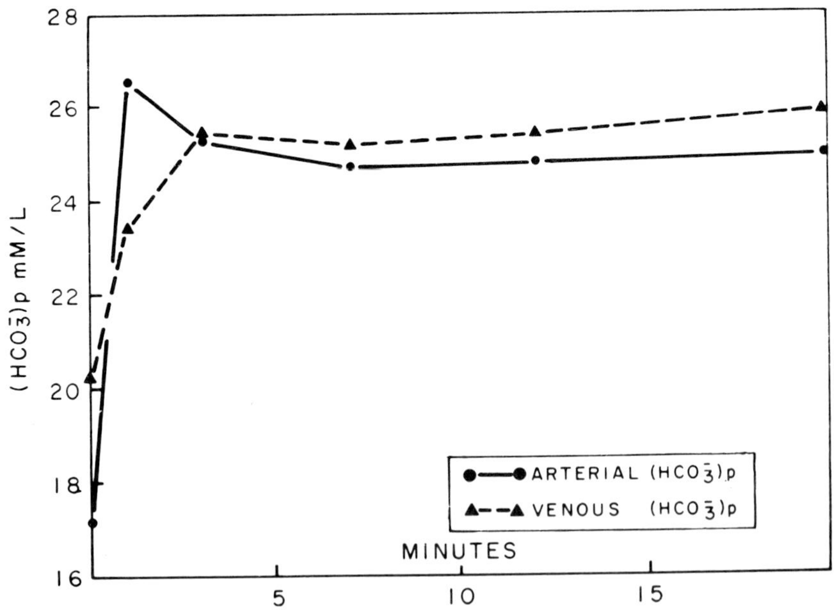

Figure 5-7. Shows plasma bicarbonate concentration in arterial and venous blood as a function of time after starting to breathe 30% CO_2. The high level attained initially in the arterial blood is similar to the level attained by an in vitro exposure of blood to 30% CO_2. However, the bicarbonate soon falls to a lower level as HCO_3- diffuses into extravascular fluid. This demonstrates the fallacy of the assumption that an in vitro whole blood buffer curve is identical with an in vivo whole body buffer curve. (From Brown, E. B., and Clancy, R. L.: In vivo and in vitro CO_2 blood buffer curves. J. Appl. Physiol. *20*:885, 1965.)

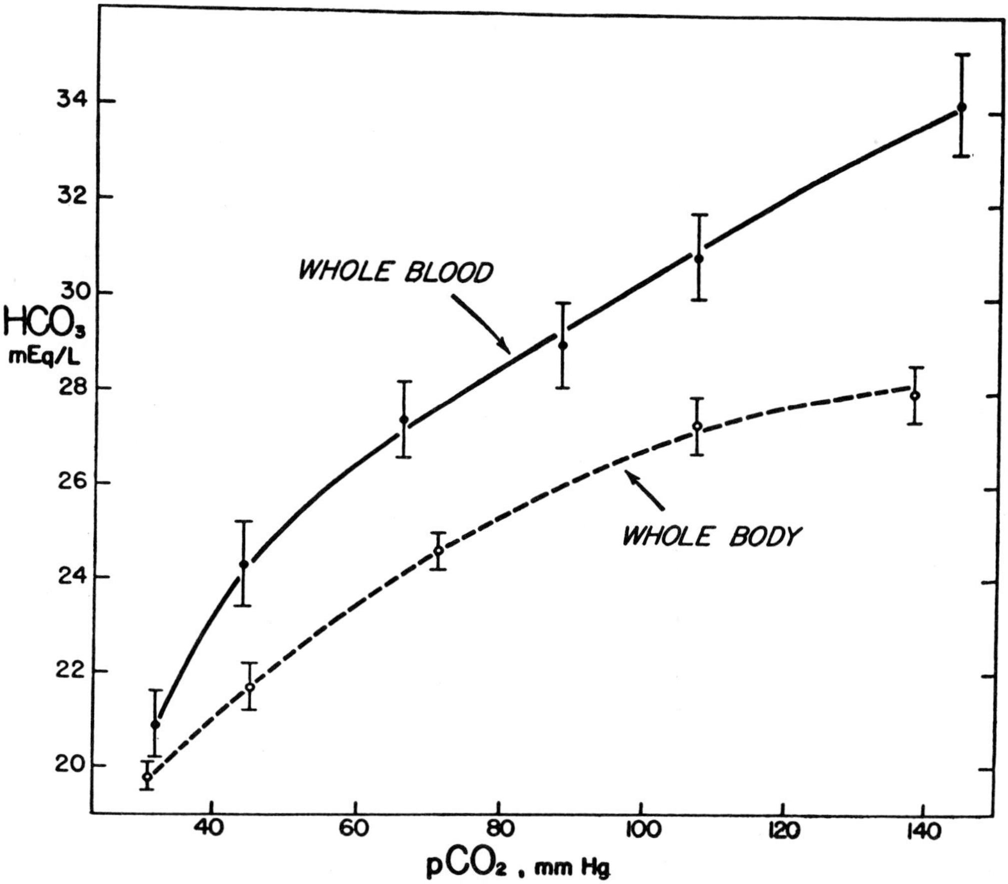

Figure 5-8. Is a plot of plasma bicarbonate in mEq/l and P_{CO_2} in mm Hg when blood is removed from a dog and equilibrated with increasing concentrations of CO_2. This upper curve for whole blood is compared with a lower curve obtained by leaving the blood in the dog while the dog breathes elevated concentrations of CO_2 and then removing the sample. It is evident that equilibration with high P_{CO_2} in vitro gives a higher value for plasma bicarbonate than equilibration in vivo. The discrepancy does not exceed about 4 mEq/l within the range of P_{CO_2} encountered clinically. (From Cohen, J. J., Brackett, N. C., and Schwartz, W. B.: The nature of the carbon dioxide titration curve in the normal dog. J. Clin. Invest. 43:777, 1964.)

Likewise, if the total animal is equilibrated with a high P_{CO_2} and a sample of blood is then removed and re-equilibrated with a 5% CO_2, the plasma bicarbonate is reduced to a remarkably low level (Fig. 5-9). This is what is done in the Astrup method and in acute hypercapnia gives rise to the erroneous impression that there is a metabolic acidosis of up to 4 mEq/l. Actually, the bicarbonate capacity of the blood is reduced because of the equilibration that occurred between blood and interstitial fluid.

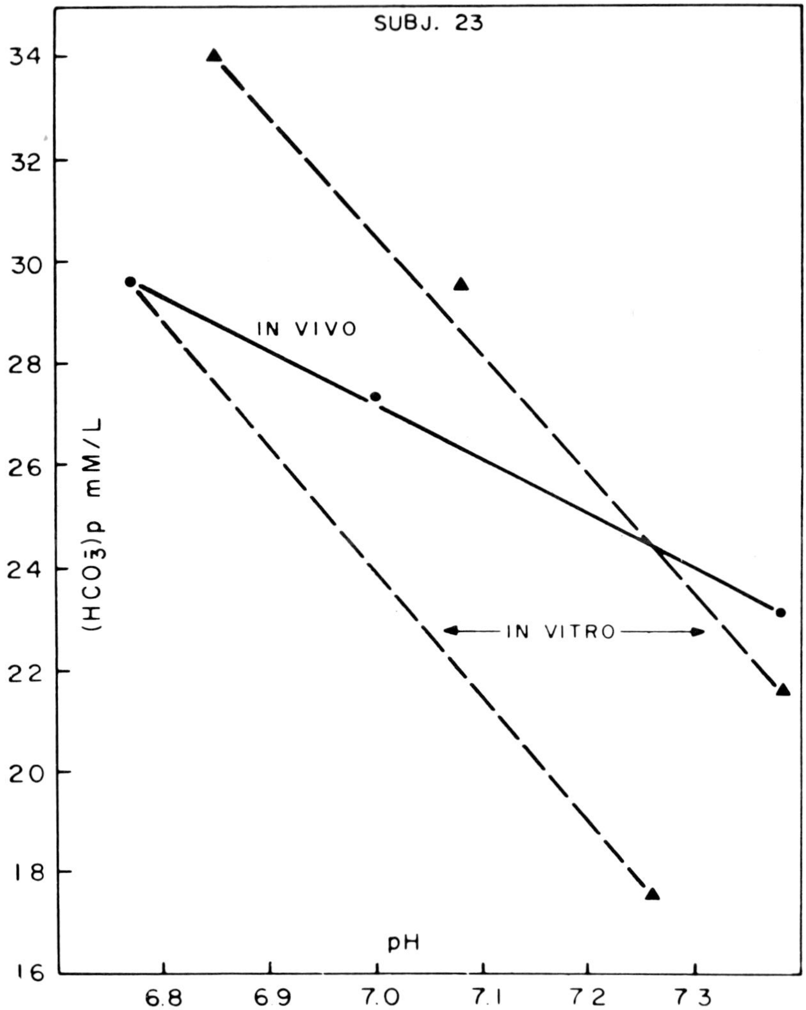

Figure 5-9. Compares the bicarbonate concentrations of blood when the whole body is exposed to a changed P_{CO_2} as compared with exposure of blood alone. The top two buffer lines are buffer curves for in vivo and in vitro. The slope is greater in vitro because bicarbonate remains in the plasma whereas in vivo it diffuses into extravascular fluids. The lower line shows the loss of bicarbonate when blood is removed from the body of an animal with a high P_{CO_2} and equilibrated with 5% CO_2. Such a sample of blood has a lowered CO_2 capacity which gives the erroneous impression that the animal has a metabolic acidosis. (From Brown, E. B., and Clancy, R. L.: In vivo and in vitro CO_2 blood buffer curves. J. Appl. Physiol. *20*:885, 1965.)

The low plasma bicarbonate of blood removed during hypercapnia and equilibrated in vitro with 5% CO_2 indicates that not only has bicarbonate diffused out of the blood in the total animal but that there has been exchange of bicarbonate for chloride and that the capacity of the removed blood for CO_2 is thereby reduced. What the Astrup method provides, as presented by Siggaard-Andersen, is a measure of the capacity of isolated blood to buffer fixed acid after a reduction to a normal P_{CO_2}. What is needed is information about the capacity of the total body to buffer fixed acid when P_{CO_2} is reduced to 40 mm Hg for the whole animal.

In red blood cells the CO_2 is hydrated to carbonic acid and then dissociates into bicarbonate and hydrogen ion, and the bicarbonate diffuses out of the blood in exchange for chloride. The erroneously high bicarbonate observed when increasing concentrations of CO_2 are used to equilibrate in vitro samples of normal blood results from the fact that the bicarbonate cannot diffuse beyond plasma when it leaves the red blood cells.

Stern and Simmons exposed animals to increasing concentrations of CO_2 and used the Astrup method to calculate the various parameters. Figure 5-10 shows the erroneous information which comes from the use of base excess, standard bicarbonate, and plasma bicarbonate as calculated. Stern and Simmons suggest the use of T40 bicarbonate, which represents the bicarbonate when the total body is equilibrated with a P_{CO_2} of 40 torr. The T40 bicarbonate should remain at 0 on such a graph indicating that acute exposure of an animal to an elevated P_{CO_2} does not change the buffer capacity of the entire body. Bunker obtained data from a patient subjected to ether anesthesia, during which the P_{CO_2} rose to 140 torr and the pH fell to 6.96. According to the Singer-Hastings nomogram (which is used in methods which extrapolate from analysis of isolated blood to whole body acid-base balance), the buffer fell to 39.5 and immediately returned to normal when the P_{CO_2} was corrected. Such a rapid fall and rise in buffer base in circumstances where renal function is minimal would be unlikely.

The Siggaard-Andersen curve or Singer-Hastings nomogram can be used to calculate the T40 bicarbonate by using a buffer line parallel to the line which would go through the normal point at pH of 7.4 and P_{CO_2} of 40 torr and the mark for a hemoglobin of 3% as suggested by Armstrong et al. This provides an estimate of what the bicarbonate would be if the hemoglobin were distributed in the entire extracellular fluid instead of limited to the vascular space. In the body, the bicarbonate formed in the red cells diffuses out into the surrounding fluid, and this includes interstitial fluid as well as plasma, so that the concentration of hemoglobin as far as this determination is concerned is the concentration which would exist if there were no cellular or endothelial barrier to the movement of hemoglobin and the hemoglobin actually were distributed in the entire extracellular fluid space.

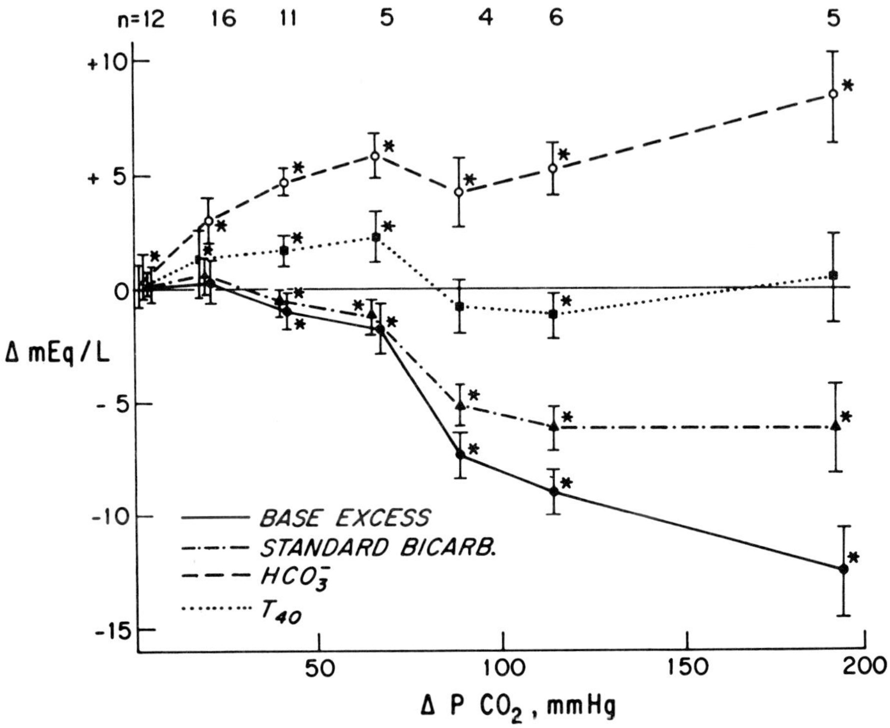

Figure 5-10. Shows the deviations from normal for various parameters calculated by the Astrup method when a dog is exposed to increasing tensions of CO_2. The T40 bicarbonate is the estimated plasma bicarbonate concentration for the animal if it is assumed that the generated bicarbonate is diluted by the interstitial fluid. There should not be any deviation from 0 for changes in T40 bicarbonate, but there is an increase in blood and interstitial fluid volume which occurs with an elevated P_{CO_2}; this was not considered in the calculation. (From Stern, L. J., and Simmons, D. H.: Estimation of nonrespiratory acid-base abnormalities. J. Appl. Physiol. *27*:21, 1969.)

RENAL COMPENSATION FOR CHRONIC HYPERCAPNIA

The patient with acute respiratory acidosis has altered function of the kidney which facilitates the excretion of hydrogen ion and retention of bicarbonate, producing a metabolic alkalosis. This is accomplished through an increased excretion of organic acid such as the conversion of monohydrogen phosphate to dihyrogen phosphate. This is referred to as an increase in titratable acidity since the urine becomes more acid and, when titrated back to the pH of plasma, reveals the excess of hydrogen in urine compared with the plasma from which the urine was formed. A more important mechanism which does require several days to reach its maximum efficiency is the excretion of ammonium ion.

The amine group is split away from amino acids in the kidney cells lining the tubule. Hydrogen ion is trapped in forming ammonium from ammonia which is excreted in the urine, and the bicarbonate derived from the carbonic acid is retained and augments total body buffer capacity. At the same time the kidney excretes chloride so that the total concentration of anions is maintained equal to the total concentration of cations in the blood. The result is a hypochloremic metabolic alkalosis.

Changes in P_{CO_2} can occur rapidly. Changes in the relative concentrations of bicarbonate and chloride require more time. A sudden return of an elevated P_{CO_2} to normal in a patient with chronic respiratory acidosis is very likely to leave the patient with a hypochloremic metabolic alkalosis. Correction of the latter requires the availability of excess chloride. Polak et al. and Schwartz et al. have shown in experiments in dogs that if a restriction in salt is imposed, the animal in unable to restore pH to normal, but that this compensation disability is corrected upon the addition of salt to the diet. Schwartz et al. published data from an experiment in which dogs were studied for 35 days with repeated measurements of P_{CO_2} and pH and during the development of chronic respiratory acidosis and recovery. Figure 5-11 is a plot of these data and demonstrates the acute hypercapnia and acidosis on day 6. The serum chloride fell and bicarbonate rose as the kidneys excreted chloride and hydrogen and reabsorbed bicarbonate, during days 6 to 10, when P_{CO_2} was elevated. On day 21, the dog was allowed room air to breathe, and the P_{CO_2} suddenly returned to normal, leaving the animal with a metabolic hypochloremic alkalosis. The dog was limited to a very low sodium chloride intake and could not correct the hypochloremic alkalosis. In fact, for a few days, ventilation was below normal and P_{CO_2} rose to 50 torr to partially compensate for the metabolic alkalosis by reestablishing a respiratory acidosis. Salt was then added to the intake and chloride was retained, bicarbonate excretion in urine increased, and pH and P_{CO_2} returned to normal. A chronically ill patient may also develop a hypokalemic hypochloremic metabolic alkalosis; correction of this may require the replenishment of total body potassium as well as chloride.

OBJECTIVES OF TREATMENT

The objectives in treating patients with acid-base disorders are to restore normal intracellular function; this is more likely to be achieved if arterial pH is restored to normal than if the P_{CO_2} is simply returned to normal. The pulmonary insufficiency obviously must be corrected if possible. In some instances improved cardiac function may be the avenue for reducing pulmonary congestion. A high P_{CO_2} may be perpetuated or increased by administration of more than 40% oxygen so that the anoxic stimulus to respiration is counteracted. Also, a high P_{O_2} may be injurious to pulmonary membranes and gas exchange.

According to Sackner, a rapid correction of chronic respiratory acidosis with a return to normal P_{CO_2} and alkaline pH can result in fatal encephalopathy. The correction should take place over 6 to 24 hours and should be to a normal pH but not necessarily a normal P_{CO_2}. With chloride replacement, correction of any potassium deficiency, correction of abnormalities in total body sodium and total body water, and with measures to improve both cardiac and respiratory function, all parameters may eventually return to normal.

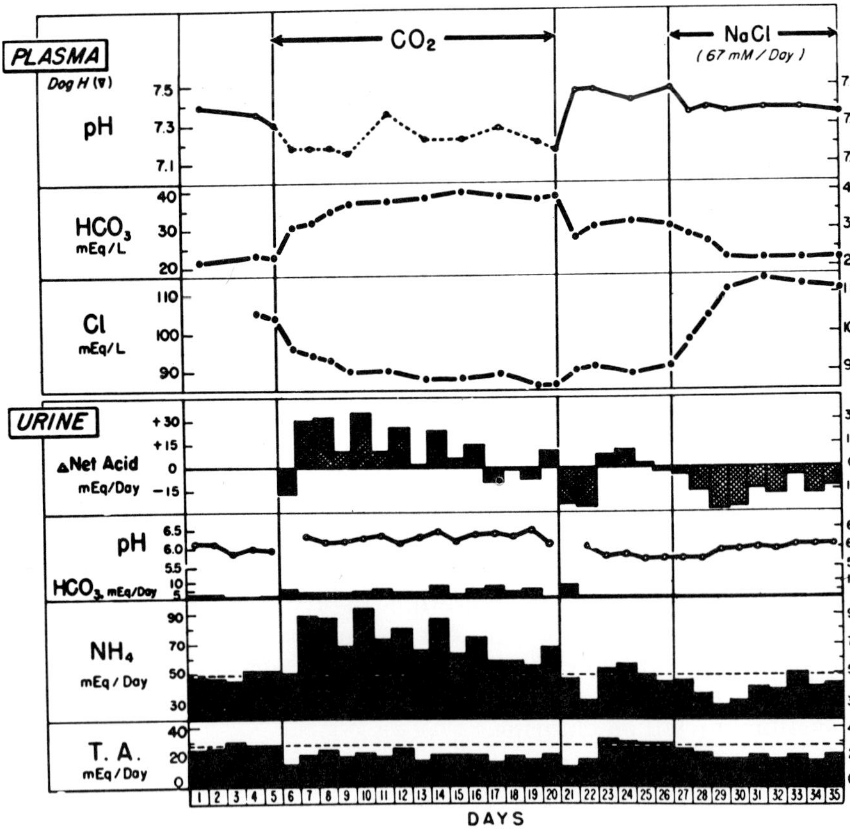

Figure 5-11. The hypochloremic alkalosis produced by the kidney in compensation for increased P_{CO_2} requires several days. When P_{CO_2} returns to normal, the kidney cannot correct the metabolic alkalosis unless additional chloride is made available. (From Polak, A., Haynie, G. D., Hays, R. M., and Schwartz, W. B.: Effects of chronic hypercapnia on electrolyte and acid-base equilibrium. I. Adaptation. J. Clin. Invest. 40:1223, 1961.)

The patient presented earlier demonstrates the complexity of acid-base abnormalities that may occur during a single illness. Respiratory acidosis was compensated by metabolic alkalosis. After improvement in ventilation, a residual metabolic alkalosis remained, due to hypochloremia or perhaps even due to a total body potassium deficiency. In Chapter 6 the sequence is reversed in that vomiting initiates a hypochloremic metabolic alkalosis and this is followed by mild compensatory respiratory acidosis. The clinician who collects data from history and physical findings as well as laboratory data and who weaves all of this information together in a logical, sequential analysis will have the best chance of restoring and maintaining normal cellular function in a normal body fluid with physiologic concentration of hydrogen ion. When data can be obtained by sampling blood before and after a change in P_{CO_2}, a better estimate of body buffer can be obtained than from a single blood sample obtained prior to the improved ventilation. There is no way to determine all that one needs to know about the past, present, and future acid-base balance of a seriously ill patient by manipulations of blood removed from the patient. These are extremely dynamic (non-steady state) problems. Better to analyze the patient's arterial blood serially and to study the data in the context of a changing pathophysiology and treatment than to retire to the laboratory with a single sample of blood.

REFERENCES

Arbus, G. S., Hebert, L. A., Levesque, P. R., Etsten, B. E., and Schwartz, W. B.: Characterization and clinical application of "significance band" for acute respiratory alkalosis. New Eng. J. Med. *280*:117, 1969.

Armstrong, B. W., Mohler, J. G., Jung, R. C., and Remmer, J.: The in-vivo carbon-dioxide titration curve. Lancet *1*:759, 1966.

Astrup, P.: A simple electrometric technique for the determination of carbon dioxide tension in blood and plasma, total content of carbon dioxide in plasma, and bicarbonate content in "separated" plasma at a fixed carbon dioxide tension (40 mm Hg). Scand. J. Clin. Lab. Invest. *8*:33, 1956.

Brackett, N. C., Cohen, J. J., and Schwartz, W. B.': The nature of the carbon dioxide titration curve in the normal dog. J. Clin. Invest. *43*:777, 1964.

Brackett, N. C., Wingo, C. F., Muren, O., and Solano, J. T.: Acid-base response to chronic hypercapnia in man. New Eng. J. Med. *280*:124, 1969.

Bronsted, J. N.: Einige bemerkungen uber den begriff der sauren und basen. Rec. Trov. Chim. Pays-Bas. *42*:718, 1923.

Brown, E. B., and Clancy, R. L.: In vivo and in vitro CO_2 blood buffer curves. J. Appl. Physiol. *20*:885, 1965.

Bunker, J. P.: The great trans-Atlantic acid-base debate. Anesthesiology *26*:591, 1965.

Campell, E. J. M.: R I pH. Lancet *1*:681, 1962.

Child, C. G.: *The Liver and Portal Hypertension.* Philadelphia: W. B. Saunders Co., 1964.

Cohen, J. J., Brackett, N. C., and Schwartz, W. B.: The nature of the carbon dioxide titration curve in the normal dog. J. Clin. Invest. *43*:777, 1964.

Davenport, H. W.: *The ABC of Acid-Base Chemistry.* 5th ed. Chicago: University of Chicago Press, 1969.

Henderson, L. J.: The theory of neutrality regulation in the animal organism. Amer. J. Physiol. *21*:427, 1908.
Huckabee, W. E.: Henderson vs. Hasselbalch. Clin. Res. *9*:117, 1961.
Kilburn, K. H.: Shock, seizures and coma with alkalosis during mechanical ventilation. Ann. Intern Med. *65*:977, 1966.
Lowry, T. M.: The uniqueness of hydrogen. J. Soc. Chem. Indust. *42*:43, 1923.
Masoro, E. J., and Siegel, P. D.: *Acid-Base Regulation: Its Physiology and Pathophysiology*. Philadelphia: W. B. Saunders Co., 1971.
Miller, F. A., Brown, E. G., Buckley, J. J., Van Bergen, F. H., and Varco, R. L.: Respiratory acidosis: its relationship to cardiac function and other physiologic mechanisms. Surgery *32*:171, 1952.
Nuttall, F. Q.: Serum electrolytes and their relation to acid-base balance. Arch. Intern. Med. (Chicago) *116*:670, 1965.
Polak, A., Haynie, G. D., Hays, R. M., and Schwartz, W. B.: Effects of chronic hypercapnia on electrolyte and acid-base equilibrium. I. Adaptation. J. Clin. Invest. *40*:1223, 1961.
Rotheram, E. G., Safar, P., and Robin, E. D.: CNS disorder during mechanical ventilation. J.A.M.A. *189*:993, 1964.
Sackner, M. A.: Management of pulmonary insufficiency. Calif. Med. *110*:355, 1969.
Schwartz, W. B., Hays, R. M., Polak, A., and Haynie, G. D.: Effects of chronic hypercapnia on electrolyte and acid-base equilibrium. II. Recovery with special reference to the influence of chloride intake. J. Clin. Invest. *40*:1238, 1961.
Schwartz, W. B., and Relman, A. S.: A critique of the parameters used in the evaluation of acid-base disorders. New Eng. J. Med. *268*:1382, 1963.
Seiger, R. G., and Hastings, A. B.: An improved clinical method for the estimation of disturbances of the acid-base balance of human blood. Medicine *27*:223, 1948.
Shaw, L. A., and Messer, A. C.: The transfer of bicarbonate between the blood and tissues caused by alterations of the carbon dioxide concentration in the lungs. Amer. J. Physiol. *100*:122, 1932.
Siggaard-Andersen, O. C.: *The Acid-Base Status of the Blood*. Baltimore: Williams & Wilkins Co., 1964.
Smith, T. C.: Editorial: Toward better management. J. Anesth. *30*:125, 1969.
Stern, L. J., and Simmons, D. H.: Estimation of non-respiratory acid-base abnormalities. J. Appl. Physiol. *27*:21, 1969.
Van Slyke, D. D., and Sendroy, J., Jr.: Line charts for graphic calculation by the Henderson-Hasselbalch equation, and for calculating plasma carbon dioxide content from whole blood content. J. Biol. Chem. *79*:781, 1928.
Winters, R. W., Engel, K., and Dell, R. B.: *Acid-Base Physiology in Medicine: A Self-Instruction Program*. Westlake, Ohio: The London Co., 1967.

Chapter 6

Nonrespiratory Defense of Neutrality

This presentation is based on the Bronsted-Lowry definitions of *acid* and *base* as donors and receptors of hydrogen ion and on the rule of electrical neutrality, which states that the concentration of anions is always equal to the concentration of cations in an electrolyte solution. The bar graph of Gamble is our canvas. Sodium concentration is the initial coat of paint. The wide variety of different illustrations of deviations from neutrality depends upon the choice of anions which come from life's palate (Fig. 6-1).

Just as the buffer anions can be divided into (1) respiratory-related bicarbonate and (2) nonrespiratory lactate, sulfate, phosphate, and proteinate, there is also a division of the acids which must be buffered in this system. Carbonic acid, when retained in excessive amounts, is buffered by hemoglobin, and the bicarbonate formed in red blood cells exchanges for extracellular chloride. Bicarbonate diffuses from plasma into the interstitial fluid. Carbonic acid is buffered by nonbicarbonate buffers. By contrast, when organic acids accumulate, or if a strong acid, like hydrochloric, is added to the body fluids, bicarbonate becomes the principal buffer. A valuable and brief review of blood and tissue buffers was presented by Brown at a symposium held at the Minneapolis V.A. Hospital in 1962, but all of the papers in this symposium provide reference material for further study.

When strong acids (or even organic acids which are weak) are added to the body fluids, the buffering by bicarbonate leads to the formation of CO_2 which is released into the alveolar air. This is a chemical reaction which does not require any change in respiratory activity. In fact, if there is no change in ventilation, the result will be an increase in the P_{CO_2}, which is defined as a respiratory acidosis. Compensatory increase in ventilation is a separate and physiologic event, not to be confused with the evolution of CO_2 as a result of chemical reactions. The separation of the explanations of chemical buffering and physiologic compensatory mechanisms is nicely presented in a programmed text by Winters et al.

The relationship between bicarbonate and other anions in the defense of neutrality can be explained in reference to the bar graph used by Gamble, which forces one to think in terms of neutrality. The bar graph representing the electrolytes in extracellular fluid is shown in Figure 6-1. Of the ions usually measured in a hospital laboratory, sodium is the chief cation and chloride the chief anion. The difference between the concentrations of chloride and sodium is made up of bicarbonate and a group of unmeasured anions. Bicarbonate is an anion of a weak acid which

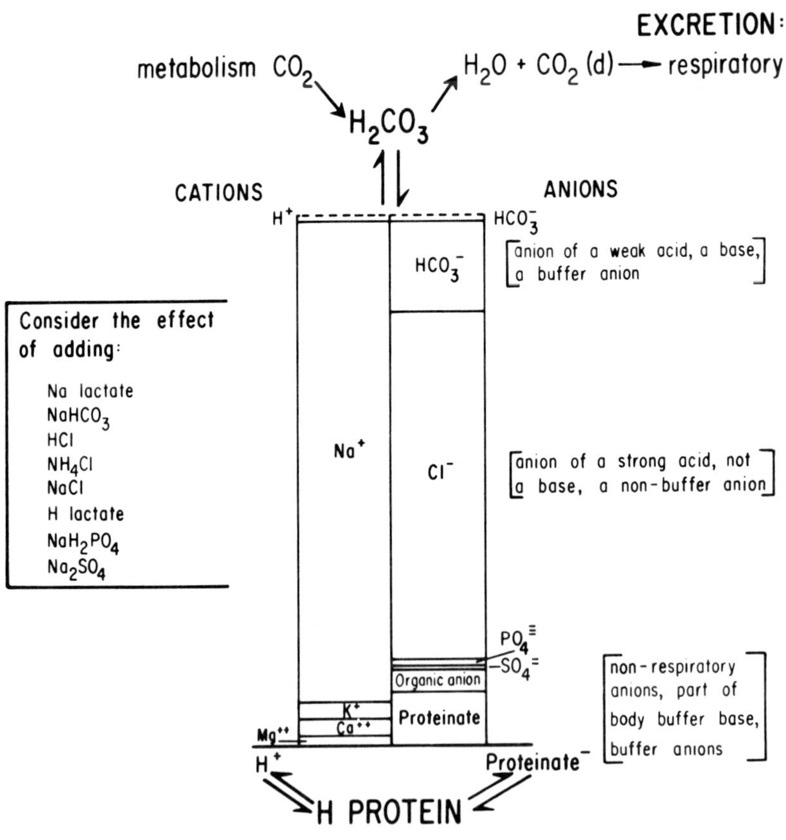

Figure 6-1. Diagrams the relationship between acid-base and electrolyte balance from the viewpoint of the clinician. Fixed cation excess (bicarbonate) indicates body buffer capacity. Carbonic acid is continually produced and excreted and is increased or decreased by rate of ventilation.

will accept hydrogen and is therefore a base. Chloride is the anion of a strong acid and might be considered as a nonbuffer anion since it is such a weak base. At the pH of the blood the unmeasured anion which is the strongest base is proteinate. If a strong acid is added to the body fluids, the hydrogen released will combine with proteinate and the combined hydrogen protein leaves the category of available buffer and becomes a weak acid. At the same time, most of the hydrogen combines with bicarbonate to form carbonic acid, which is dehyrated to provide additional dissolved CO_2, which in turn is released into alveolar air.

To the left of the bar graph are listed a number of substances that may enter body fluids or accumulate in the body fluids and which will have an effect on the hydrogen ion concentration. When sodium lactate is administered, the lactate is metabolized and H^+ is consumed. The result is the same as if sodium bicarbonate had been administered, an addition to the sodium in the body fluids on the cation side of the ledger and an increase in bicarbonate which increases the ratio of bicarbonate to chloride and provides more buffer capacity, producing what can be described as a hypochloremic alkalosis.

If hydrochloric acid or ammonium chloride is added, the hydrogen combines with bicarbonate forming more carbonic acid with release of CO_2 and a reduction of bicarbonate, together with an increase in concentration of chloride. The addition of hydrogen creates an increase in hydrogen ion concentration which is minimized by the bicarbonate buffer but nevertheless represents a hyperchloremic acidosis. Ammonium chloride releases hydrogen, leaving ammonia which is converted to urea, so that this in essence is the same as the administration of hydrochloric acid. Sodium chloride solutions cause a hyperchloremic acidosis by virtue of the fact that equal amounts of sodium and chloride are placed into the system which normally has less chloride than sodium. This increases the concentration of chloride and since the electrical equivalence of anions and cations must be maintained, the concentration of bicarbonate decreases by forming carbonic acid and dehydrating to CO_2. According to Muntwyler, a solution of physiologic saline with a P_{CO_2} less than 40 torr has a pH of 5.0 or less. Following infusion of such a solution, the kidneys excrete the excess chloride and hydrogen so as to produce an appropriate balance of fixed cations and anions to accommodate that concentration of bicarbonate which will reestablish a normal hydrogen ion concentration. If the kidneys are not functioning normally as is frequently the case in seriously ill patients, then infusion of saline will produce a hyperchloremic acidosis.

Both weak and strong acids dissociate into hydrogen and an anion. In the case of the strong acid, this is a nearly complete dissociation, and as an example, hydrochloric acid dissociates so completely that the chloride will not accept more than an extremely small amount of hydrogen to reform hydrochloric acid as a nonionized molecule and therefore the chloride cannot be considered as a significant base. On the other hand, a weak acid, such as carbonic acid, has less of a tendency to dissociate into hydrogen and bicarbonate. The anion bicarbonate is a base because it will accept hydrogen and in the presence of the salt of that acid a buffer is created. If more hydrogen ion is added to the solution, more of the undissociated carbonic acid is formed. On the other hand, if hydrogen is removed from the solution by the addition of an alkaline substance, the weak acid dissociates providing additional hydrogen. A buffer therefore prevents wide fluctuations in hydrogen ion concentration, whereas a strong acid or a strong base causes fluctuations in hydrogen ion concentration. The rule of electrical neutrality requires that if an anion such as chloride, which is neither acid nor base is added to an electrolyte solution, there must be some positively charged ion to balance the ledger. Hydrogen is continuously formed as a result of metabolic processes, just as CO_2 is continuously being formed, and hydrogen could make up the difference on the cation side of the ledger except that this would increase the acidity.The bicarbonate buffer and other buffers take up the hydrogen with removal of bicarbonate and other anions from the buffer pool.

One of the ways of explaining nonrespiratory changes in acid-base balance is to refer to a discrepancy between fixed anions and fixed cations. The term "fixed" signifies that the ions so designated cannot be released through changes in ventilation. The only nonfixed anion is therefore bicarbonate. A change in plasma bicarbonate concentration can be designated as a change in the fixed cation excess or a change in the fixed anion deficit. This sort of terminology is a semantic solution to the problem of talking about changes in chloride concentration as causing changes in acid-base balance. If there were no other anions besides bicarbonate and chloride, then the terms "fixed cation excess," "fixed anion deficit," and "base bicarbonate" would all be interchangeable terms.

"Anion gap" is a term used to designate all of the anions besides chloride and bicarbonate. $(Na^+ + K^+ + Ca^{++} + Mg^{++}) - (HCO_3^- + Cl^-) =$ anion gap. A decrease in anion gap indicates laboratory error. An increase in anion gap requires some disease process such as diabetic ketosis, uremia, severe infection, or shock which could cause an increase in the anions which are not usually measured: lactate, sulphate, phosphate, beta-hydroxybutyrate or acetoacetate.

Kappagoda et al. have criticized the use of the Henderson-Hasselbalch equation and related nomograms in estimating the requirements in treating nonrespiratory acid-base derangements and feel that a trial of therapy with repeat analysis of pH, P_{CO_2} and HCO_3^- after a known dose of acid or alkali and with P_{CO_2} maintained close to 40 mm Hg provides the most accurate prediction of the total requirement. They observe that if such an in vivo titration is performed, mixed venous blood will provide the best sample of total body buffering. If P_{CO_2} cannot be controlled at a level near 40 mm Hg and especially if the patient's alveolar P_{CO_2} is in question, then arterial blood is required. Arterial blood comes from the alveolar tonometer, whereas mixed venous blood mirrors the body buffer capacity.

Critics of the use of nomograms for interpretation of data from isolated blood samples have emphasized the need for evaluating the response of the entire body to changes in P_{CO_2} and have introduced data from groups of patients who were in a supposed well-defined steady state of some specified deviation from neutrality. Such data are presented graphically as the 95% confidence limits for that condition. Any attempt to simplify the problems of acid-base balance will be open to criticism. These are not steady state conditions. There is a time lag in the response of extracellular buffers to an alteration in alveolar P_{CO_2} or to the administration of ammonium chloride or sodium lactate. There is a greater time lag in the response of cellular buffers. Pierce et al. have described this time lag in ventilatory response to acute base deficits in humans and have reported it may last for 11 to 24 hours. What appears to be a mixed disorder may represent only a lag in readjustment between cellular and extracellular buffers. The best approach is to follow patients closely and to watch the response to treatment. Acute change can usually be corrected fairly rapidly. Chronic abnormalities require a more prolonged treatment. Each patient requires special study and repeated observation of the response to treatment as a part of the evaluation.

For the clinician at the bedside the calculation of the magnitude of a hypochloremic alkalosis or a metabolic acidosis can be based upon the estimated size of the extracellular fluid. This is a conservative estimate. In the more severe and prolonged deviations from neutrality, a large portion of the acid or alkaline load is accommodated by intracellular buffering and possibly even by other mechanisms. Peters and Dart found that mild metabolic acidosis stimulated CO_2 production, whereas with high doses of

HCl, CO_2 production was severely depressed. They calculated that up to one-third of HCl could be buffered intracellularly and as much as one-half of a large dose of NaOH could be buffered outside of the extracellular fluid.

Lemann et al. gave large loads of acid or alkali over a period of days. They could not account for all of the acid or alkali. They suggest that it may be buffered by bone or perhaps hydrogen can combine with an electron and cease to function as an ion. There is no accurate way of predicting exactly how much acid or alkali will be required to correct a patient, especially when the abnormality is longstanding. Calculations should be conservative, and treatment must be closely monitored with appropriate laboratory assistance.

NONRESPIRATORY ALKALOSIS

A hypochloremic, nonrespiratory alkalosis can result from either addition of sodium bicarbonate or subtraction of hydrochloric acid. In both situations there is an increase in the ratio of bicarbonate to chloride and, in the Henderson-Hasselbalch equation, an increase in the ratio of bicarbonate to carbonic acid. The most common alkalosis observed by surgeons is one of subtraction, in that the patient is secreting hydrochloric acid in his gastric juice which is lost from either vomiting or suction. There is still controversy as to whether the parietal cell actively secretes hydrogen ion or chloride or both. If it is an active secretion of hydrogen ion, then the chloride goes along to maintain electrical neutrality. If the secretion is an active transport of chloride, the hydrogen could move along passively. Whatever the actual mechanism, hydrogen is lost from the body fluids and whenever hydrogen ion is formed hydroxyl ion is also formed, which would be buffered in the body fluids by carbonic acid, thereby increasing the concentration of bicarbonate in the tissue fluids and blood that leave the region of actively secreting parietal cells. The amount of hydrochloric acid secreted into the lumen of the stomach can be measured by titration of the hydrogen ion in gastric juice. The amount of acid secreted into the stomach has also been estimated by measuring the decrease in hydrogen ion concentration of the blood. For all of the acid which is secreted there is left behind an equal alkalosis or increase in the body's capacity to buffer acid.

When acid gastric juice is secreted, it normally passes on into the duodenum where it stimulates secretin; this in turn stimulates the production of bicarbonate in both the bile and pancreatic juice so that the acid is neutralized in the duodenum. Then all of this fluid with its electrolytes is reabsorbed. The alkaline wave in the body economy is usually transient. Alkalosis occurs only when the secreted acid juice leaves the body, as in a patient with hypertrophic pyloric stenosis or an obstructing duodenal ulcer.

Patients with severe vomiting and with chloride and bicarbonate approaching the same concentration become progressively more difficult to care for. They are unreasonable and confused. Eventually stupor and coma supervene. Goldman et al. described two patients with stupor and convulsions. The problem is more complex than a disturbed hydrogen ion concentration. Usually they have some elevation in the serum creatinine and blood urea nitrogen, and there is likely to be a contraction of extracellular fluid and expansion of intracellular fluid, if the vomiting is severe and of recent onset. Such an acute onset with loss of isotonic electrolyte solution and ingestion of water leads to salt deficiency with a low concentration of serum sodium.

Graham studied muscle biopsy water and electrolytes in 18 adults with pyloric obstruction. In patients vomiting once a day for several months, extracellular fluid was slightly increased. With patients whose vomiting had been more marked but who were not otherwise very ill, the extracellular fluid volume was below normal, and in both the chronic and subacute forms of vomiting and alkalosis, total body water was normal. In the acute and severely ill patient who is confused or semicomatose, there is an internal shift of fluid and a deficit of extracellular electrolyte. Cells, including the central nervous system, are expanded and extracellular fluid, including plasma volume, is contracted. The concentration of sodium is usually below normal. The stupor, coma, and convulsions could be due to the severe alkalosis or the internal shift of fluids or in most instances a combination of both.

In Chapter 5, there was discussion of a patient who had chronic retention of carbonic acid; compensation for this was the excretion of chloride and retention of bicarbonate to create a hypochloremic metabolic or nonrespiratory alkalosis. In the patient who has normal respiratory function and whose primary disturbance is loss of acid gastric juice and a hypochloremic alkalosis, it might be anticipated that the compensation for this would be a retention of carbonic acid. Roberts et al., from data available in the medical literature and from a study of dogs with hypochloremic alkalosis, concluded that no respiratory compensation occurred. The explanation provided for this was that in order to have an increase in P_{CO_2} there would need to be a decrease in P_{O_2} and the hypoxia would drive the respiratory center, thus preventing the retention of carbonic acid.

Reeves and Brown produced hypochloremic alkalosis in dogs and observed that there was an elevation in P_{CO_2} whether the

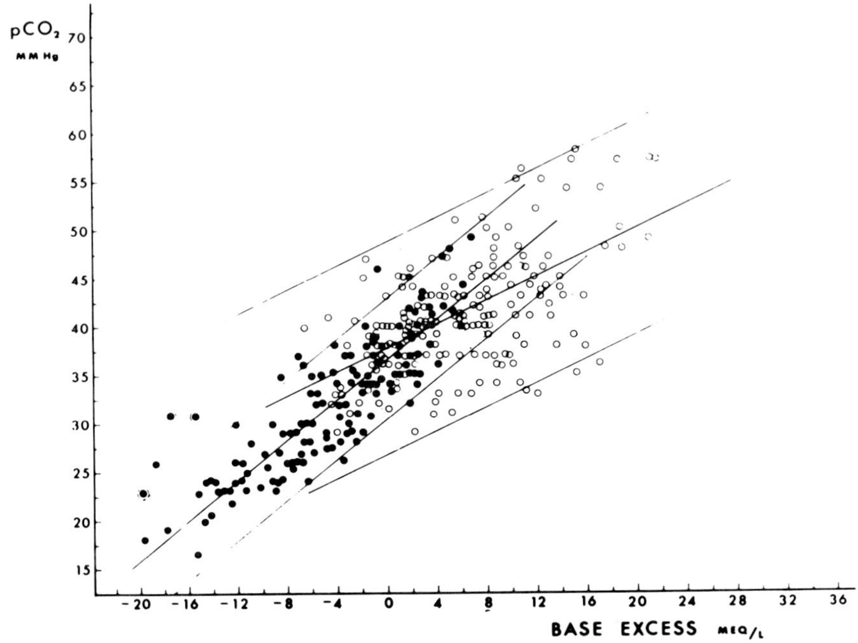

Figure 6-2. A plot of P_{CO_2} in mm Hg and base excess in mEq/l for infants with pyloric stenosis (open circles) and for infants with nonrespiratory acidosis (black dots). The lines indicate the means and standard deviations for the regression equations. There is respiratory compensation in nonrespiratory alkalosis, but it is neither as great nor as predictable as for nonrespiratory acidosis. (From Kildeberg, P.: *Clinical Acid-Base Physiology*. Baltimore: Williams & Wilkins Co., 1968.)

animals were provided oxygen-enriched air or not. Kildeberg found an elevation in P_{CO_2} in patients with nonrespiratory alkalosis and published a scattergram in which data from patients with both metabolic acidosis and alkalosis were plotted against P_{CO_2}. This illustration indicates that there is a respiratory compensation for metabolic alkalosis but that the compensation is not as great as the respiratory compensation for metabolic acidosis (Fig. 6-2). In addition to a lesser slope of the regression line, the standard deviation is greater or, in other words, the elevation of P_{CO_2} is less predictable in metabolic alkalosis than the decrease of P_{CO_2} in metabolic acidosis.

Fuller and Mehdi studied three patients and found reports of five in the literature in whom severe metabolic alkalosis was accompanied by extreme hypercapnia. As the alkalosis was corrected P_{CO_2} returned to normal in these patients suggesting that the hypercapnia was secondary or perhaps compensatory. However, in each instance there was azotemia and/or dehydration, and perhaps the hypercapnia was due to depression of the respiratory center rather than a vigorous compensatory response. These were adults with normal pulmonary function.

Kildeberg's data are of particular interest in that his patients are children and one would suppose that most of them probably had normal lungs. In an adult with pulmonary emphysema and an obstructing duodenal ulcer with loss of acid gastric juice and a hypochloremic alkalosis, and with a P_{CO_2} above 40 torr, there may be pulmonary insufficiency as a primary cause of the elevation in carbonic acid. If the P_{O_2} is below 70 torr, then an elevated P_{CO_2} is probably primary and not compensatory. The differential diagnosis between primary pulmonary disease and primary nonrespiratory disease in such a patient obviously requires data from the history and physical examination and cannot be made from a set of laboratory data. The physician will need to reconstruct the sequence of events.

In the course of treatment of a patient with a low serum chloride and high bicarbonate concentration, there should be a response to treatment with isotonic saline or rarely arginine chloride. In the days before the flame photometer, failure of the chloride and bicarbonate to return to normal levels after treatment with sodium chloride indicated the need for the administration of potassium. Now with the flame photometer the serum potassium concentration can be measured and if the high serum bicarbonate and hypochloremia are related to a potassium deficiency, this can be recognized and treated with a combination of potassium chloride and sodium chloride.

Total body potassium deficiency is associated with the movement of two sodium ions and one hydrogen ion into the cell for each set of three potassium ions that are deficient. This creates an intracellular acidosis and an extracellular alkalosis. The increased acidity of the renal tubular cells causes the urine to be more acid than would be expected in a patient with hypochloremic alkalosis. The loss of acid urine containing high concentrations of chloride serves to perpetuate the hypochloremic alkalosis in extracellular fluid. In the presence of a potassium deficit, all of the filtered bicarbonate is reabsorbed by the renal tubule and some chloride is excreted, even though the serum chloride concentration is below normal. Renal conservation of potassium is poor even when that ion is deficient, in contrast to sodium which is conserved by the kidney when body sodium is depleted. If the alkalosis is on the basis of a deficiency of total body potassium, the administration of potassium chloride should correct the alkalosis. As potassium moves into the cells, the hydrogen moves out into the extracellular fluid, and the kidney begins to excrete bicarbonate and to conserve chloride (Fig. 6-3).

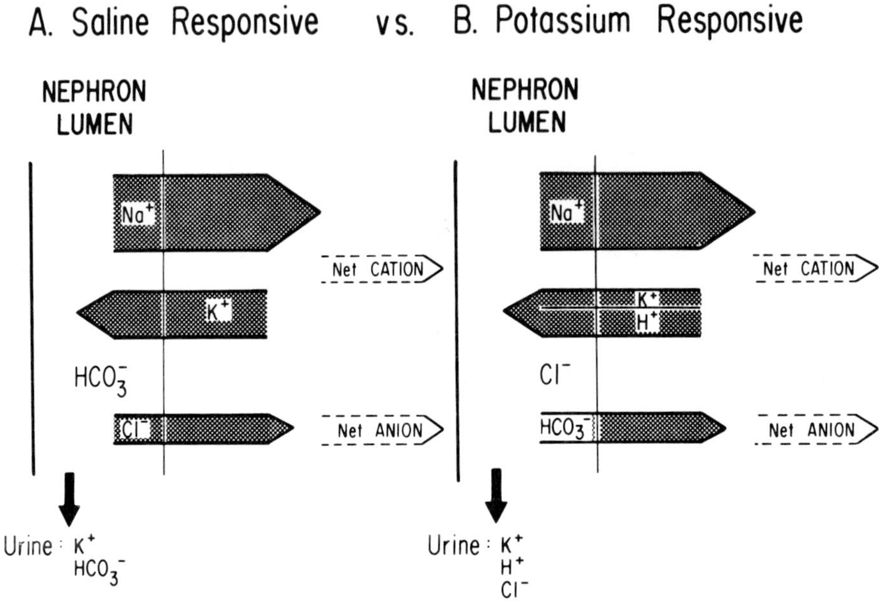

Figure 6-3. Compares two types of hypochloremic alkalosis and their perpetuation by renal tubular reabsorption of chloride when simple chloride deficiency is at fault and by reabsorption of bicarbonate when total body potassium is deficient.

The treatment of simple hypochloremic alkalosis where there is no potassium deficiency is usually carried out by the administration of isotonic saline. In comparison to extracellular fluid, isotonic saline has approximately 50 mEq/l of excess chloride, which serves to correct the chloride deficiency. A calculation of the requirement of chloride, to return chloride concentration to normal and to bring the concentration of bicarbonate back to normal, should be based on the desired change in concentration times the liters of estimated extracellular fluid. For example, a 60-kg lean man has approximately 12 liters of extracellular fluid. If his serum chloride concentration is to be raised by 12 mEq/l, then he needs 144 mEq of excess chloride which will require nearly 3 liters of 0.9% NaCl. The sodium bicarbonate is rapidly excreted by the kidney and the chloride is reabsorbed, as is shown in Figure 6-4. The patient who is secreting extremely acid gastric juice and who has a markedly lowered concentration of serum chloride may need to receive some of his correction fluids in the form of arginine chloride. The arginine is metabolized, leaving behind hydrogen which combines with the bicarbonate and thereby reduces the concentration of bicarbonate at the same time that the concentration of chloride is increased.

If loss of gastric juice leading to hypochloremic alkalosis were simply a loss of HCl, then replacement should be arginine chloride, NH_4Cl, or HCl in the amount calculated to correct the total body deficit. Actually gastric juice loss is usually a mixture of secretions and not pure HCl from parietal cells. Isotonic saline with added potassium chloride usually corrects the abnormality even though it might seem to have an excessive amount of sodium and no hydrogen. Patients with hypochloremic alkalosis have lost large volumes of extracellular fluid. As a result, the kidney conserves sodium by reabsorption in the renal tubule. Anions must also be reabsorbed from the glomerular filtrate, and since chloride concentration is low the bicarbonate is reabsorbed. Therapeutic expansion of extracellular fluid permits some of the sodium to be excreted together with bicarbonate but the chloride is retained, provided there is no potassium deficiency. Kurtzman demonstrated that extracellular fluid volume was an important determinant of renal HCO_3^- reabsorption. Cohen, in reviewing the effect of expanding extracellular fluid upon correction of alkalosis, observed that expansion without chloride would not correct the alkalosis because of the constraints of electrical neutrality. If bicarbonate is to be excreted, some anion must take the place of the bicarbonate. Although correction may be accomplished in some patients with saline alone, the more severe alkalosis usually requires addition of potassium as soon as renal function is adequate.

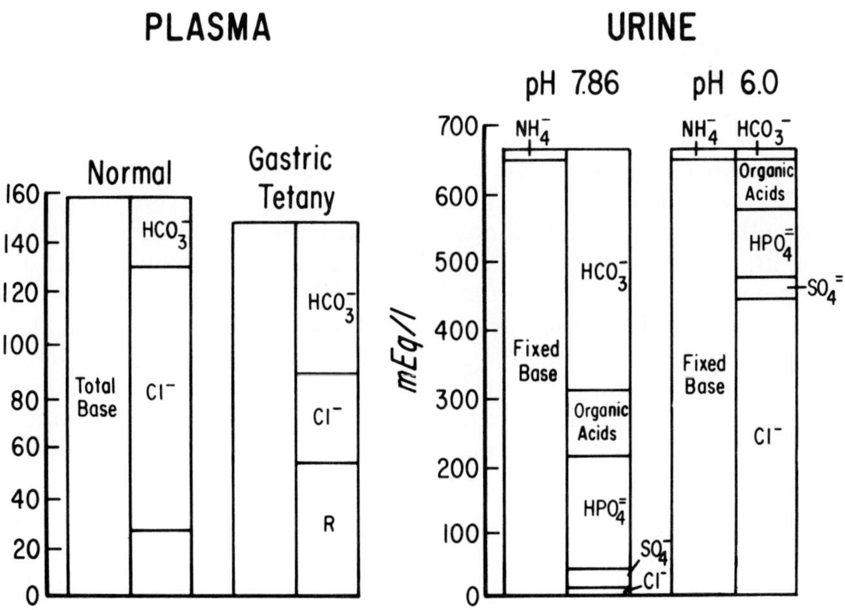

Figure 6-4. Shows bar graphs of the ionic composition of plasma in a patient with hypochloremic alkalosis from vomiting as compared with normal. Also shown are bar graphs for alkaline and acid urine demonstrating how the kidney corrects acid-base inbalance. Gastric tetany requires excretion of bicarbonate and conservation of chloride.

It is extremely important to consider all of the different aspects of fluid replacement, including the fluids for urine and insensible loss, the replacement of ongoing abnormal fluid loss in both its volume and composition, plus the fluids necessary for correction of any existing dehydration or extracellular fluid deficit. Failure to take into consideration all aspects of the patient's needs may allow the patient to remain chronically dehydrated and uremic. Such patients are often nutritionally depleted and as soon as the major correction in their fluid, electrolyte, and acid-base balance has been accomplished, they may need a period of feeding with intravenous glucose, amino acids, and vitamins, such as will be discussed in Chapter 7. The turnover of large volumes of fluid is actually an advantage in that the concentration of glucose does not need to be as high in the administered fluids, and there is less risk of phlebitis. It may even be possible to administer the nutrients through a peripheral vein if they are diluted with the replacement solutions.

Berry in 1960 and Judd et al. in 1970 have used the term *third kidney phenomenon,* which is descriptive of some patients with large volumes of fluid loss from vomiting or gastric suction and in whom large volumes of intravenous fluids are required. There is nothing qualitatively different about these patients, and successful treatment by withholding fluids seems inappropriate. What these patients need is careful replacement of any deficits and then early institution of feedings with central venous nutrient plus adequate amounts of potassium, magnesium, calcium, and any other items that are deficient. Kozoll et al. in a series of papers about obstructing gastroduodenal ulcers showed that prior to 1965 mortality rates were related to the duration of symptoms, the degree of emaciation, the presence of hemoconcentration from extracellular fluid deficiency, and the elevation of creatinine. Mortality was especially high if gastric siphonage had to be continued longer than 5 days and reduced if a period of oral feeding could be used prior to operation. The way to avoid high mortality and morbidity in such patients is to restore plasma and body proteins by use of intravenous replacement and nourishment before operation is attempted. If bleeding from the ulcer bed supervenes, an emergency operation may be required in spite of suboptimal nutrition.

NONRESPIRATORY ACIDOSIS

"Nonrespiratory acidosis" can be defined as any mechanism which reduces total body buffer capacity. In terms of the Henderson-Hasselbalch equation, such a mechanism acts to decrease the bicarbonate or numerator of the equation. There are two ways in which body buffer may be reduced: by loss and by buffer action. There may be loss of buffer from the body, as occurs in a duodenal fistula where bicarbonate is in high concentration in bile and pancreatic juice. The loss of bicarbonate together with sodium results in a reduction in the concentration of plasma bicarbonate and an increase in the concentration of the chloride in the extracellular fluid. This is a subtraction of base causing a metabolic acidosis.

Body buffer may also be used up in buffering acid, as for example in uremia, where acid radicals produced by metabolic activities are retained. In shock where there is poor circulation through the tissues and inadequate provision of oxygen, the metabolism becomes anaerobic and produces an excessive amount of lactic acid. Lactic acid is buffered by the bicarbonate buffer, the hydrogen ion combining with the bicarbonate to produce carbonic acid which, with the help of red blood cell carbonic anhydrase, leaves the solution as carbon dioxide. A similar type of metabolic acidosis occurs in uncontrolled diabetes where there is an accumulation of acetoacetic and beta-hydroxybutyric acid. Any increase in the amount of acid which is buffered by bicarbonate buffer will result in an evolution of CO_2. This is a chemical reaction and does not require any change in ventilation. In the plot of P_{CO_2} and pH, the accumulation of fixed acids reduces body buffer and causes a shift of the buffer line to the left (B in Fig. 6-5). Compensation occurs due to stimulation of the respiratory center by increased intracellular concentration of hydrogen ions, and there results an increased rate of ventilation with a lowering of P_{CO_2} below 40 torr. This can be observed as a shift along the buffer line (C in Fig. 6-5). The compensation is always incomplete so that a normal pH is not reached. The compensatory hyperventilation accentuates the loss of CO_2 which is produced by the chemical buffering interactions discussed above and shown below.

H^+ added results in a loss of gaseous CO_2

$$\downarrow \qquad\qquad\qquad\qquad\qquad\qquad \uparrow$$

$$H^+ + HCO_3^- \rightleftharpoons H_2CO_3 \rightleftharpoons H_2O + CO_2$$

Addition of acid results in loss of CO_2 from this open system which decreases the capacity of the bicarbonate buffer.

The estimation of magnitude of nonrespiratory acidosis is customarily made by obtaining the product of the bicarbonate deficit in mEq/l multiplied by the estimated liters of extracellular fluid. This is a conservative estimate since there is also intracellular buffering, as demonstrated by Peters and Dart. The agent used most often in the treatment of metabolic acidosis is an isotonic solution of sodium lactate. Frequently there is concern about giving 1/6 molar sodium lactate to a patient who may have some elevation of lactic acid as a result of circulatory insufficiency. It is argued that the lactate has to be metabolized before the acidosis will be corrected by conversion of lactate to bicarbonate. Actually lactate is still metabolized even when serum lactate concentration is elevated, and in most patients sodium lactate is as effective as sodium bicarbonate. There are rare patients with extreme retention of lactic acid in whom sodium bicarbonate should be used and may be required in large quantities. In the treatment of cardiac arrest, it is customary to use sodium bicarbonate so as to obtain an immediate correction of the acidosis which has resulted from impaired circulation. It is customary to administer 44 mEq of sodium bicarbonate without having obtained an arterial pH, but further administration of sodium bicarbonate ideally should be governed by measurements of arterial pH. The objective is to establish and maintain a normal hydrogen ion concentration.

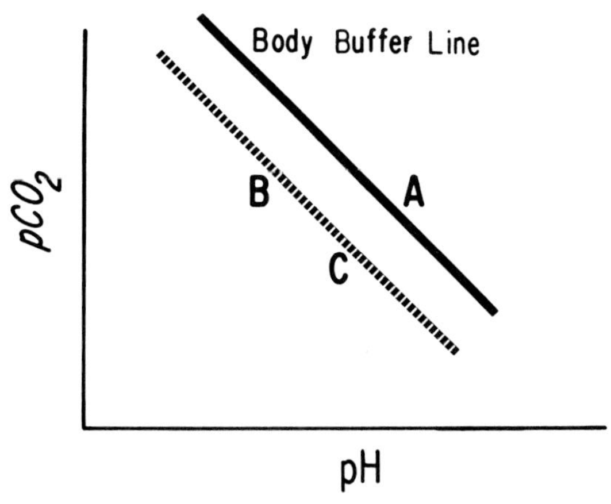

Figure 6-5. If a normal person had arterial blood drawn at various times while breathing different concentrations of CO_2, the solid body buffer line would be obtained. After accumulation of nonvolatile (fixed) acids, repetition of the experiment (breathing different concentrations of CO_2) would produce the dotted body buffer line shown as shifted to the left. While breathing room air, such a person (with a nonrespiratory acidosis) would hyperventilate and reduce his P_{CO_2} so that instead of having data at B his data would be at C.

The abnormality in concentration of chloride is of limited help in estimating the magnitude of the depletion of body buffer. If the kidneys are functioning well, chloride may have been excreted in compensation for retention of other anions. Usually renal function is impaired, and chloride excretion by the kidneys is inadequate. In fact, a high chloride concentration in a patient with acidosis suggests renal insufficiency. Patients who are uremic or otherwise ill and retaining nonbuffer anions frequently are also nauseated and vomiting or have a nasogastric suction tube with removal of excessive chloride. While this is not a predictable compensatory mechanism, the loss of acid gastric juice may correct what would otherwise be a nonrespiratory acidosis. The low concentration of chloride in a patient who is retaining unmeasured anions may permit the patient to have a normal pH. As long as the pH is normal, it is permissible for the patient to have a low concentration of chloride. There is nothing deleterious in a hypochloremia as long as the cellular pH is normal.

Patients who have severe metabolic acidosis are otherwise ill and may have impaired circulation and metabolism, so that the sodium pump is functioning poorly and so that cellular potassium tends to diffuse out of the cell, increasing the extracellular fluid potassium concentration. There is in addition to this a specific effect of extracellular acidosis in causing an elevation of extracellular potassium concentration. Hydrogen, when increased in extracellular fluid as compared to intracellular fluid, tends to diffuse into the cell in exchange for potassium. Brown and Groott found that an increase in P_{CO_2} caused a greater increase of hydrogen ion concentration in extracellular fluid than in intracellular fluid so that hydrogen moved into cells in exchange for potassium. Impairment of kidney function in such patients impairs excretion of excessive potassium. The relationship between hydrogen ion concentration and potassium concentration in the extracellular fluid provides an emergency measure for reduction of dangerous levels of plasma potassium concentration. Lowering the extracellular hydrogen ion concentration by the administration of sodium bicarbonate or sodium lactate will cause potassium to move back into the cell in exchange for cellular hydrogen.

LACTIC ACIDOSIS

Lactic acidosis has been mentioned as an example of an increase in the anion gap and is to be distinguished from diabetic ketoacidosis, uremic acidosis, and other causes of an increase in unmeasured anions. Any sudden increase in metabolism, such as vigorous muscular exercise, will cause an increase in lactic acid. Lactic acid is a product of anaerobic metabolism. Normal muscular activity produces lactic acid which circulates to the liver where it is converted to pyruvate and thence either to glucose or, through oxidative decarboxylation in the Krebs cycle, it provides additional energy and CO_2.

Lactic acidemia is common, transient, and seldom requires treatment. It is self-regulating in that accumulation of lactic acid and CO_2 causes the individual to stop excessive physical activity and allow the oxygen debt to be paid. In circulatory collapse lactate accumulates in the poorly perfused tissues. In theory, such an acidosis would be corrected by the complete metabolism of the lactate, and the administration of sodium bicarbonate would be unnecessary. However, before the lactate can be metabolized a normal circulation is required, and acidosis may interfere with the very cardiovascular function required to re-establish normal tissue perfusion.

Cardiac arrest is the most dramatic situation in which sodium bicarbonate is required in the correction of lactic acidemia. Silberschmid found that increased hydrogen ion concentration causes a decrease in blood pressure, decreased cardiac output, sinus bradycardia, increased central venous pressure, and an increase in peripheral resistance. Campbell found an augmentation of vagal inhibition of the heart by acidosis. Campbell et al. found a depressed pressor response to epinephrine in the presence of acidosis. Observations of the deleterious effects of acidosis strongly suggest that correction of any existing acidosis should be a part of resuscitation measures in treating cardiac arrest as well as in the treatment of less dramatic forms of circulatory insufficiency.

Chazan reported upon 22 patients studied during treatment of cardiac arrest. In many the acidosis is predominantly respiratory, and improvement in ventilation is essential to successful treatment. In 8 patients metabolic acidosis required a moderate amount of sodium bicarbonate, but even in these patients lowering of P_{CO_2} was of help in correcting the acidosis. Close monitoring of arterial P_{CO_2} and pH is essential to appropriate treatment. There is nothing to be gained from massive doses of $NaHCO_3$ if the patient does not have a nonrespiratory acidosis. A normal pH and P_{CO_2} should be provided to make other measures optimum in their effect.

CELLULAR pH

Abnormalities of acid-base balance can be avoided by providing nutrients, water, and normal concentrations of cations and anions through a normal circulation so that cellular metabolism is normal. Hydrogen is a product of oxidation-reduction reactions which produce energy. Protons are not free but attach to water molecules to form hydronium, H_3O^+. Oxidative metabolism involves movement of electrons. Hydrogen becomes an ion by the removal of an electron. Just as there is a hydrogen concentration there is an electron pressure. Dormandy has reviewed the relationship rH between pH and Eh. In less abstract terms, this is the relationship between concentration of hydrogen and concentration of free electrons in equilibrium with the concentration of hydrogen atoms. Measurements of pH are means of determining the health of these relationships. We usually infer the intracellular pH from what can be more easily measured, the arterial blood pH. Schloerb has used an indicator dye to measure cellular pH in dogs and finds the normal to be 6.84 ± 0.06 in skeletal muscle with a simultaneous venous blood pH of 7.40 ± 0.03. Not all organs had the same cellular pH. Liver cell pH was 6.52 ± 0.247 and heart was 6.77 ± 0.09. In the presence of an alkalosis from loss of gastric juice the intracellular pH was 6.92 ± 0.07. In three moribund patients intracellular pH was 6.57, 5.92, and 5.70.

Wolpert et al. have implanted a pH electrode into the tissues as a means of monitoring pH at a site closer to cells in patients. This may be a means of obtaining earlier warning of impending acid-base imbalance.

The ultimate objective is to maintain a normal pH in cells. Homeostatic mechanisms are functioning best when cellular pH is normal regardless of what changes may be required of extracellular fluid. Dormandy observed that patients die because they were not "acidosed" enough; their cells had failed to extrude excess hydrogen into the extracellular fluid.

REFERENCES

Berry, R. E. L.: The "third kidney" phenomenon of the gastrointestinal tract. Arch. Surg. (Chicago) *81*:193, 1960. Symposium.

Brown, E. B.: Blood and tissue buffers. Arch. Intern. Med. (Chicago) *116*:665, 1965.

Brown, E. B.: and Groott, B.: Intracellular hydrogen ion changes and potassium movement. Amer. J. Physiol. *204*:765, 1963.

Campbell, G. S.: Cardiac arrest: further studies on the effect of pH on vagal inhibition of the heart. Surgery *38*:615, 1955.

Campbell, G. S., Houle, D. B., Crisp, N. W., Jr., Weil, M. H., and Brown, E. G., Jr.: Depressed response to intravenous sympathomimetic agents in humans during acidosis. Dis. Chest *33*:18, 1958.

Chazan, J. A.: The acidosis of cardiac arrest. New Eng. J. Med. *278*:360, 1968.

Cohen, J. J.: Correction of metabolic alkalosis by the kidney after isometric expansion of extracellular fluid. J. Clin. Invest. *48*:1181, 1968.

Dormandy, T. L.: Body pH. Lancet *1*:755, 1966.

Fuller, M. A., and Mehdi, F.: Compensatory hypoventilation and hypercapnia in primary metabolic alkalosis. Amer. J. Med. *50*:281, 1971.

Gamble, J. L., and Ross, S. G.: Paradox of aciduria in the presence of hypochloremic alkalosis. J. Clin. Invest. *1*:403, 1924-1925.

Garella, S., Chazan, J. A., and Cohen, J. J.: Saline-resistant metabolic alkalosis or "chloride-wasting nephropathy." Ann. Intern. Med. *73*:31, 1970.

Goldman, M. A., Lisak, R., Matz, R., and Davidson, F. Z.: Hypochloremic alkalosis with symptoms of seizure disorder. N. Y. State J. Med. *70*:306, 1970.

Graham, J. A.: Muscle water and electrolytes in pyloric stenosis. Lancet *1*:386, 1970.

Judd, D. R., Simmons, R. D., Kelley, W., and Newton, W. T.: Gastric outlet obstruction due to peptic ulcer. Arch. Surg. (Chicago) *100*:90, 1970.

Kappagoda, C. T., Linden, R. J., and Snow, H. M.: An approach to the problems of acid-base balance. Clin. Sci. *39*:169, 1970.

Kildeberg, P.: Metabolic alkalosis in hypertrophic pyloric stenosis: clinical significance and treatment. Acta Paediat. *53*:132, 1964.

Kildeberg, P.: *Clinical Acid-Base Physiology*. Baltimore: Williams & Wilkins Co. 1968.

Kozoll, D. D., and Meyer, K. A.: Obstructing gastroduodenal ulcer symptoms and signs. Arch. Surg. (Chicago) *89*:491, 1964.

Kozoll, D. D., Mittelpunkt, A., and Meyer, K. A.: Laboratory findings in obstructing gastroduodenal ulcer. Arch. Surg. (Chicago) *91*:347, 1965.

Kozoll, D. D., Mittelpunkt, A., and Meyer, K. A.: Obstructing gastroduodenal effects of treatment on morbidity and mortality. Arch. Surg. (Chicago) *91*:431, 1965.

Kurtzman, N. A.: Regulation of renal bicarbonate reabsorption by extracellular volume. J. Clin. Invest. *49*:586, 1970.

Lemann, J., Jr., Lemon, E. J., Goodman, A. D., Litzow, J. R., and Relman, A. S.: The net balance of acid in subjects given large loads of acid or alkali. J. Clin. Invest. *44*:507, 1965.

Lockey, E., Longmore, D. B., Ross, D. N., and Sturridge, M. F.: Potassium and open heart surgery. Lancet 1:671, 1966.

Muntwyler, E.: *Water and Electrolyte Metabolism and Acid-Base Balance.* St. Louis: C. V. Mosby Co., 1968.

Peters, R., and Dart, C. H., Jr.: Metabolic alterations in CO_2 production in acid-base derangement. Ann. Surg. *170*:128, 1969.

Pierce, N. F., Fedson, D. S., Brigham, K. L., Mitra, R. C., Sack, R. B., and Mondal, A.: The ventilatory response to acute base deficit in humans: time-course during development and correction of metabolic acidosis. Ann. Intern. Med. *72*:633, 1970.

Reeves, J. L., and Brown, E. G., Jr.: Respiratory compensation to metabolic alkalosis in dogs: influence of high oxygen concentration. J. Appl. Physiol. *13*:179, 1958.

Roberts, K. E., Popell, J. W., Beals, R., and Randall, H. T.: Evaluation of respiratory compensation in metabolic alkalosis. J. Clin. Invest. *35*:261, 1965.

Schloerb, P. R.: A new approach to the DMO intracellular pH method. Surg. Forum *15*:70, 1963.

Siggaard-Andersen, A.: The pH, log P_{CO_2} blood acid base nomogram revised. Scand. J. Clin. Lab. Invest. *14*:598, 1962.

Silberschmid, M.: Circulatory effects of acute lactic acidosis in dogs prior to and after hemorrhage. Amer. J. Surg. *112*:175, 1966.

Winters, R. W., Engel, K., and Dell, R. B.: *Acid-Base Physiology in Medicine: A Self-Instruction Program.* Westlake, Ohio: The London Co., 1967.

Wolpert, P. W., Noller, K., Shaughnessy, D., Houchin, D. N., Baccari, M. E., and Miller, F. A.: Tissue pH: a new clinical tool. Arch. Surg. (Chicago) *101*:308, 1970.

Chapter 7
Nutrition

To achieve the lowest possible rate of mortality and morbidity in the care of complicated problems in surgery requires close attention not only to the balance of fluid and electrolytes but also, at the same time, to the patient's nutrition. The retention and distribution of fluid and electrolytes are influenced by the patient's state of nutrition. Surgeons have special skills in managing nutrition by virtue of the types of patients that they care for, the uses that they make of central venous catheters in the administration of nutrient solutions, and their ability to establish gastrostomy and enterostomy sites for tube feedings.

THE METABOLIC POOL

Food consists mainly of plant and animal cells which are ingested intermittently and from which nutrients are slowly released and absorbed into the metabolic pool of glucose and amino acids. The absorbed glucose replenishes glycogen in the liver, supplies current energy requirements, stimulates release of insulin (which in turn blocks amino acid release) and, in excess, glucose is converted to glycerol and fatty acids which form triglycerides for storage in the fat depots. Amino acids absorbed from the intestine are used to synthesize albumin in the liver and protein in muscle and in all cells. Fatty acids, derived from the digestion of micelles (composed of triglycerides, bile salts, cholesterol, and digestive enzymes) in the intestinal lumen, are re-esterified in the cells of the intestinal mucosa, and these triglycerides are packaged as lipoprotein-coated, water-soluble chylomicrons which pass into the intestinal lymphatics and thence into the systemic circulation by way of the thoracic duct. Peripheral and small vessel activation of lipoprotein lipase by heparin releases the fatty acids at sites of utilization for energy or for storage in the fat depots.

Between meals glucose is supplied to a small degree by the glycogen stores, but in larger measure by release of the nonessential amino acid alanine from muscle. Alanine is converted to glucose in the liver. Other amino acids and the kidney participate in the production of glucose to a lesser degree. Fatty acids are also mobilized during periods of fasting and are burned in preference to glucose by most tissues. Fatty acids supply the energy in the liver for conversion of lactate and pyruvate to glucose. The lactate comes from glycolysis in muscle and passes through the circulation to the liver where reconversion to glucose provides a renewed source of substrate for muscle glycolysis. This transformation of lactate to glucose to lactate to glucose is the Cori cycle, which provides a means by which the aerobic metabolism of fat in the liver provides energy by the anaerobic metabolism of glucose in peripheral muscle. According to Owen et al., about one-half of the glucose produced in the liver comes from the lactate and pyruvate, and the other half of glucose supplied by the liver comes from glycerol and amino acids.

GLUCOSE METABOLISM

Glucose is the preferential substrate for energy in all cells when it is available. Glucose stimulates insulin production, and under the influence of insulin, glucose enters cells and at the same time seems to block the entrance of fatty acids into cells so that the energy metabolism comes from glucose and not fatty acids. At the same time, some of the glucose upon entrance into fat is converted into glycerol phosphate, which provides a basis for re-esterification of fatty acids thereby maintaining the fatty acids in fat depots. Whereas most tissues derive energy from fatty acids, the brain requires glucose in quantities of 100 to 150 gm a day. The renal medulla and reparative cells such as fibroblasts and macrophages are also dependent upon a supply of glucose. Some glucose is required at all times for complete combustion of fatty acids and for the prevention of ketoacidosis.

The supply of glucose in the blood is very limited, as it is estimated to be around 40 calories; added to this is glycogen in the liver sufficient to supply some 200 additional calories. The large reservoir of functional muscle protein is mobilized whenever blood glucose levels are low. Amino acids, predominantly alanine from muscle, are converted to glucose in the liver; two-carbon fragments from fatty acids supply the energy for this conversion. Fatty acids are not converted to glucose but are used directly as an energy source when glucose concentrations are low. In prolonged starvation the brain adapts to the burning of ketones so that less glucose is required from the protein stores. Owen et al. have gathered evidence from various sources to suggest that elevation of serum insulin blocks peripheral mobilization of amino acids.

The hormonal control of catabolism has remained a mystery. Schimmel and Knobil noted that gluconeogenesis begins before there is a fall in insulin concentration or a rise in free fatty acid concentration. We have known for over thirty years that, if a starving patient is provided glucose in an amount above 150 gm a day, there is a reduction in urinary nitrogen loss from the starvation level of approximately 12 gm to as little as 1 gm per day. In a normal man, much of the catabolic effect of an operative procedure is the result of the associated starvation, unless this minimal glucose requirement is supplied in the intravenous fluids.

A normal person may be able to metabolize as much as 600 gm of intravenously administered glucose per day, but there is no need to provide 2400 calories a day to a patient who is well nourished and only ill for a few days. The patient who is markedly undernourished, grossly obese, severely traumatized, or elderly is less tolerant of large amounts of glucose. The amount of glucose actually required will depend upon the objectives of treatment. Six hundred calories a day may be sufficient to prevent excessive catabolism, but if amino acids are administered for synthesis of protein, larger amounts of glucose are needed.

FATTY ACID METABOLISM

In contrast to glucose and amino acids which provide 4 calories per gram, fat provides 9 calories per gram. A kilogram of body fat supplies 9000 calories whereas a kilogram of muscle or lean nonfat tissue supplies only 1200 calories per kilogram. This is because 70% of the weight of these lean tissues is made up of water.

Whenever blood glucose and insulin levels are low, the glucose no longer enters fat cells to provide a substrate for formation of glycerol phosphate and the re-esterification of fatty acids. As a result the fatty acids which are continuously being released within the fat cells leave the fat depot and enter the circulation. The hydrolysis of triglycerides in the fat cell releases glycerol, which also leaves the cell since there is no mechanism in the cell for reutilization of the glycerol which has been released (Fig. 7-1).

Randle et al (1963) noted competition between glucose and fatty acids to gain entrance into most tissues except for the obligatory glucose-burning tissues such as the nerve cells. Whenever glucose concentration is high, the glucose enters cells, and fatty acid is blocked from entrance to cells. By contrast when the fatty acid levels are high, the fatty acids gain ready access to body cells, and glucose is blocked and preserved for use by the brain. The bulk of energy during the day is derived from combustion of fatty acids since glucose is not available in excess except following a meal.

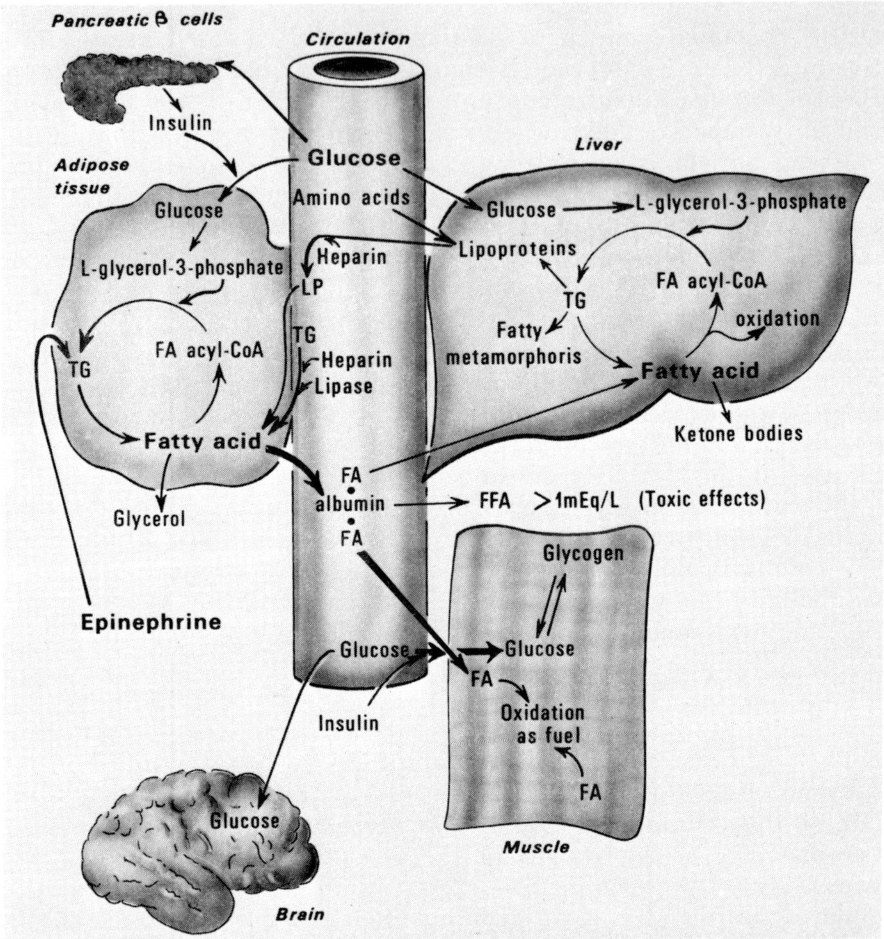

Figure 7-1. Shows the interrelationships of glucose and fatty acid metabolism. When glucose is in adequate concentration, it is used by all cells for energy and in the liver and adipose tissue for formation of L-glycerol-3-phosphate. When glucose levels fall, fatty acid is released from fat stores and is burned as fuel, blocking entrance of glucose into most tissues and leaving the remaining glucose for use in the brain. Epinephrine causes lipolysis. Fatty acids are carried by albumin in the blood, but at high levels free fatty acids are present to cause platelet agglutination, blood clotting, and other toxic effects.

ETHYL ALCOHOL

In the early days of parenteral nutrition, the difficulties in providing an adequate caloric intake were attributed to the lack of a high-calorie substance which could be given intravenously. One of the solutions to this supposed problem was the use of alcohol which provides 7 calories per gram. Moore and Karp reviewed the experience prior to 1945 and reported that in 150 patients who were given 1 to 3 liters of a 5% to 10% solution of alcohol they did not observe the nausea, vomiting, acidosis, and headache from the administration of alcohol intravenously which was observed when similar amounts of alcohol were given by mouth. A normal average adult can burn 10 gm of alcohol per hour. Alcohol is burned in preference to glucose. Nitrogen balance cannot be achieved if alcohol is the sole source of calories.

Rice, Orr, and Enquist reported the use of a solution of amino acids, invert sugar, and alcohol in which about a third of the calories were supplied by the alcohol. This reduced the osmolality of the solution so that it could be given through a needle in peripheral veins. It was still productive of phlebitis, and the site of infusion had to be changed frequently. As plastic catheters became available, these permitted the infusion to be given into central and larger veins, but a long plastic catheter in a peripheral vein still caused phlebitis. Phlebitis has been minimized by introduction of the subclavian catheter which has minimal contact with the endothelium and by the administration of solutions with a high concentration of glucose into a central venous pool where there is rapid mixing with a large amount of blood. As long as glucose can be provided in sufficient amounts to supply the needed calories, the impetus to finding a high-calorie molecule such as alcohol no longer exists. Alcohol removes plasticizer from some of the catheters that are in use and increases the brittleness of these catheters.

AMINO ACIDS

Amino acids are normally absorbed from the proximal 100 cm of small bowel. They enter the metabolic pool and are thence incorporated into muscle protein, plasma proteins, and other proteins in the body. There are 20 different amino acids, 8 of which cannot be formed in the body and therefore must be obtained from the diet. Such amino acids were referred to in 1914 by Osborne and Mendel as essential amino acids. The sequence of events leading to the establishment of the amino acid needs of man has been reviewed by Rose. If any one of the essential amino acids is deficient in a protein food or in an infusion of amino acids, the excess of all other amino acids is converted to energy use rather than the building of protein. A food which has exactly the proportion of essential amino acids required for the building of body protein is said to have a high biological value. In the past much attention has been paid to the ratio of essential amino acids to nonessential amino acids in the food and in the plasma as an index of biological value.

Recently the nonessential amino acid alanine has become the focus of attention in states of starvation and increased catabolism. Early in starvation, alanine is released from the muscle and is taken up by the liver where it is converted to glucose. During periods of negative nitrogen balance, protein synthesis in the liver is sustained or even increased while muscle protein production is markedly decreased. Waterlow observed that a much greater proportion of the amino acids entering the metabolic pool during starvation are reutilized. Even in a well-nourished individual there is a continual turnover of amino acids within the body, so that at any one time the amino acids in the metabolic pool come mostly from the turnover of protein in the body rather than from recently ingested food. In prolonged starvation the amino acid levels, which initially may have risen to above normal levels, fall to subnormal levels since all of the amino acids available have to be derived from the breakdown of other proteins in the body.

There is no storage of protein in the body analogous to the storage of triglycerides in globules of fat. All of the protein is functional. About 5% of the body protein in a well-nourished person is rapidly lost during fasting and is therefore considered to be the most readily available or labile protein. Some 25% of body protein may be lost at a somewhat slower rate. At any point during starvation nitrogen equilibrium can be maintained at a suboptimal level. Muscle and skin contribute the major portion of protein nitrogen lost during the earlier stages of depletion, although all of the organs contribute to some degree. Allison and Wannemacher found that the RNA decreased in all organs as the protein content diminished, indicating that a decrease in protein synthesis occurred when circulating amino acids were not available in adequate amounts. Trauma and infection increase the demands for energy and may increase the utilization of muscle and skin protein for glucose production and for production of cells involved in the area of injury and repair. If an injury is not too massive, then an adequate dietary supply of calories and amino acids can promote positive nitrogen balance. After a period of negative nitrogen balance, as the proper diet is increased, muscle, skin, and other proteins are replenished.

ALBUMIN

Plasma albumin is of particular interest, because when it is in decreased concentration it represents an index of the poor nutritional state. Also the colloid osmotic pressure of albumin in the vascular space is an important factor in maintaining a normal plasma volume. Life without albumin has been noted in those patients with a congenital deficiency in production of albumin. Such people have a high rate of gamma globulin synthesis and high concentrations of serum globulin, cholesterol, and phospholipids. They have increased sedimentation rates. They have a tendency to develop mild to moderate edema. They fatigue easily and tend to develop anemia and occasional diarrhea. If the person with analbuminemia is given an infusion of albumin, dextran, or polyvinylpyrrolidone, the elevated serum cholesterol and phospholipid levels return to normal. The importance of albumin in maintaining normal volumes of water in the body is illustrated in the shark with its low concentration of albumin and high concentration of urea when living in sea water. When the shark is transferred to a fresh-water environment, the urea concentration decreases and the concentration of albumin rises. From these observations it is apparent that albumin has an important function as an osmotic agent. This function can be performed by other molecules in a healthy body, but in a starved individual a decrease in concentration of albumin represents a serious depletion which may require early correction in order to re-establish adequate circulation and function of the various organs.

Albumin also functions as a carrier for many electrolytes, hormones, small molecules normally present in the body, and various drugs. Thyroxine, calcium, copper, zinc, fatty acids, bilirubin, uric acid, acetylcholine, cholinesterase, vitamin C, Chloromycetin, Aureomycin, barbiturates, and Dicumarol are among the many and varied substances which are carried by albumin. In most instances the sites of adsorption are different for each of the items listed, so that they do not compete with each other for position on the albumin molecule. The concept of albumin as a carrier of other molecules can be generalized even to the property of its colloid osmotic pressure since this is dependent upon its ability to bind water. Rankin has observed that albumin binds less water per gram when the concentration of albumin is reduced.

Albumin is synthesized in the hepatocytes of the liver on rough endoplasmic reticulum which is formed under the stimulus of branched chain amino acids and under the stimulus of a deficit in total body albumin. Albumin synthesis can be stimulated, therefore, by catabolic states which cause a rise in the amino acid concentration in the blood, if total body protein is not too severely depleted. Synthesis of albumin is stimulated by thyroid hormone and cortisone, probably because these hormones mobilize protein from the muscle, connective tissue, and lymphocytes and thereby increase the amino acids in the metabolic pool. Albumin also moves into the vascular space under cortisone influence. The albumin produced in the hepatocytes is extruded into the space of Disse, which is separated from the vascular sinusoids by an endothelial layer containing large pores. Hepatic lymph is from the space of Disse and therefore high in concentration of albumin, but much of the newly produced albumin enters directly into blood circulating through the liver.

The normal adult has 4.5 to 5.0 gm/kg of total body albumin. When the total body albumin is in normal quantity, 60% of the albumin is located outside of the vascular space; most of this is in the skin. When albumin stores are depleted to the extent that plasma albumin concentration falls below normal, then all available albumin is present in the vascular space, and it can be surmised that the total body albumin is less than normal. When a healthy individual loses blood acutely, there is a rapid movement of albumin into the vascular space from extravascular areas, so that blood volume is restored. This mechanism for the restoration of blood volume after hemorrhage would of course be impaired in a patient whose total body albumin was also greatly depleted.

Albumin is sequestered after major operations. Mouridsen found that at least one-third of the drop in concentration of serum albumin which is observed after a major operation in rabbits can be accounted for by sequestration in the albumin-rich fluid in the wound. The wound becomes another compartment which is not in equilibrium with the rest of the body. About 6% of the intravascular albumin can be sequestered in the wound. After six to eight days the lymphatics are re-established, and the normal rate of removal of albumin from the wound is resumed. It is not unusual to observe a 1 gm/100 ml decrease in concentration of albumin following a gastric resection. Gump et al. also found an increase in extravascular albumin-containing fluid in the lungs of traumatized people.

Ravdin, in 1940, called attention to the impairment of wound healing and the edema which occurred even weeks or months following wound healing at the site of the gastrointestinal anastomosis when animals were acutely depleted of albumin by plasmapheresis. Administration of plasma in volumes 6 times the normal plasma volume over a 2-week period in such protein-depleted dogs caused a rise in plasma proteins, allowed normal healing of wounds, and relieved previously anastomosed sites of their edema. Circulation, oxygenation, and a generous supply of glucose and amino acids are all necessary for normal wound healing. Poor nutrition has an invidious influence upon all of these.

A serum albumin level below 3 gm/100 ml is indicative of a state of malnutrition of sufficient severity so as to warrant energetic efforts at correction before attempting an elective operation. A normal concentration of serum albumin does not signify that the total body protein is normal since circulating serum albumin levels may be maintained in the poorly nourished individual even while extravascular albumin and muscle protein are being depleted.

UNDERNUTRITION

The recognition of poor nutrition is sometimes difficult unless it is suspected and specifically looked for. The signs and symptoms of malnutrition may be obscured by the very disease which caused the malnutrition. Taylor and Keys studied a group of healthy young men who, for a 6-month period, were restricted to 45% of their estimated normal caloric intake. The diet contained 1570 calories, 55 gm of protein, and 25 gm of fat per day. These men lost 24% of their body weight. The subjects became depressed and developed edema, anemia, polyuria, bradycardia, and weakness. Their oxygen consumption was decreased even more than the decrease in cell mass. The reduction in oxygen consumption was estimated to be due to both a reduction in cell mass (accounting for about two-thirds of the decrease) and a reduction in metabolic rate of the remaining cellular mass (accounting for one-third of the decrease). There was minimal change in the concentration of serum proteins, and the decrease observed could be accounted for by an increase in plasma volume of 8%. The extracellular fluid volume was increased by 4.3%. Taylor and Keys were under the impression that fat, muscle, liver, and skin lost a great deal of substance whereas the brain, skeleton, and serum proteins were maintained. They found that the work of the heart was decreased by 50%, a reduction of 20% more than could be accounted for by lowered oxygen intake. A starved person survives for a time without adequate food by consuming cellular substance, preserving serum proteins, and expanding plasma and interstitial fluid volume.

Haxhe created a 27% weight loss in dogs and found decreases in red cell volume of 26%, in exchangeable potassium of 27%, in total cardiac output of 30%, and in red blood cell cardiac output of 41%. This is in contrast to the compensatory increase in cardiac output which may be observed in a patient who has an acute anemia without weight loss. The red blood cell cardiac output is depressed even more than the body cell mass in starvation or undernutrition. This confirms the observation of Taylor and Keys that there is a decrease in function of the remaining cellular cytoplasm in addition to the decrease in actual cell mass. Alleyne, in a study of severely malnourished Jamaican children, also found a reduced cardiac output with both bradycardia and reduced stroke volume.

Moore and Ball refer to the extreme changes which occur in starvation as "skin and bones cachexia." Moore, Olesen et al. have measured the decrease in exchangeable potassium, which is an index of reduced cellular mass, and the increase in exchangeable sodium, which documents an expansion of extracellular fluid. These changes are similar to those diagrammed in Figure 4-1 in which the total body water is shown to be normal or decreased, but there is a shift in fluid with a decrease in intracellular space and an increase in the extracellular sodium-containing fluid. The reduction of intracellular fluid is more in muscle than it is in the visceral areas, as is indicated by a decrease in urinary creatinine excretion which is an index of muscle mass.

The cachectic patient has few reserves. He is able to survive by virtue of a slowing in substrate consumption, decreased cardiac output, bradycardia, shift of fluid into the extracellular space (which helps to maintain extracellular fluid volume), and the localization of all of the available albumin in the vascular space (which helps to preserve a circulating blood volume). If an operation is performed, infection occurs, loss of fluid results from diarrhea or intestinal fistula, or some other serious complication develops, then the poorly nourished individual is likely to have inadequate circulation with sludging, thrombosis, poor wound healing, infection, and death.

Malabsorption is exaggerated by undernutrition, since all of the digestive functions including motility and the production and secretion of digestive enzymes are impaired. Neale et al., in a study of patients with malnutrition after partial gastrectomy, observed that they all had diarrhea with bulky, offensive stools, emaciation, edema, and profound weakness, with low serum albumin levels. Two of the patients had a marked deficiency in excretion of digestive enzymes by the pancreas. Liver function was impaired.

After the administration of 25 gm of albumin a day for 6 days, Neale et al. observed that the total body weight was decreased from 50 to 38 kg from loss of edema fluid. The liver function improved, and the concentration of fat in the feces dropped from 50 to 12 gm a day. Tandon et al. have described recovery in the production of pancreatic enzymes that occurs after restoration of body proteins. The depleted patient is anorexic and apathetic about taking pancreatic extract as well as food. Even if the patient is treated with central venous infusions of nutrients, the pancreas may for a time be incapable of producing sufficient insulin, and therefore extra insulin must be made part of the treatment.

OVERNUTRITION OR OBESITY

Not all of the nutritional problems which surgeons face are due to an inadequate intake of food. Extreme obesity has been so resistant to medical treatment that surgeons have been developing operations which will help the obese patient lose weight. One justification for such aggressive treatment comes from data, as published by Marks, which indicate a higher mortality rate as obesity increases and also a greater incidence of many surgical and nonsurgical diseases in the obese at the time of death.

Obesity also makes the recognition of extracellular fluid depletion more difficult, since the subcutaneous fat preserves the normal contour of the skin and obviates the use of skin turgor as an index of extracellular fluid volume. Thermal regulation is impaired, and cooling blankets may be needed to control excessively high fever. Wound infections are more common. The obese individual is more likely to develop incisional hernias, just as he more commonly has umbilical, esophageal hiatus, and inguinal hernias. Hypertension, diabetes mellitus, and degenerative arthritis are accelerated.

The overweight patient may also have a deficiency in body protein. Obesity is the result of the ingestion of more calories than are expended for work and the consequent storage of triglycerides. A patient who is eating more fat and carbohydrate than is required may at the same time be taking an inadequate amount of protein in the diet. A state of unhealthy protein-deficient obesity may result also from injudicious and overzealous regimens designed to produce weight loss. There is a limit to how rapidly fat can be mobilized and burned as a part of the patient's daily energy requirements. An average dieting adult should still receive 50 gm of protein a day as well as enough carbohydrate to bring the total caloric intake to a 1000 calories. Total starvation increases the weight loss, but the additional loss is due to breakdown of muscle and lean body tissue so as to provide the glucose that is necessary for metabolism of the endogenous fat.

FATTY ACID TOXICITY

The excessive mobilization of fat in starvation, or in starvation plus trauma, results in an elevation in serum fatty acid levels (Fig. 7-1). Fatty acids, which are a major source of energy supply, are also potentially toxic. There is evidence which was reviewed by Mason et al. that excessive levels of fatty acid may be a cause of death in patients who are in a negative caloric balance. Fatty acids are attached to albumin during their transit from sites of liberation to sites of utilization. At concentrations of albumin of 4 gm/100 ml and fatty acid levels of 1.1 mEq/l, it has been estimated that 3% of the unesterified fatty acids are free (or in excess of what can be carried by the albumin). The free fatty acids adsorb to platelets and increase platelet stickiness. The free long-chain saturated fatty acids also form micelles to which the Hageman factor adsorbs and unfolds, exposing a surface of the Hageman factor which activates blood clotting. Fatty acids, when in excess, are also taken up by the alveolar lining cells of the lung and interfere with the production of surfactant, so that this may contribute to the production of atelectasis. The injection of long-chain fatty acids into dogs has caused death from disseminated intravascular coagulation. If clotting was prevented by heparinization, the animals still died with rhythm disturbances observed in the electrocardiograms prior to death. Fatty acids also have been shown to depress myocardial contractility and to interfere with coronary blood flow.

Acute starvation causes mobilization of fatty acids to borderline toxic levels. Adrenaline, growth hormone, and ACTH also cause mobilization of fat. The starved patient, particularly if he is extremely obese, is likely to develop dangerous elevations of serum fatty acids during and following a major operation unless special attention is paid to supplying glucose and promoting glucose utilization in order to tie up the fatty acids in fat cells. It is not enough for the patient to have a normal or slightly elevated blood glucose concentration. Blood glucose levels rise during and after operations even when glucose is not provided. The important objective is to promote entrance of glucose into cells. This requires the administration of glucose intravenously so that insulin production is stimulated. If glycosuria occurs insulin can be given.

Allison, Hinton and Chamberlain studied patients with burn injuries and observed changes in insulin production and effectiveness. In milder injuries the patients merely became resistant to the effects of insulin so that higher serum insulin levels were required. In more severe injuries there was an initial failure in insulin secretion which over subsequent days was corrected, and then was followed by a decreased responsiveness to insulin. Similar increases in resistance to insulin have been observed following other types of injury. The hypercatabolic state would seem to involve insulin intolerance and a shift from glucose to fat metabolism with mobilization of both muscle protein and fat, sometimes resulting in a dangerously high level of serum fatty acids.

Certain amino acids stimulate the release of insulin and theoretically should promote entrance of glucose into fat cells, thereby reducing serum fatty acid levels. This hypothesis was tested by Rollins comparing serum fatty acid levels during operative treatment of our extremely obese patients who were randomized into three experimental groups. It appears from this study that there is no significant difference in the serum fatty acid levels whether the patients receive 5% glucose, 10% glucose, or 5% glucose and 5% casein hydrolysate. All were effective in preventing excessive elevation of serum free fatty acids.

FAT EMBOLISM

Fatty acid toxicity and fat embolism have certain common denominators, but they are not the same thing. Fat embolism is thought to be a movement of fatty tissue through the blood stream with globules of fat lodging in the small vessels in the lung and elsewhere, obstructing blood flow during the initial mechanical phase. Later on the fat is hydrolyzed, releasing fatty acids which have a local toxic effect including a severe inflammatory reaction. Some of the effects of excessive concentrations of fatty acid would probably be similar whether they occurred following fat embolism or whether they resulted from the excessive mobilization of fatty acids from fat stores.

During the chemical phase of fat embolism, the toxic effects of fatty acids are located in the areas of fat lodgment, whereas in mobilization of excessive free fatty acids a more generalized effect is observed, but in both instances the lungs are involved and intravascular coagulation may be a major factor in the ultimate outcome.

The treatment of fat embolism is directed towards supporting the respiration and circulation and reducing the inflammatory reaction in the lung by the administration of cortisone. The management of fatty acid toxicity is directed toward prevention of excessive mobilization of fatty acids by making sure that the patient has an adequate supply of glucose in his intravenous fluids and by promoting the utilization of glucose when necessary by the administration of exogenous insulin. Both fat embolism and fatty acid toxicity can cause death without being detected or even suspected. Fat embolism has usually occurred before the patient comes to the hospital. Fatty acid toxicity from excessive mobilization of fat is a potential hazard which should be obviated by prevention of the hypercatabolic state.

PREVENTION OF UNDERNUTRITION

Patients who are unable to eat are given intravenous fluids with the idea of maintaining a normal fluid and electrolyte balance. They should also receive glucose in these fluids to reduce the loss of protein from the body. It was mentioned that the nitrogen loss could be reduced from 12 to 1 gm per day by supplying as little as 600 calories of glucose. The preservation of 11 gm of nitrogen would be equal to the preservation of 69 gm of protein, and since muscle and lean body nonfat tissue is 70% water, this is equivalent to the preservation of 230 gm of muscle. A patient who requires 3000 calories per day and receives fluids without thought directed toward the calories required may after ten days be deficient of some 25,000 calories which he might have received if the physician had simply considered the possibilities of maintaining his nutrition during the convalescent period.

Madden et al. presented detailed studies in 1946 of several patients treated with intravenous amino acids and mentioned a young man who was fed (by Albright and Reifenstein) for 26 days with parenteral Amigen and glucose. This latter patient was thereafter given a full meal by mouth and was able to eat this without disturbance. They observed that if a 26-day fast had been induced without supplying amino acids, thereby allowing a depletion of body proteins and development of enzyme deficiencies, this man would not have been able to secrete normal amounts of digestive juices and enzymes. Therefore he would not have been able to eat and digest a full meal. The use of high calorie and amino acid nutrient solutions intravenously carries some hazard, makes additional work on the part of the staff, and should not be used for every patient who undergoes a major operation. Every patient should receive at least 600 calories a day. If the patient is already depleted before the operation or if the operation is a complex one from which he may not recover within a few days, and if it is anticipated that there may be a prolonged period of time during which intravenous fluids will be the only source of nutrients, then a complete and hypertonic infusion of amino acids and glucose by central venous catheter is indicated. Healing will be better, convalescence will be smoother and shorter, and infections and fistulae will be less likely to occur and more readily taken care of if they do develop.

Wilmore and Dudrick showed in puppies that if intravenous nutrient solutions are given following extensive resection of the small bowel, hypertrophy and hyperplasia of intestinal villi in the remaining small bowel will be increased, and absorption will be more normal even after the animal is subsisting on ingested food. Those patients requiring a major operative procedure who are depleted in body proteins may benefit from a preoperative period of forced feeding, even if the feeding has to be given by the intravenous route and even though the operation is intended to make it possible to eat normally. Complications which develop in the poorly nourished individual may lead to death, whereas in the partially restored patient the same complications, if they occur, are more easily dealt with. In some instances a gastrostomy, or feeding enterostomy, can be performed as an initial brief operation, and the patient's nutrition can be corrected by the administration of tube feedings in preparation for a more extensive abdominal operative procedure.

Following an operation the energy requirements are increased, and the production of positive nitrogen balance may be somewhat more difficult. In 1936 Cuthbertson described what he called "the catabolic state," and for three decades it was thought by the majority of physicians that such a state could not be reversed. Clark and Bruschwig in 1942 demonstrated that positive nitrogen balance could be induced by the intravenous route using a solution of dextrose, emulsified fat, and Amigen. Elman had given intravenous amino acids to dogs in 1937 and to human beings in 1940 and published a book on the intravenous use of amino acids in 1947. In 1947 there were at least three different reports showing that a positive nitrogen balance could be produced even during the immediate postoperative period. These reports by Riegel et al., Holden et al., and Werner related to patients undergoing moderate and uncomplicated operative procedures. Werner used a solution composed of pure essential amino acids, but most of the work was done with protein hydrolysates made from casein. Rice et al. in 1950 used alcohol to augment the caloric levels without producing such a high osmolarity and therefore with less injury to the small peripheral veins. The traumatized patient needed as much as 30 calories per kilogram per day to assure utilization of the amino acids and to induce a positive nitrogen balance.

Even with these reports, however, there remained a general scepticism as to whether these patients were really building protein or whether the amino acids were being sequestered in some labile storage area from which the nitrogen was lost after the short-term experiment was completed. Werner demonstrated that the metabolic response to stress was not necessarily one of obligatory negative nitrogen balance but rather an increase in metabolic rate and nitrogen turnover so that if adequate nutrients were supplied, anabolism could be accelerated to the point where it would equal or exceed the increased rate of catabolism. Holden et al. observed that it was easier to establish a positive nitrogen balance in women than in men. They also showed that androgens would increase the accumulation of nitrogen when the caloric intake was modest, but that if the caloric intake were high, nothing was to be gained from administration of androgens.

Wilmore, Curreri, et al. in 1971 randomized a comparison of dietary intakes of 600, 3000, and 6000 calories in patients with extensive thermal injury, sepsis, weight loss, and poor wound healing. The 6000 calorie diet was given half by vein and half by parenteral tube feedings. Metabolic rates were not influenced by the different caloric intakes, but the 600-calorie intake produced a respiratory quotient of 0.80, whereas 3000 calories produced an RQ of 0.89, and 6000 calories produced an RQ of 1.01. Respiratory quotient is the ratio between the volume of carbon dioxide expired and the volume of oxygen inspired in a given time. The RQ's for carbohydrate, fat, and protein are respectively 1.00, 0.707, and 0.801. The respiratory quotient can therefore be used as an index of the type of fuel which the body is burning. The change in respiratory quotient observed by Wilmore indicates that when the caloric intake is low, the individual burns protein and fat from his body stores and that as the carbohydrate intake is increased, body energy is derived from burning carbohydrate. Wilmore's study provides additional evidence that efforts to maintain a neutral or positive nitrogen balance by providing adequate calories are worthwhile, even in the extensively injured patient.

There is an increase in requirement for calories beginning at the time of injury and extending until healing is well established. Massive injury, sepsis, and major complications add to the caloric requirements. If these increased needs are met, positive nitrogen balance can be maintained, healing will be more certain, and complications are less frequent and more easily dealt with. There are many instances in which the judicious use of insulin, albumin, and blood, as well as correction of fluid and electrolyte imbalance, may improve the utilization of glucose so that the necessary amounts of these nutrients can be safely given.

Emphasis upon high-caloric feedings in the burned or traumatized patient requires a warning as well. Evans and Butterfield in 1951 and Arney et al. in 1960 have called attention to "stress diabetes," which is most likely to be a problem in those extensively burned patients who are being force fed. A failure to recognize this condition will lead to acute dehydration from osmotic diuresis as well as shock, hyperpyrexia, coma, and death, as described in Chapter 2. Urinary glucose levels of 1 or 2+ are often correctly attributed to the overzealous use of intravenous glucose infusion and are of no serious consequence. The infusion rate can be reduced or insulin given on a sliding scale to correct the problem. When 4+ glucose appears in the urine, however, this no longer should be explained as simply due to the intravenous infusion of glucose producing blood glucose levels slightly above the renal threshold. Once the urinary glucose is 4+, the urinary sugar is no longer an index of the blood level, and extremely high blood glucose levels may develop. As soon as a 4+ test is observed in the urine, the patient should not only be treated with insulin and a reduction of the rate of glucose infusion, but in addition blood glucose levels should be followed until returned to normal.

Physicians have been inclined to administer incomplete nutrient solutions and have found less than optimum utilization of the contents of these solutions because they were incomplete. Lockhart and Elman in 1949 demonstrated that glucose utilization was increased when amino acids were given simultaneously with the glucose. Habif et al. in 1951 found an improvement in nitrogen balance when both potassium and phosphate were added to an infusion of amino acids and glucose, although addition of phosphate alone was not effective. Strickler and Rice in 1953 were under the impression that the administration of 12% invert sugar,

6% amino acids, and 4% alcohol during the early postoperative period made it much easier to maintain normal fluid and electrolyte balance. In 1949 Ellison et al. gave 3 liters a day of 5% amino acids to a series of patients and varied the caloric intake. They found that serum albumin levels increased when the caloric intake was raised to 30 to 45 calories per kilogram body weight per day. In 1969 J. W. Anderson et al. observed that patients who weighed more than 170% of ideal body weight and who were depleted of potassium during fasting had an abnormal glucose tolerance test, whereas similarly obese and fasted patients who were given potassium showed an improvement in their ability to secrete insulin. The conclusion from these observations would seem to be that treatment with intravenous nutrients should be complete and should be patterned so as to correct any specific deficiencies that exist. The excellent nitrogen retention and growth demonstrated by Dudrick (1968) through the use of the intravenous solutions containing all of the necessary nutrients, minerals, and vitamins support this conclusion. There is one seemingly contradictory study by Kaess et al., in which a 3% to 11% total body potassium deficiency was created in six *normal* males with no effect upon glucose tolerance, fatty acid levels, or plasma insulin levels during either oral or intravenous glucose tolerance tests.

In the seriously ill patient undergoing major operative treatment the administration of a nutrient solution should be at a steady rate and a constant composition insofar as calories, amino acids, and minerals are concerned. This is more logical than the administration of a liter of amino acid solution, followed by a liter of hypertonic glucose, and then a separate infusion of the day's electrolytes. This latter approach plus an inadequate supply of calories probably accounted for some of the discouragement and scepticism when amino acids were used thirty years ago in the treatment of patients.

Albumin production in hepatocytes is resumed as the central venous nutrient infusion is increased, but in the severely depleted patient it is occasionally desirable to administer 25 to 50 gm of albumin a day, for a 5- to 10-day period, during early treatment in order to restore a normal colloid osmotic pressure and normal plasma volume and to withdraw edema fluid from the tissues, so as to improve circulation and permit better utilization of the nutrients that are being given. If a marked anemia exists, whole blood or washed red blood cells should also be given. Cachectic patients may lose as much as 10% of their body weight as their body protein stores are repleted. The amount of weight loss depends upon the amount of nutritional edema. Following the weight loss there is a period of stable weight and finally a gradual increase in body weight without any evidence of edema, which is an indication (along with the maintenance of a normal serum albumin without albumin infusions) that the patient's nutrition has improved to the extent that any needed major operative procedure can be undertaken.

CENTRAL VENOUS CATHETERS

Wilmore and Dudrick have provided evidence that proper insertion and care of a catheter in the subclavian vein will make for a low rate of infection and other complications. There needs to be rapid mixing of the highly concentrated and therefore potentially irritating nutrient solution. This at the present time is best accomplished by having the end of the catheter in the superior vena cava. There should be a minimum of contact between the catheter and the endothelium, with a minimal obstruction to blood flow past the catheter. This cannot be achieved by a peripheral cannulation and a long catheter which runs from some area in the arm to the superior vena cava.

There are three ways in which catheters are placed so as to discharge their contents into the superior vena cava: (1) a cutdown cannulation of the external or internal jugular vein; (2) a percutaneous puncture and cannulation of the internal jugular vein; and (3) a percutaneous cannulation of the subclavian vein. The cutdown is usually used in infants. The vein is exposed through a small skin incision above the clavicle and lateral to the sternocleidomastoid muscle. A long large-bore needle is used to pass the Silastic catheter through a long subcutaneous tunnel extending from behind the ear to the site of entrance into the vein. The cutdown incision is closed.

In the other two techniques the patient is placed in steep Trendelenburg position so as to distend the neck veins making them easier to puncture and reducing the risk of air embolism. A pillow or folded sheet is placed beneath the dorsal spine and the head is extended without a pillow. In all of these approaches the skin is prepared as for an operative procedure. The operator wears cap, mask, and sterile gloves and drapes the field with sterile towels. All equipment must be laid out on a sterile field and ready for use. The sternocleidomastoid is grasped in the sternal notch with the index finger and the thumb laterally encircles the origin of the muscle and lifts it up. The skin is injected with local anesthetic in a small amount so as to raise a small wheal as if placing a skin test, and the large-bore needle is inserted through the wheal which is placed 1 cm lateral to the muscle and about 1 cm above the thumb grasping the muscle. The needle is advanced aiming at a point 1 cm lateral to the ipsilateral manubrio-clavicular joint. A 10-ml syringe is attached to the needle, and slight suction is applied as the needle is advanced. As soon as blood is obtained in the syringe the needle is advanced another 2 or 3 mm and 5 ml of blood aspirated and reinjected. The syringe is removed holding the needle in position, an 8″ catheter is inserted through the needle and the needle is removed from the skin, the hub of the needle and expanded end of the catheter are engaged, and the sterile micropore filter and intravenous tubing are attached. A stiff plastic guard is placed around the sharp end of the needle and the catheter to prevent shearing of the catheter and embolization, and the guard and catheter are taped to the neck. If, during the insertion of the catheter, there is some obstruction, the plastic catheter must not be withdrawn without at the same time withdrawing the needle because the catheter can be cut by the sharp edge of the needle creating a catheter embolus.

Cannulation of the subclavian vein requires placement of the patient and preparation of the skin as in the above description except that nothing is placed beneath the shoulders and the head is turned sharply toward the opposite side. The neck is kept at a 90-degree angle with the shoulder which helps to keep the catheter from going into the opposite subclavian or ipsilateral jugular vein. The point of puncture is halfway between the two ends of the clavicle and 2 cm below the clavicle. The needle is aimed at the sternal notch. If the aim is too far cephalad, the subclavian artery will be punctured; if too dorsal, the brachial plexus (or the thoracic duct on the left side); and if too caudad and dorsal, the pleural cavity will be entered.

Common to the jugular and subclavian vein cannulation are the following: (1) A 14-gauge, 8″ long polyethelene intracath is used for all patients nine years old or older. (2) The skin must be prepared with all the care that would be used for a formal operation using a defatting agent, scrub, and antiseptic solution. Landmarks such as the sternal notch should be included in the sterile field. (3) The local anesthetic should be limited to the epidermis. Injection of deeper tissues is not necessary and will obliterate landmarks and flatten the vein that is to be cannulated. (4) If the needle is inadvertently advanced too far and possibly through the opposite wall of the vein, light suction is applied through the syringe as the needle is withdrawn until blood appears in the syringe. Then after advancement for a few millimeters, blood is aspirated again, reinjected, and the rest is as outlined above. (5) When the guard has been placed, a sterile fluid-filled micropore filter and the intravenous tubing are attached, and reflux of blood and free flow of fluid are again tested by lowering and raising the intravenous bottle. (6) Tincture of benzoin is poured over the skin around the area so as to make a thick film. This keeps the skin dry and thus discourages bacterial growth. It also helps immobilize the catheter. A small dressing is applied, and the catheter and intravenous connections are taped to the chest wall with wide tape. (7) The dressing is changed every three days using cap, mask, sterile gloves, and a repeat of the preparation of the skin and application of a dressing as outlined above. (8) The Silastic catheter used in infants can be used for months. The other catheters should be changed every three weeks to the opposite side. Of course, if there is unexplained fever, the catheter should be changed sooner. (9) Immediately after insertion of a central venous catheter an upright chest roentgenogram should be obtained to make sure the catheter is properly positioned and that there is no pneumothorax. If the tip of the catheter is in the jugular or opposite subclavian vein, then it must be removed in order to obviate thrombosis of that vein.

Silicon rubber catheters are recommended by Filler et al., and Teflon catheters are recommended by Freeman and MacLean as being less likely to cause sepsis. Daily urine and blood cultures are recommended with a special search for candida if sepsis is suspected. Otherwise cultures should be taken once a week. If the suspicion of sepsis is strong, the catheter should be removed even without a positive culture. Whenever the catheter is removed, it should be cultured by snipping the tip of the catheter into a culture tube. If the catheter fails to return blood when the dressing is changed and if minor adjustments do not permit aspiration of blood, this, according to Freeman and MacLean, is an indication of fibrin on the tip of the catheter and is an indication for removal of the catheter. Formation of fibrin may be deterred by the addition of heparin to the solution at the concentration of 1 u/ml.

Initially the infusion rate needs to be limited to prevent glycosuria. In the severely depleted patient 1000 calories per day during the first few days are as much as should be attempted. The subcellular organelles require time for regeneration before massive infusions of amino acids and glucose can be efficiently used in replenishing depleted albumin, red blood cells and muscle protein. Cellular potassium, magnesium and phosphate are needed and all of the coenzymes produced from vitamins. Overzealous treatment in initial stages may cause such distortion of fluid, substrate, and body electrolytes and may so impair cellular function as to cause coma and death. The deterioration in the patient's condition may be accompanied by glycosuria. Silvis and Paragas (1971) observed a profound fall in concentration of serum phosphate, but the administration of insulin, phosphate, or other supposedly deficient electrolytes did not lead to recovery. The infusion of central venous nutrient should be stopped, and a slower infusion of 5% glucose substituted. When the patient has recovered, the central venous nutrient can then be resumed at a greatly reduced rate.

If glycosuria or signs of the fatal hyperalimentation syndrome (paresthesias, weakness, seizures, and hypophosphatemia) do not appear, the rate of infusion may be increased to 2500 to 3000 ml per day. After these higher rates of infusion have been in force for a number of days, there is danger of hypoglycemia should the infusions suddenly be stopped, and the nursing staff should be alerted to this danger. The nursing staff should also be instructed not to increase the infusion rate in order to try to make up for a period when the rate was too slow. The prescribed infusion rate should be re-established. Attempts to catch up will simply overload the patient with glucose, with the danger of an osmotic diuresis, dehydration, and all of the potential regulatory difficulties that this implies. When the time comes to discontinue the infusion, a less concentrated glucose solution should be provided for twelve hours, while insulin production is adjusting to the lower requirements.

The patient's requirements for vitamins B and C should be given at least once a day. Vitamin K should be given every three to four days. Folic acid is given twice a month and vitamin B-12 once a month. There are trace elements and essential fatty acids that are probably required and which can be supplied by giving a unit of plasma once or twice a week. Plasma and whole blood needed should be given through another site.

Rea et al. have suggested that severe heart failure is the only contraindication to the use of the central venous nutrient solution. Abnormal liver function is usually more of an indication for improved nutrition than a contraindication to the use of amino acids. One should not hesitate to supply this kind of nutrient to a patient who has had a recent extensive liver resection or who has undergone a portal systemic shunt for bleeding varices secondary to cirrhosis of the liver. The objective should be to create a state of protein building which will thereby minimize the amount of ammonia and other wastes. Such patients need a rebuilding of their muscle protein so that they will have sufficient strength to ventilate their lungs. Essential amino acids in ideal concentration would be better than a crude hydrolysate for patients with liver or renal disease.

CENTRAL VENOUS NUTRIENT

Dudrick et al. in 1968 demonstrated that long-term parenteral nutrition would promote positive nitrogen balance and normal growth. Short-term positive nitrogen balance had been produced

20 years earlier, and Rice et al. were strong advocates of maintaining positive nitrogen balance throughout the early postoperative period with a solution containing amino acids, invert sugar, and alcohol. There were centers in this country where surgeons used such a solution for a few years, but they gradually gave up the practice because of lack of sufficient conviction of its value to override the problems attendant upon the administration of a hypertonic solution. The revival of this type of therapy promises to persist and may even be extended to the care of the permanently disabled patient who needs an artificial gastrointestinal tract. Rhoads and Scribner et al. have written about the possible administration of central venous nutrients or infusion into an arteriovenous fistula as a means of permanent care of patients. The increasingly common care by chronic hemodialysis of patients who are anephric has demonstrated that it is possible to maintain intravenous cannulation of various sorts for prolonged periods of time.

Commercially produced intravenous nutrient solutions are now available. Until recently the technique of preparation of such solutions has been similar to that of 20 years ago, when the physician or his nursing staff began with a liter bottle of 5% glucose and 5% casein hydrolysate. Two hundred ml were removed from the bottle and replaced with 150 ml of 50% glucose and 50 ml of 95% ethyl alcohol so that the solution provided a calorie per ml. Additions also were made of multiple vitamin preparations, potassium chloride, and on occasion other additives. Such a technique of mixing on the ward increases the chance for contamination, and therefore the mixing was done as close to the time of administration as possible. If a laminar flow hood was available, it was used to decrease the risk of contamination. The use of a micropore filter in the intravenous line adds a safety factor and is advocated by some because, in addition to the possibility of contamination, the solution is an excellent culture medium for fungi.

Alcohol is no longer used by most physicians because it causes hardening of some of the plastic catheters, and there is concern about the use of alcohol in patients with fatty liver, cirrhosis, or pancreatic disease. Also there no longer seems to be the necessity to find a high-calorie substitute for part of the glucose, since the central venous infusion site decreases the likelihood of injury to the endothelium. Without the use of alcohol a mixture of 500 ml of 5% Amigen and 5% glucose plus 200 ml of 50% glucose will provide a basic solution to which the complex of vitamins B and C, the potassium, calcium, and magnesium salts can be added.

Heat sterilization of a *mixture* of amino acids and glucose cannot be used because of a chemical reaction which takes place.

Commercial solutions are available now in two interconnected bottles which have been separately sterilized. The mixing of the amino acids and glucose still needs to be performed prior to administration. These hydrolysates of casein and fibrin contain some short-length peptides in addition to the amino acids. Both of these amino acid hydrolysates are satisfactory at concentrations recommended. With a pure amino acid preparation it would undoubtedly be possible to use a solution with a lower concentration of amino acids. Such a solution with a minimum of waste and appropriate concentrations of essential amino acids has been used for the treatment of anephric patients by Wilmore and Dudrick, demonstrating that patients could be maintained for much longer periods of time without dialysis. There was even the impression that some of the nonessential amino acids could be produced in the body from urea. Richards et al. administered the carbon skeleton alpha-keto-acid analogues of amino acids to healthy and uremic men and found that these were converted to amino acids, suggesting that a no-protein diet might be designed for anephric patients and still make available essential amino acids.

The ideal composition of amino acids for intravenous use is not known and may be at variance with an ideal composition for use in the digestive tract. The gut and liver are important in regulating peripheral plasma amino acid composition. Stegink and DenBesten found that plasma cystine level was maintained if a cysteine-free elemental diet was given by gastric gavage for two weeks, but the plasma cystine level was not maintained if the same diet was infused intravenously. Such observations will have an important bearing on the choice of constituents for the ideal intravenous solution.

Another consideration in the compounding of an ideal intravenous diet relates to the effect upon acid-base balance as reviewed by Heird et al. Protein and amino acids are amphoteric; they function as both cations and anions, acids and bases depending upon the pH of the solvent. Also different amino acid solutions and protein hydrolysates have varying proportions of organic and inorganic anions (Fig. 7-2). If after the utilization of the solution in protein production or for energy, there is a residue of fixed anions in excess of fixed cations then the patient will be more acid. On the other hand if the residue provides an increment in anion gap the patient will be more alkaline. An ideal intravenous amino acid infusate should have no effect upon acid-base balance or at least the effect should be known so that it can be counteracted by addition of either ammonium chloride or sodium lactate. If this is unclear, perhaps you should refer again to this paragraph after rereading Chapters 5 and 6.

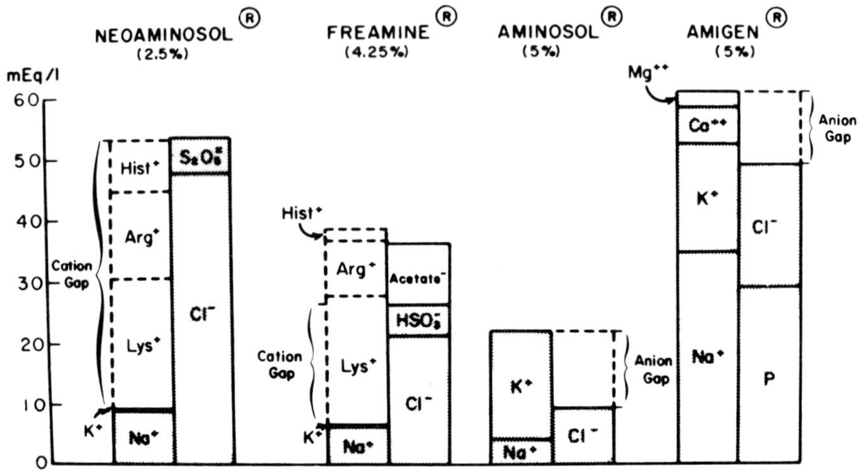

Figure 7-2. Shows the relationship of fixed anions to fixed cations and the cation or anion gap which could cause either acidosis or alkalosis depending upon the solution used. (From Heird, W. C., Dell, R. B., Driscoll, J. M., Jr., Grebin, B., and Winters, R. W.: Metabolic acidosis after intravenous alimentation with amino acids. New Eng. J. Med. *287*:943, 1972.)

The preparations in use have a minimal amount of potassium so that the physician can use this solution even in a patient who has a high normal serum potassium concentration. For the majority of patients, additional potassium must be added to the solution, usually 40 mEq/l, which brings the total potassium content to 55 mEq/l. This means that if the patient is given 3 liters a day, he will receive 165 mEq of potassium. Even this may not be sufficient in some patients if there is a deficiency of total body potassium.

RISKS OF CENTRAL VENOUS TREATMENT

Some patients tolerate total parenteral alimentation for a month or more without complications, but there are complications that do arise. Rea et al. have referred to allergic reactions, hyperosmolar coma, catheter sepsis, clotting of the catheterized vein, and pneumothorax. I have mentioned the hypoglycemic reactions following discontinuation of the infusion and there are occasional occurrences of metabolic acidosis which will be discussed later.

Following World War II, prisoners liberated from concentration camps were provided nourishing foods in quantity and showed a surprisingly high mortality rate. In recent years with the reintroduction of intravenous feedings there have been illnesses and deaths which were due to overvigorous treatment, but usually unrecognized as such. These patients have complicated illnesses and the development of paresthesia, weakness, seizures, coma, and death is likely to be attributed to their serious illness rather than to the treatment.

Silvis and Paragas (1972) observed three patients with paresthesias, convulsions, and coma, one of whom died. The symptoms began four to seven days after beginning infusions of amino acids and high concentrations of glucose. They ruled out any hyperosmolar, uremic, or keto-acidotic basis for the coma and other symptoms. In a separate paper they described the production of this same syndrome in dogs that became malnourished following intestinal resection and wherein treatment was started after the animals had lost 50% of their body weight. The administration of an intravenous solution containing 140 calories/kg/day led to drowsiness and in some animals, coma, with death occurring on an average of 5.4 days after the start of treatment. This same sequence was produced also in rats that were starved and then suddenly subjected to high-calorie infusion. If, after starvation and weight loss, the animals were provided enough feed to maintain them at their reduced weight for a while after weight loss and before treatment was started, the mortality rate was reduced. The mortality rate could also be reduced by starting out with infusions containing fewer calories.

The cause of symptoms and death could not be determined from this study, but it was observed in both the patients and the animals that there was a marked fall in concentration of serum phosphorus which might be used as a laboratory finding, warning the physician that such a syndrome might develop. The addition of phosphate to the infusions did not prevent death. Extreme hyperventilation has been observed in patients developing this reaction. Travis et al. found a decrease in red blood cell 2,3-diphosphoglyceric acid which they thought might explain the hyperventilation. A reduction in 2,3-DPG in the red blood cells causes the oxygen to be retained more avidly so that it is not available to the tissues and could cause the individual to be anoxic as far as his tissues were concerned, even though the oxygen content of the blood was normal.

The cells of the body under conditions of starvation require some time to activate their ribosomes and to produce the cellular enzymes that are necessary for the increase in metabolism. A chronically, severely malnourished patient who is to receive infusions of central venous nutrient should have these started at less than 50 ml per hour. The infusion rate should be increased slowly over at least a week; if the infusion rate is increased more rapidly, or to higher than usual levels, the serum phosphorus concentration should be monitored. If this falls, it is a warning that the infusion of nutrients should be reduced in dosage until the patient has had a chance to accommodate. The only treatment known thus far for the hyperalimentation syndrome is to decrease or discontinue the infusion and resume treatment at a slower rate.

In spite of care to avoid contamination of the solutions and the special care in the insertion and management of the central venous catheters, occasional infections occur. These occur not only in debilitated patients but also in patients who have received multiple broad-spectrum antibiotics so that the normal flora have been suppressed and antibiotic-resistant, opportunistic bacteria and fungi are present in the mouth, colon, and unhealed wounds.

Candidemia developing in debilitated patients requires treatment with amphotericin B. If a patient is not debilitated, removal of the catheter may solve the problem without specific treatment. Otherwise amphotericin B should be given intravenously over a 6-hour period each day for five to ten days. The dose is 0.25 mg/kg body weight the first day, with an increase to 1 mg/kg during the next two to three days. If the diagnosis of sepsis is correct, a response should be observed within 48 hours. Renal toxicity is almost uniformly observed and should be monitored. Mycostatin can be given by mouth for overgrowth of candida in the GI tract and is safe since it is not absorbed. Five-fluorocytosine looks promising but is not yet available.

Candida albicans grows rapidly if introduced into hypertonic glucose solutions. Its growth is inhibited by normal serum. A frequent nidus for candidemia is the indwelling catheter. Brennan et al. have solved this problem by flushing the catheter with 0.6 mg of a 1 mg/ml solution of amphotericin B followed by a second dose which is allowed to remain in the catheter for 5 to 10 minutes before the central venous nutrient solution is restarted. This flush is performed twice a week when the catheter site is being reprepped and dressed. This provides a sterilizing concentration locally for candida but is an infinitesimal dose for the patient. Anderson and Yardley published a photomicrograph of a catheter-related thrombus with yeast forms and pseudohyphae growing in it which illustrates why candidemia may be relieved simply by removal of a catheter and prevented by a periodic amphotericin flush.

Thrombosis is another potential hazard of prolonged catheterization. The risk is greatly increased if the position of the catheter is not checked roentgenographically immediately after insertion. Raffensperger and Ramenofsky reported thrombosis and massive necrosis in the liver of an infant, which led to death. This was due to the catheter passing from the subclavian vein through the vena cava and into the hepatic vein. McDonough and Altemeier reported subclavian vein thrombosis in four patients with propagation into the heart in two. They warn against use of the subclavian catheter in patients with body surface burns and feel that it has the same dangers that arise from prolonged use of catheters in peripheral veins. One of their patients had frequent and multiple punctures of the subclavian vein which led to a thick narrow subclavian vein which could no longer be cannulated even when exposed through an incision.

Fatal air embolism has caused death during insertion of subclavian catheters when the patient was in a semi-Fowler's position instead of in the recommended steep Trendelenburg position. There are instances of pneumo-, hydro-, and hemothorax. Catheter embolization has occurred because of insecure fixation or from shearing of the catheter by the needle. Such embolized catheters have been removed from the heart, and others have been found at autopsy. Catheters have become knotted inside the vena cava or heart, requiring surgical removal.

The risks are reduced by proper attention to the details outlined earlier but they are always present, and therefore if the patient can be fed by some other route or if high osmotic intravenous feedings are not really needed, they should not be used. For many patients, peripheral vein infusion of a less concentrated solution over a short period of time and with frequent changes of intravenous sites may suffice. A small-bore needle should be used if concentrated solutions are given peripherally, so that the blood flow will be maximum past the site of infusion as suggested in 1947 by Elman. Plastic catheters used peripherally lead to an extremely high incidence of phlebitis and may cause serious sepsis requiring excision of the vein, in addition to appropriate antibiotics. There are many causes for postoperative fever, but one of the first places to look currently is at the site of a plastic catheter placed in a peripheral vein in the operating room and used for several days.

TUBE FEEDINGS

Sometimes tube feedings can be administered by a nasal gastric tube or a gastrostomy or enterostomy tube in a patient who otherwise might receive central venous nutrient. Use of the gastrointestinal tract decreases the risk and improves the efficiency of nutrient administration. Some of the same potential hazards exist for tube feedings as have been mentioned above. The formula can be contaminated and is a good growth medium for bacteria. Also, diarrhea can result from a too rapid administration or from use of a feeding with too high an osmotic load, with resultant dehydration. As with any concentrated feeding the urinary output needs to be monitored and specific gravities checked periodically to make sure that the supply of water is sufficient to take care of the daily solute load.

A debilitated patient may be able to stand a brief operation for the insertion of feeding and suction tubes, whereas a more extensive procedure needs to be deferred until the nutrition has improved. Patients with emergency operations in whom severe pancreatitis, fistulae in the duodenum or other problems are found, which might impair the ability to eat in a normal fashion, can often be provided with feeding and suction tubes which simplify subsequent management and make it possible to use at least part of the gastrointestinal tract during a prolonged and complex illness, while keeping the upper gastrointestinal tract at rest. Witzel gastrostomies and enterostomies are generally preferable because the long channel in the bowel wall helps to seal the lumen at the catheter site when the catheters are finally removed. The Witzel tunnel also helps to prevent leakage in a patient who is debilitated and may have poor healing initially.

In patients who are having difficulty with secretions and require tube feedings, it may be possible to use a suction gastrostomy to keep the stomach empty and a feeding gastrostomy with the end of the catheter threaded down into the duodenum so that the tube feeding can be given below the pyloric sphincter; or a feeding enterostomy can be used in combination with a suction gastrostomy. Patients with neurological diseases involving swallowing are especially benefited by such management. We have attempted to nourish patients with severe tetanus this way while they have been curarized, but two patients have developed massive small bowel necrosis. Although the mechanism is obscure, it seems unwise to attempt further use of enterostomy in the treatment of curarized tetanus patients.

The tube feedings can be given by syringe into the stomach or by drip. Some of the feedings tend to settle out and do not drip at a steady rate. Then if the tubing is opened up so that the feeding will flow at a satisfactory rate, it may run too rapidly when not attended, overloading the intestine, and causing the patient to have diarrhea. An enterostomy catheter is often temporarily occluded by the peristaltic action of the gut, which in addition to the settling out in the gravity container, adds to the problems of regulating flow. Barron et al. have designed a food pump which solves the problem by forcing the feeding in at a slow constant rate. The use of such a pump requires careful monitoring to make sure that air is not pumped into the intestinal tract when the bottle runs empty or that formula is not forced into a patient who develops some intolerance to feedings. Periodic aspiration of the tubing will help alert the nursing staff to the latter type of problem. Use of collapsible plastic bags for formula will obviate pumping air into the patient when containers are empty.

The diet for tube feedings should be prepared so that the ratio of protein calories to total calories is not above 20%. Ideally the protein calories should be around 15%. The latter ratio provides 74 gm of protein in 2000 calories. Use of a higher protein content increases the solute load requiring excretion in the urine and may lead to dehydration if the water intake is inadequate, as has been discussed in Chapter 2.

Milk is frequently used as the protein source in tube feedings. Cows' milk contains 4.8% of the disaccharide lactose (7% in human milk). Lactase is present in the intestinal mucosal cells of most infants but is absent or deficient in many adults. This enzyme splits lactose into glucose and galactose. Without the enzyme the lactose remains in the gut where it (1) undergoes fermentation and (2) causes an osmotic effect, both of which may produce diarrhea. If the enzyme deficiency is partial, the patient may tolerate milk in a normal diet taken by mouth but develop diarrhea if tube feedings are given into the duodenum or jejunum. Intolerance to lactose is found in people coming from cultures where milk has never been used. Simoons has published a world map of these areas. People from around the Mediterranean, Eastern Asia, Japan, Indochina, and Western Africa have a 60% to 70% rate of intestinal lactase deficiency. In Europeans the incidence is around 6%. The symptoms produced by milk in such people are bloating, cramping, flatulence, and diarrhea.

A meat-base formula or one with lactose excluded should be used in any patient who shows an intolerance for milk either by history or when tube feedings are begun. Formulas are available which have a lower protein content and also a lower concentration of electrolytes and therefore a lower osmolarity, so as to obviate the problems of dehydration from an excessively high solute load. The physician should review the composition of the formulas available and seek to choose one which has a protein concentration of around 15%. If higher concentrations of protein and salt are used, then special attention must be given to supplying an adequate amount of water and to monitoring of the urine volume and specific gravity, body weight, and serum sodium so as to prevent serious water depletion and hypertonicity. Table 7-1 compares some of the currently available formulas.

There are also available elemental diets prepared from pure amino acids and glucose, which may be useful in selected patients. Bury et al. have described the beneficial effects of the use of such diets in the management of fistulae of the alimentary tract. No digestion is required but the rate of administration of elemental diets must be slow and steady so that the high osmolarity will not cause diarrhea. Bounous et al. observed that a significant proportion of the amino acids used by cells of the intestinal mucosa come from the gut lumen rather than through

TABLE 7-1. COMPARISON OF TUBE FEEDINGS

	Fortified Skim Milk	Doyle's Meritene	Gerber's Meatbase	Vivonex Standard	Vivonex 100 HN
Percentage of calories from protein	33	24	20	8.5	18.3
Total calories/liter	360	1000	822	1000	1000
Osmolality (mOsmol/liter)	290	608	270	760-1200*	844
Lactose containing	yes	yes	no	no	no
Sodium mEq/l	26	39	17	37.4	33.5
Potassium mEq/l	37	43	15	29.9	17.9
Calcium mEq/l	71	70	72	22.1	13.3
Phosphate mEq/l	64	121	55	43.1	25.8
Magnesium mEq/l	No data	24	4	16.0	9.6
Cost per liter $	0.23	1.40	1.25	5.33	10.00

*Dependent upon flavor

the blood perfusing the area. There is a peptidase in the normal intestinal mucosa which completes protein digestion and makes amino acids available. This peptidase is deficient in patients treated with 5-fluorouracil. Intestinal ulceration in such patients can be prevented by providing an elemental diet by mouth for four days prior to and during 5-fluorouracil treatment according to Bounous.

Medium-chain triglycerides composed of 8 to 10 carbon fatty acids can be used as a source of calories when there is impairment of fat digestion or obstruction of intestinal lymphatics. Medium-chain triglycerides are absorbed without hydrolysis and directly into the portal circulation, in contrast to the longer-chain triglycerides which require hydrolysis by pancreatic lipase in the intestinal lumen, re-esterification and formation into chylomicrons in the mucosa, and discharge into the intestinal lymphatics.

It cannot be overemphasized that when high-caloric feedings are forced upon a patient by either gavage or the intravenous route, the urine must be monitored frequently so as to prevent dehydration from glycosuria and solute diuresis. This requires observation not only of urine volume and specific gravity, but also of urine sugar. If the urinary sugar rises, the infusion rate must be reduced or insulin administered, and if the sugar concentration in the urine rises to 4+, then additional measures must be taken to make sure that the blood sugar has not risen to extraordinary heights. Blood sugars must then be measured. Not only should insulin be administered but the intravenous glucose or tube feedings may need to be given at a slower rate or in some instances discontinued until the blood glucose has returned to normal. There are patients with high renal thresholds for glucose in whom urinary glucose levels of 1 to 3+ may also indicate a need for more frequent analyses of blood glucose. Rosenberg et al. have presented details of a patient and reviewed five other case reports from the literature where sudden coma, hyperglycemia, dehydration, and hypertonicity occurred in burned patients from overzealous feeding. Wyrick et al. have reported hyperosmotic coma from the use of intravenous hyperalimentation and observed that the death rate reported for such complications is 41% to 45%. These same risks exist with tube feedings.

REFERENCES

Alleyne, G. A. O.: Cardiac function in severely malnourished Jamaican children. Clin. Sci. *30:*553, 1966.

Allison, J. B., and Wannemacher, R. W., Jr.: The concept and significance of labile and overall protein reserves of the body. Amer. J. Clin. Nutr. *16:*445, 1965.

Allison, S. P., Hinton, P., and Chamberlain, M. J.: Intravenous glucose-tolerance, insulin, and free-fatty-acid levels in burned patients. Lancet *2:*1113, 1968.

Anderson, A. O., and Yardley, J. H.: Demonstration of candida in blood smears. New Eng. J. Med. *286:*108, 1972.

Anderson, J. W., Herman, R. H., and Newcomer, K. L.: Improvement in glucose tolerance of fasting obese patients given oral potassium. Amer. J. Clin. Nutr. *22:*1589, 1969.

Arney, G. K., Pearson, E., and Sutherland, A. B.: Burn stress pseudodiabetes. Ann. Surg. *152:*77, 1960.

Barron, J., Prendergast, J. J., and Jocz, M. W.: Food pump: new approach to tube feeding. J.A.M.A. *161:*621, 1956.

Bounous, G., Gentile, J. M., and Hugon, J.: Elemental diet in the management of the intestinal lesion produced by 5-Fluorouracil in man. Canad. J. Surg. *14:*312, 1971.

Bounous, G., Hugon, J., and Gentile, J. M.: Elemental diet in the management of the intestinal lesion produced by 5-Fluorouracil in the rat. Canad. J. Surg. *14:*298, 1971.

Brennan, M. F., Goldman, M. H., O'Connell, R. C., Kundsin, R. B., and Moore, F. D.: Prolonged parenteral alimentation: candida growth and the prevention of candidemia by amphotericin instillation. Ann. Surg. *176:*265, 1972.

Bury, K. D., Stephens, R. Y., and Randall, H. T.: Use of a chemically defined, liquid, elemental diet for nutritional management of fistulas of the alimentary tract. Amer. J. Surg. *121:*174, 1971.

Cahill, G. F., Jr., Felig, P., and Marliss, E. B.: Some physiological principles of parenteral nutrition. In *Body Fluid Replacement in the Surgical Patient.* Fox, C. L., Jr., and Nahas, G. G., eds. New York: Grune & Stratton, 1970.

Clark, D. E., and Brunschwig, A.: Intravenous nourishment with protein carbohydrate and fat in man. Proc. Soc. Exp. Biol. Med. *49:*329, 1942.

Cuthbertson, D. P.: Further observation on the disturbance of metabolism caused by injury with particular reference to the dietary requirements of fracture cases. Brit. J. Surg. *23:*505, 1936.

Dudrick, S. J., Rhoads, J. E., and Steiger, E.: Intravenous hyperalimentation. Med. Clin. N. Amer. *54:*577, 1970.

Dudrick, S. J., Wilmore, D. W., Vars, H. M., and Rhoads, J. E.: Long-term total parenteral nutrition with growth, development, and positive nitrogen balance. Surgery *64:*134, 1968.

Dudrick, S. J., Wilmore, D. W., Vars, H. M., and Rhoads, J. E.: Can intravenous feeding as the sole means of nutrition support growth in the child and restore weight loss in an adult? Ann. Surg. *169:*974, 1969.

Ellison, E. H., McCleery, R. S., Zollinger, R. M., and Case, C. T.: The influence of caloric intake upon the fate of parenteral nitrogen. Surgery *26*:374, 1949.
Elman, R.: *Parenteral Alimentation in Surgery.* New York: Paul B. Hoeber, 1947.
Evans, E. I., and Butterfield, W. J. H.: The stress response in the severely burned: an interim report. Ann. Surg. *134*:588, 1951.
Filler, R. M., Eraklis, A. J., Rubin, V. G., and Das, J. B.: Long-term total parenteral nutrition in infants. New Eng. J. Med. *281*:589, 1969.
Freeman, J. B., and MacLean, L. D.: Intravenous hyperalimentation: a review. Canad. J. Surg. *14*:180, 1971.
Gump, F. E., Mashima, Y., Ferenczy, A., and Kinney, J. M.: Pre- and post-mortem studies of lung fluids and electrolytes. J. Trauma *11*:474, 1971.
Habif, D. V., Randall, H. T., and Lockwood, J. S.: The effect on nitrogen retention as the result of administering phosphate ion with amino acids intravenously. Surg. Forum *458*:1950-1951.
Haxhe, J. J.: Experimental undernutrition. I. Its effects on cardiac output. Metabolism *16*:1086, 1967.
Heird, W. C., Dell, R. B., Driscoll, J. M., Jr., Grebin, B., and Winters, R. W.: Metabolic acidosis after intravenous alimentation with amino acids. New Eng. J. Med. *287*: 943, 1972.
Holden, W. D., Krieger, H., Levey, S., and Abbott, W. E.: The effect of nutrition on nitrogen metabolism in the surgical patient. Ann. Surg. *146*:563, 1957.
Kaess, H., Schlierf, G., Ehlers, W., von Mikulicz-Radecki, J.-G., Hassenstein, P., Walter, K., Brech, W., and Hengstmann, J.: The carbohydrate metabolism of normal subjects during potassium depletion. Diabetologia *7*:82, 1971.
Lockhart, C. E., and Elman, R.: The effect of intravenous glucose and amino acids on glycosuria and urinary output in humans. Surg. Gynec. Obstet. *88*:97, 1949.
Madden, S. C., Bassett, S. H., Remington, J. H., Martin, F. J. C., Woods, R. R., and Shull, F. W.: Amino acids in therapy of disease: parenteral and oral administrations compared. Surg. Gynec. Obstet. *82*:131, 1946.
Marks, H. H.: Influence of obesity on morbidity and mortality. Bull. N.Y. Acad. Med. *36*:296, 1960.
Mason, E. E., Gordy, D. D., Chernigoy, F. A., and Printen, K. J.: Fatty acid toxicity. Surg. Gynec. Obstet. *133*:992, 1971.
McDonough, J. J., and Altemeier, W. A.: Subclavian venous thrombosis secondary to indwelling catheters. Surg. Gynec. Obstet. *133*:397, 1971.
Moore, D. C., and Karp, M.: Intravenous alcohol in the surgical patient. Surg. Gynec. Obstet. *80*:523, 1945.
Moore, F. D., and Ball, M. R.: *The Metabolic Response to Surgery.* Springfield, Ill.: Charles C Thomas, 1952.
Moore, F. D., Olesen, K. H., McMurrey, J. D., Parker, H. V., Ball, M. R., and Boyden, C. M.: *The Body Cell Mass and Its Supporting Environment.* Philadelphia: W. B. Saunders Co., 1963.
Mouridsen, H. T.: The extravascular retention of albumin in wound tissue and its contribution to the postoperative hypoalbuminaemia in rabbits. Clin. Sci. *37*:431, 1969.
Neale, G., Antcliff, A. C., Welbourn, R. B., Mollin, D. L., and Booth, C. C.: Protein malnutrition after partial gastrectomy. Quart. J. Med. *36*:469, 1967.
Osborne, T. B., and Mendel, L. B.: Amino acids in nutrition and growth. J. Biol. Chem. *17*:325, 1914.
Owen, O. E., Felig, P., Morgan, A. P., Wahren, J., and Cahill, G. F., Jr.: Liver and kidney metabolism during prolonged starvation. J. Clin. Invest. *48*:574, 1969.
Raffensperger, J. G., and Ramenofsky, M. L.: A fatal complication of hyperalimentation: a case report. Surgery *68*:393, 1970.
Randle, P. J., Garland, P. B., Newsholme, E. A., and Hales, C. N.: The glucose fatty acid cycle: its role in insulin sensitivity and the metabolic disturbances of diabetes mellitus. Lancet *1*:785, 1963.
Randle, P. J., Garland, P. B., Newsholme, E. A., and Hales, C. N.: The glucose fatty acid cycle in obesity and maturity onset diabetes mellitus. Ann. N.Y. Acad. Sci. *131*:324, 1965.
Rankin, E. M.: Colloid osmotic pressure and body water distribution. In *Body Fluid Replacement in the Surgical Patient.* Fox C. L., Jr., and Nahas, G. G., eds. New York: Grune & Stratton, 1970.

Ravdin, I. S.: Symposium on fluid and electrolyte needs of surgical patients; hypoproteinemia and its relation to surgical problems. Ann. Surg. *112:*576, 1940.

Rea, W. J., Wyrick, W. J., Jr., McClelland, R. N., and Webb, W. R.: Intravenous hyperosmolar alimentation favorable experience in 54 patients. Arch. Surg. (Chicago) *100:*393, 1970.

Rhoads, J. E.: Long-term parenteral alimentary support. Transplantation Proc. *3:* 1503, 1971.

Rice, C. O., Orr, B., and Enquist, I.: Parenteral nutrition in the surgical patient as provided from glucose, amino acids and alcohol. Ann. Surg. *131:*289, 1950.

Richards, P., Brown, C. L., Houghton, B. J., and Thompson, E.: Synthesis of phenylalanine and valine by healthy and uremic men. Lancet *2:*128, 1971.

Riegel, C., Koop, C. E., Drew, J., Stevens, L. W., and Rhoads, J. E.: Nutritional requirements for nitrogen balance in surgical patients during early postoperative period. J. Clin. Invest. *26:*18, 1947.

Rollins, D. M.: Reducing plasma free fatty acids in obese females during gastric operations. Unpublished master's thesis. Iowa City, Iowa: University of Iowa, 1972.

Rose, W. C.: The sequence of events leading to the establishment of the amino acid needs of man. Amer. J. Public Health *58:*2020, 1968.

Rosenberg, S. A., Brief, D. K., Kinney, J. M., Herrera, M. G., Wilson, R. E., and Moore, F. D.: The syndrome of dehydration, coma and severe hyperglycemia without ketosis in patients convalescing from burns. New Eng. J. Med. *272:*931, 1965.

Schimmel, R. J., and Knobil, E.: Insulin, free fatty acids, and stimulation of hepatic gluconeogenesis during fasting. Amer. J. Physiol. *218:*1540, 1970.

Scribner, B. H., Cole, J. J., Christopher, G., Vizzo, J. E., Atkins, R. C., and Blagg, C. R.: Long-term total parenteral nutrition. J.A.M.A. *212:*457, 1970.

Silvis, S. E., and Paragas, P. V., Jr.: Fatal hyperalimentation syndrome animal studies. J. Lab. Clin. Med. *78:*918, 1971.

Silvis, S. E., and Paragas, P. V., Jr.: Paresthesias, weakness, seizures and hypophosphatemia in patients receiving hyperalimentation. Gastroenterology *62:*513, 1972.

Simoons, F. J.: Primary adult lactose intolerance and the milking habit: a problem in biologic and cultural interrelations. II. A culture historical hypothesis. Amer. J. Dig. Dis. *15:*695, 1970.

Stegink, L. D., and DenBesten, L.: Synthesis of cysteine from methionine in normal adult subjects: effect of route of administration. Science *178:*514, 1972.

Strickler, J. H., and Rice, C. O.: An approach toward the ideal in parenteral nutrition. Minn. Med. *36:*221, 1953.

Tandon, B. N., Banks, P. A., George, P. K., Sama, S. K., Ramachandran, K., and Gandhi, P. C.: Recovery of exocrine pancreatic function in adult protein-calorie malnutrition. Gastroenterology *58:*358, 1970.

Taylor, H. L., and Keys, A.: Adaptation to caloric restriction. Science *112:*215, 1950.

Travis, S. F., Sagerman, H. J., and Ruberg, R. L.: Alteration of red cell glycolytic intermediates and oxygen transport as a consequence of hypophosphatemia in patients receiving hyperalimentation. New Eng. J. Med. *285:*763, 1971.

Waterlow, J. C.: Observations on the mechanism of adaptation to low protein intakes. Lancet *2:*1091, 1968.

Werner, S. C.: The use of a mixture of pure amino acids in surgical nutrition. I. Certain pharmacologic considerations. Ann. Surg. *126:*169, 1947.

Wilmore, D. W., and Dudrick, S. J.: Safe long-term venous catheterization. Arch. Surg. (Chicago) *98:*256, 1969.

Wilmore, D. W., and Dudrick, S. J.: Effects of nutrition on intestinal adaptation following massive small bowel resection. Surg. Forum *20:*398, 1969.

Wilmore, D. W., and Dudrick, S. J.: Treatment of acute renal failure with intravenous essential L-amino acids. Arch Surg. (Chicago) *99:*669, 1969.

Wilmore, D. W., Curreri, P. W., Spitzer, K. W., Spitzer, M. E., and Pruitt, B. A.: Supranormal dietary intake in thermally injured hypermetabolic patients. Surg. Gynec. Obstet. *132:*881, 1971.

Wyrick, W. J., Rea, W. J., and McCelland, R. N.: Rare complications with intravenous hyperosmotic alimentation. J.A.M.A. *211:*1697, 1970.

Chapter

8

Bypass Operations in Obesity and Hyperlipidemia

There are operations for the treatment of obesity and hyperlipidemia which are relatively new additions to the procedures of surgeons. Two of these operations consist of bypassing part of the intestine, and the other bypasses most of the stomach and the duodenum. Although used for the treatment of patients who have an excess of fat or excessively high concentrations of serum cholesterol and triglyceride, the intestinal operations have the potential for creating certain deficiencies in fluid, electrolytes, vitamins, and proteins.

INTESTINAL BYPASS IN OBESITY

In 1954, Kremen et al. published their experimental evaluation of the relative importance of jejunum and ileum for maintaining normal nutrition. They designed an experiment in dogs in which 50% of the small bowel was bypassed, the segment at rest being made into a Thiry-Vella fistula. Weight loss was greater when the ileum was bypassed. The animals were able to accommodate to bypass of one-half of the small bowel, but the accommodation was best if the ileocecal valve was left in the digestive stream. Comparisons of two levels of fat in the diet indicated that with bypass of the distal small bowel and the ileocecal valve, there was increased loss of nitrogen in the stool, and this was greatly exaggerated if the fat intake was high.

The stimulus to this study came from patients requiring extensive intestinal resection and for whom the surgeon did not have a choice as to how much and what segment of intestine would be removed. Kremen's experiment was designed to provide surgeons with a basis for a prognosis should they be confronted with the necessity of resecting a large amount of intestine. It was suggested, however, that intestinal bypass might be used in treating obesity, and in the published discussion of his paper Kremen described an obese patient in whom the proximal 36 inches of jejunum had been anastomosed to the terminal 18 inches of ileum end-to-end. The bypassed two-thirds of small bowel was anastomosed so as to drain into the transverse colon. This patient did not have diarrhea and gradually lost weight. Because of the presence of a foot and a half of terminal ileum, there was no defect in absorption of vitamin B12.

Other surgeons, who undertook intestinal bypass for the treatment of extreme obesity, did not at first adopt the specific operation used by Kremen but instead anastomosed the proximal jejunum to transverse colon, thus eliminating the ileocecal valve. An excellent example is the work described by Lewis et al. in eleven extremely obese patients. Three of these patients had the proximal 20 inches of jejunum and the other 8 patients had 30 inches of jejunum anastomosed to transverse colon or cecum. One of these patients died suddenly on the fifth postoperative day; the cause of death could not be determined. The patient did have severe coronary atherosclerosis and a very fatty liver. Another patient died at home 8 months postoperatively from a massive pulmonary embolus which arose from a recent venous thrombosis in a leg. The authors commented that the experience in management of these patients would discourage them from recommending this procedure. Postoperative complications required hospitalization for correction of electrolyte deficiencies in 6 of the 11 patients. It was observed in these patients that there was a marked decrease in the serum cholesterol level. In one of the patients a cholesterol absorption test was performed before and after the intestinal bypass and showed that the operation eliminated cholesterol absorption. This was subsequently exploited in the surgical treatment of hypercholesterolemia.

Payne et al. also attempted to use an anastomosis between proximal jejunum and colon, bypassing most of the small bowel and the ileocecal valve. One of their patients, a 20-year-old woman began at 307 pounds and within 6 months had reached 204 pounds and seemed well, but then she died suddenly of pulmonary embolism which originated in the pelvic veins. They reestablished continuity in the surviving patients and abandoned this particular form of intestinal bypass as being unsafe. Payne subsequently resorted to an anastomosis between proximal jejunum and the side of the distal ileum. This was a safer procedure and effective in causing weight loss in the majority of patients. There were, however, some patients in whom weight loss did not occur and in whom it was possible to demonstrate that there was regurgitation of chyme from the site of anastomosis retrograde into the bypassed segment of small bowel. This allowed absorption of sufficient food so as to sustain an excessive weight.

During 1971 at least three different papers appeared, one by Salmon, another by Scott et al., and a third by Buchwald and Varco, describing an operation for obesity in which the proximal short segment of jejunum was anastomosed end-to-end to the terminal ileum. The bypassed segment of bowel was drained into the colon in either the cecum, transverse or sigmoid colon. This is, in essence, the operation as originally described by Kremen. Kremen demonstrated that the use of the ileocecal valve allows the animal to accommodate sufficiently with regard to absorption of fluids and electrolyte so as to survive. There is also much less opportunity for material to reflux into the bypassed segment.

Buchwald and Varco have concentrated on those very obese patients who also have hyperlipidemia, and they recommend that the segment of ileum retained should be only 3 or 4 cm in length so as to minimize absorption of bile salts and cholesterol. Others who have been treating obesity in patients with normal serum lipids have been less concerned about the serum cholesterol level and have allowed a longer segment of terminal ileum. Scott uses 12 inches of jejunum and 12 inches of ileum; Varco recommends 40 cm of jejunum and 4 cm of ileum; Salmon recommended 10 inches of jejunum and 20 inches of ileum. In all of these reports, the majority of patients have lost a satisfactory amount of weight. There are occasional patients who do not lose weight or who, having lost weight, regain it as the intestine hypertrophies and as the intestinal mucosa undergoes hyperplasia.

The early and late mortality rate has decreased with the less radical procedures. Occasional patients remain who have excessive diarrhea and negative nitrogen balance and who develop fluid and electrolyte imbalance, protein malnutrition, and enlargement of the liver from extreme fatty metamorphosis. Such patients are predisposed to anasarca and liver failure. Phlebitis and pulmonary embolism are mentioned occasionally. It is difficult to bypass the intestine in sufficient extent to cause weight loss in the majority of patients without causing protein malnutrition and fatty liver in some of the patients. All of these patients have fatty metamorphosis at the time of their operation but, in contrast to simple dieting, the fatty liver after intestinal bypass does not improve initially and for 6 months to a year there may be an increase in the amount of fat in the liver. By the end of the first year, most of the patients have a decrease in fat in the liver indicating that with sufficient time, the intestine accommodates and nitrogen balance is finally maintained at a more satisfactory level.

In a patient whose body composition was studied in detail

during the course of weight loss after intestinal bypass, Moore and others showed that the patient remained unhealthy in terms of a low total body potassium in spite of a reduction in total body fat. The patients studied by Scott et al. showed low serum protein concentrations as well as low serum calcium, phosphorus, and cholesterol levels, all of which suggested a state of malnutrition rather than the desired loss of fat stores and preservation of protein cellular mass.

My personal experience with intestinal bypass in treating obesity was limited to two patients operated upon shortly following the experience of Kremen. My first patient had an end-to-side anastomosis between proximal jejunum and distal ileum and balance studies showed no impairment in digestion and absorption probably because of regurgitation of chyme into the bypassed small bowel. The second patient was therefore subjected to an anastomosis of proximal small bowel to transverse colon, and a severe diarrhea followed. After some 6 weeks of intravenous fluid therapy additional small bowel was added to the functioning segment but the anastomosis still was made so as to bypass the ileocecal valve. Diarrhea continued. Hypocalcemia was a temporary problem. Some 5 years later it was necessary to remove bilateral staghorn calculi from the kidneys probably resulting from chronic dehydration and highly concentrated urine. Further knowledge of this procedure has come from the literature and care of a few patients operated upon elsewhere.

The patient with intestinal bypass is a patient with a short gut syndrome. Wright and Tilson have divided the course of such patients into three stages. Stage 1 is the period of nausea, vomiting, and diarrhea which may last for a month before the bowel becomes sufficiently enlarged, hyperplastic, and functionally augmented so as to allow the patient to begin to take fluids and food by mouth without increasing the diarrhea. Stage 2 is a period of either gradual improvement in nutrition or progressive deterioration, hypercalcemia, nutritional edema, and in some instances death from hepatic failure, infection, or other complications. Stage 3 is a period of return to a productive life. According to the literature, the type of intestinal bypass now in use for treating obesity does not pose such severe problems in most patients. Nevertheless there are some in whom early fluid and electrolyte balance and later protein malnutrition are a problem.

For patients with resection or bypass of large segments of bowel the early postoperative management should be centered upon intravenous infusion. Nothing should be given by mouth until the diarrhea is less than 2 liters or less than 7 to 8 bowel movements per day. Replacement of fluid should be quantitative and of similar composition to the fluid lost. Usually the pH will be neutral or alkaline and a ratio of isotonic saline to isotonic sodium lactate of 2:1 will be appropriate. Forty mEq of KCl should be added to each liter, and each liter should contain 10% glucose. Additional glucose and amino acid solution should be given during the day so that the patient is maintained in an optimum nutritional status as detailed in the preceding chapter. If diarrhea persists, then calcium, magnesium, and phosphate will also be required but these become deficient only if neglected for several weeks. The intravenous feedings should be continued during the time of early trials at oral feeding so that the patient remains in balance even if diarrhea is stimulated by the trial. If fluid and electrolytes are tolerated, then glucose may be added. Protein is added next and finally fat.

Fat is the most difficult food to digest when the intestine is shortened, in spite of its being absorbed 90% in the duodenum and upper jejunum. There is a failure of absorption of bile salts in the lower ileum, and the pool of bile salts becomes so deficient that a micellar solution is not formed with fat in the duodenum. If more than 100 cm of small bowel is absent, then administration of bile salts by mouth may help to reduce the steatorrhea. If less than 100 cm of terminal ileum are absent from the food stream, persistent diarrhea may actually be caused by bile salts entering the colon. In such patients, Hofmann and Poley have found that up to 16 gm per day of cholestyramine may be effective in controlling the diarrhea by removing bile salts from solution before they enter the colon. Another index of whether to consider adding or removing bile salts in the management of diarrhea is the amount of fat in the stool. If there are more than 20 gm of fat, try bile salts. If the stool fat is less than 20 gm, then perhaps the diarrhea is due to bile salts entering the colon in excessive concentrations and cholestyramine should be tried.

The terminal ileum and ileocecal valve are important in preventing diarrhea not only because of the absorption of bile salts. This is the water wringer of the gastrointestinal tract. Electrolytes and other solutes are absorbed actively at higher levels and water follows passively, but normally a rather fluid chyme reaches the terminal ileum only to be converted to soft stool before it enters the cecum. Richardson and Griffen have observed that the absence of the ileocecal valve also allows colonic bacteria to reflux into the small bowel. With a short small bowel such bacteria may reach the upper jejunum and duodenum and deconjugate bile salts, thereby adding to the deficiency in formation of a micellar solution of fat and adding to the steatorrhea. A similar situation occurs in large duodenal diverticuli where colonic bacteria cause deconjugation of bile salts and steatorrhea.

PARTIAL ILEAL BYPASS FOR HYPERCHOLESTEROLEMIA

Gomes et al. have reviewed the use of ileal bypass in the treatment of hyperlipidemia. This operation is based on the premise that a high serum cholesterol level contributes to the production of atherosclerotic changes which eventually will lead to coronary occlusion, cerebral vascular accidents, and other complications. An additional part of the premise is that, for patients with high serum cholesterol, if something can be done to bring the cholesterol to normal, the formation of atherosclerotic plaques will be prevented. Of all of the different types of hyperlipidemia, the most common, and the type most amenable to this sort of treatment, would seem to be the Frederickson type II which is a familial, mendelian dominant disease in which the serum cholesterol is in the range of 300 to 400 mg%. The homozygote has levels twice as high but is relatively rare. It is common even for heterozygotes to die of myocardial infarction or stroke by the age of 40, and it is thought that if the serum cholesterol can be reduced and maintained at less than 200 mg% that the atherosclerotic disease will be delayed. Partial ileal bypass has as its purpose the interruption of the enterohepatic circulation of both cholesterol and bile acids. In addition, secretion of cholesterol in the bypassed segment of intestine continues. Bile salts and cholesterol are lost in the stool. Also with the shortened bowel there is some acceleration of transit which contributes to decreased absorption of cholesterol and bile salts.

Acetate is a precursor of cholesterol, and there are some 26 steps in the chemical transition between these two substances. The feedback inhibition of cholesterol formation has been so organized in the liver that if serum cholesterol concentration is lowered, it is to be anticipated that there will be an increased rate of formation of cholesterol. Cholesterol also is a precursor of bile acid which has an inhibitory effect on its own formation so that if bile acid is removed from the system, it is to be anticipated that there also will be an increased rate of transformation of cholesterol to bile acid. The removal of bile acid from the system by preventing its reabsorption in the intestine will therefore augment the removal of cholesterol.

Twelve grams of bile salts are present in the body pool, and 5 to 10 gm are secreted with each meal but the bile acids are reabsorbed so that although 20 to 30 gm of bile salt may be secreted each day, only 800 mg is normally lost in the stool. Bile acids participate in the formation of micelles composed of fatty acids, triglycerides, and cholesterol. The cholesterol is water insoluble but is carried down the gastrointestinal tract through the action of the bile salts. The reduction in bile salt pool, therefore, has another effect in impairing the absorption of cholesterol and triglycerides.

In view of the considerable influence that Varco has had in the development of intestinal bypass operations through his early conversations with Kremen and his later work with Buchwald, it is of interest to note that in 1947 Varco described the use of intermittent external biliary drainage for the relief of pruritus in certain chronic disorders of the liver. It is also of historical interest that Carey, who was an internist at the University of Minnesota, together with Williams described the use of a resin which forms a complex with bile acids and removes them from the enterohepatic circulation; a substitute for T-tube drainage in patients with pruritus. This resin which was subsequently called "cholestyramine" represents the currently most effective nonsurgical way of reducing serum cholesterol levels.

Buchwald in 1964 reviewed the experimental bases for partial ileal bypass in the treatment of hypercholesterolemia. He has shown in a number of different experimental animals as well as in a large series of humans that elevated levels of serum cholesterol can be lowered and that as long as the patients are given injections of 1000 units of vitamin B12 every month, they do not develop any signs of deficiency and most do not have any sustained diarrhea. These patients also do not lose weight unless the bypass is more extensive than is usually used for the operative treatment of hyperlipidemia. The operation for hyperlipidemia consists of anastomosing the proximal two-thirds of the small bowel to the cecum, thus bypassing the ileocecal valve and the distal one-third of small bowel. If the patient is also obese, a more extensive intestinal bypass is used but an end-to-end anastomosis is made to the terminal ileum, using 3 or 4 cm of the latter, and the bypassed bowel is anastomosed to the cecum so as to provide an outlet for its content.

Aoki et al. found in 50 adults and 7 children with Frederickson type II hyperlipidemia that cholestyramine is effective in lowering the serum cholesterol levels. In 30 adults a 23% average reduction was obtained by giving 22 gm of cholestyramine a day in three divided oral doses. With similar treatment in 20 adults with tendon xanthoma, there was a 26% average fall in serum cholesterol from 393 to 293 mg/100 ml. These figures were for follow-up periods ranging from 12 to 24 months. In the 7 children, ages 4 to 17, cholestyramine was given in a dose of 14 gm per day for 3 months, and the serum cholesterol level was reduced from an average of 319 to 271 mg/100 ml. The cholestyramine is unpleasant to take by mouth and would need to be continued for an indefinite period of time which makes it a rather expensive treatment.

Buchwald (1968) has been able to lower the serum cholesterol concentration to less than 200 mg/100 ml in 61% of his patients. In 5 patients the cholestyramine was added to the treatment in patients with partial ileal bypass in doses of 32 gm/day for 3 weeks. This failed to have any further effect on lowering of the serum cholesterol concentration. Diet alone in the hands of Buchwald lowered serum cholesterol 11%. An additional 40% drop occurred after partial ileal bypass. The combination of diet and partial ileal bypass is the most effective method so far developed for the treatment of type II hyperlipidemia.

It would appear that partial ileal bypass and the administration of cholestyramine have similar effects. Since the terminal ileum is the site of greatest absorption of bile salts and cholesterol, it seems to be unnecessary to bypass more than that amount of bowel recommended by Buchwald and Varco. Dowling, Mack, and Small studied monkeys whose bile was diverted in varying amounts and found that maximum synthesis of bile acid occurred when 20% of the bile was diverted, at which point bile acid synthesis was 10 times its normal rate. They found that resection of the distal one-third of the small bowel resulted in about the same decrease in bile salt secretion as a 50% diversion of bile by T-tube drainage.

The Minnesota group has studied the incorporation of *tritium* into cholesterol and has found that cholesterol synthesis is increased by a median value of 5.6 times with a range of 1.6 to 12.8 when studied three months after partial ileal bypass. After one year, the cholesterol synthesis rate remained at an estimated 40 mg/kg as compared with the preoperative value of around 10 mg/kg. There is a marked increase in loss of both bile acid and cholesterol in the stool. Although the body's synthesis pathways compensate in part for this loss, there is a decrease in the total body cholesterol pool and a significant decrease in the concentration of cholesterol in the plasma.

Buchwald and colleagues have not been able to demonstrate that partial ileal bypass has reversed atherosclerotic changes in these patients. Ideally, patients should be subjected to this operation early in life before their atherosclerosis has progressed to any degree of severity. Buchwald and Varco have treated a group of children from families with type II hyperlipidemia. As with so many surgical and other types of treatment used in serious diseases, there is no randomized study comparing the complications and longevity in patients with and without partial ileal bypass. There is no randomized study of the effects of cholestyramine on hyperlipidemia. Both treatments will lower elevated serum cholesterol levels. The partial ileal bypass seems to be more effective in lowering serum cholesterol than the administration of cholestyramine, but which treatment will be the most beneficial in the prolongation of life and in decreasing morbidity is not evident.

The review of earlier studies and the effect of a cholesterol-lowering diet in male survivors of myocardial infarction reported by Leren provide evidence that a lowering of serum cholesterol is effective in reducing the risk of recurrent myocardial infarction. When this is coupled to the evidence that partial ileal bypass will reduce serum cholesterol levels, it would seem that there must be many patients who could benefit from such an operation.

The reduction of the bile salt pool as a consequence of disturbed ileal function is conducive to the secretion of an abnormal bile supersaturated with cholesterol according to Dowling, Bell, and White. It may be that an increase in incidence of gallstones may be an unwanted side effect of ileal bypass.

GASTRIC BYPASS AND OBESITY

The treatment of obesity by shortening the intestine is based upon the thesis that reducing a patient's ability to digest and absorb food will cause loss of weight. If such a patient overeats, and especially if the intake of fat is high, according to Kremen et al. there will be an excessive loss of nitrogen in the stool. This will lead to protein malnutrition, one manifestation of which is a large fatty liver. Such changes may progress to liver failure or intractable edema along with other manifestations of malnutrition, giving the picture of an adult with kwashiorkor. In the course of 9 to 12 months, the intestine becomes sufficiently hypertrophied and intestinal mucosa becomes sufficiently hyperplastic that most patients have an improvement in their absorption and the restoration of the liver to a more normal histology.

The ideal operation for obesity should limit the amount of food ingested and should allow normal digestion and absorption of that food. Gastric bypass was introduced for the treatment of obesity in 1966 (Fig. 8-1). It is patterned after a subtotal gastric resection, except that nothing is removed. As an intern at the University of Minnesota, the first operation that I participated in was a two-thirds gastric resection with a short-loop retrocolic gastroenterostomy for the treatment of duodenal ulcer. This was considered the treatment of choice for peptic ulcer at the time and was effective in that 97% of patients were relieved of their ulcer disease. However, a third of the patients had dumping symptoms, and the majority of patients failed to return to their usual body weight. Wangensteen suggested on more than one occasion that the reduced weight might be an unrecognized and unappreciated advantage and might reduce the risk of atherosclerotic heart disease. But in the minds of most physicians and patients, gastric resection was considered undesirable in the effect it had on body weight. A search was made for other procedures which would eliminate the ulcer diathesis and permit a more "normal" body weight.

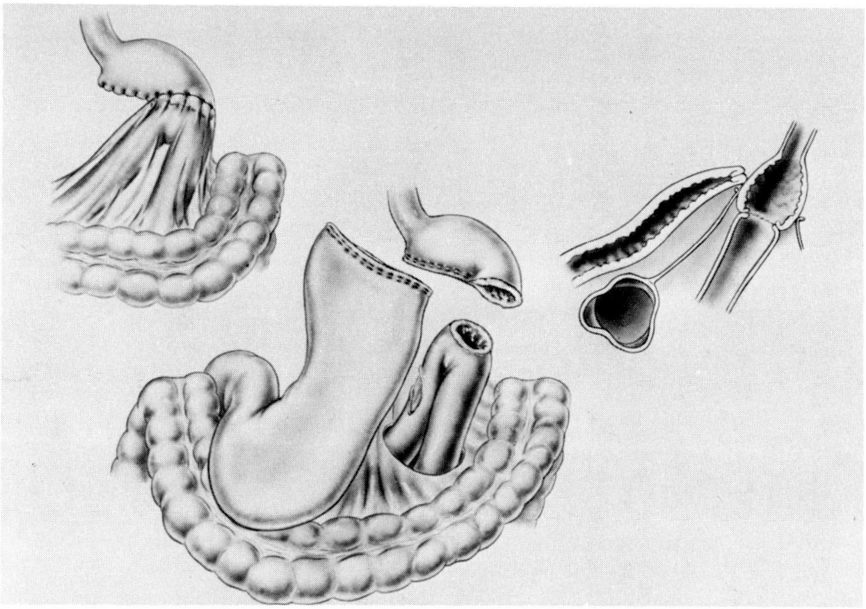

Figure 8-1. Illustrates the potentially reversible 90% gastric bypass operation with a short-loop retrocolic gastroenterostomy. The ligament of Treitz is divided. The mesocolon is secured to the 10% stomach pouch, and the closed distal 90% of excluded stomach is attached to the anterior wall of the fundic segment. These steps are important in preventing proximal loop stasis. (From Mason, E. E., and Ito, C.: Gastric bypass. Ann. Surg. *170*:329. 1969. By permission of the J. B. Lippincott Company.)

The severity of the supposed disability was related to the extent of the gastric resection. Patients who had a total gastric resection were the thinnest. It was also observed that a Billroth II type of operation caused a lower weight than a Billroth I. There was evidence of impaired mixing of food, bile, and pancreatic juice and an increased loss of fat in the stool with the Billroth II operation, in which the food bypassed the duodenum. It was generally agreed, however, that the chief cause of reduced weight after gastric resection was the inability of the patient to eat more than a small amount of food at one time.

The original thoughts about gastric bypass were in terms of a possible operation for the treatment of duodenal ulcer. Exclusion operations were tried early in the history of the treatment of duodenal ulcer and discarded because of the high incidence of stomal ulcer formation. According to the thesis behind gastric bypass, sufficient stomach would be excluded with the antrum so that whenever any acid was formed, part of it would wash over the antrum and duodenum, thus inhibiting secretion of gastrin and stimulating the secretion of secretin. There would be less acid secretion, and because of secretion of bicarbonate in the pancreatic juice and bile, the acid which came from the excluded stomach would be neutralized in the duodenum. With this arrangement, the normal feedback regulation of acid secretion by gastric acid would be maintained. In fact, it might even be more effective in its inhibition of acid secretion because there would be little or no food mixed with the acid secreted in the excluded stomach.

Early in this experience, there were 8 thin patients with severe duodenal ulcer who were subjected to a two-thirds gastric bypass for the treatment of duodenal ulcer. All of these patients seemed to have an immediate relief of their symptoms, and in 6 of the patients there has been no further evidence of acid peptic disease. However, in 2 of these patients whose primary disease was a duodenal ulcer, stomal ulcers have developed, requiring resection of the excluded stomach and vagotomy. Since we do not have any means for determining ahead of time which patients with ulcer disease will respond to this operation, gastric bypass is not recommended for the treatment of acid peptic disease. There are other methods which are more effective and more predictable.

Before any operations were performed on patients, a series of experiments were undertaken in the laboratory to help determine whether gastric bypass would be ulcerogenic or protective. These were reported by Mason and Ito in 1967. Dogs were prepared with a Pavlov pouch, and their response to a standard meal was studied with collection of pouch juices and analysis for acid (Fig. 8-2). A two-thirds gastric bypass was performed leaving the pouch in place, and after recovery the dogs were again studied with the standard meal. A marked reduction in acid secretion resulted. The dogs were then subjected to a resection of the acid-secreting portion of the excluded stomach but leaving the excluded antrum. With this, a standard meal caused a steady increase in acid secretion over the 3½ hours that the dogs were followed, indicating that the excluded and uninhibited antrum would cause stimulation of acid secretion. Finally, the antrum was resected, and the feeding experiments then showed almost no acid secretory response to a meal. Comparison of two-thirds gastric bypass and two-thirds gastric resection in these experiments showed a similar effect in suppression of gastric secretion except that the bypass operation allowed a little more acid secretion than did the distal resection. These and other laboratory experiments indicated that gastric bypass was protective rather than ulcerogenic and, together with the experience in the patients with duodenal ulcer, encouraged us to go ahead with a study of patients who were extremely obese.

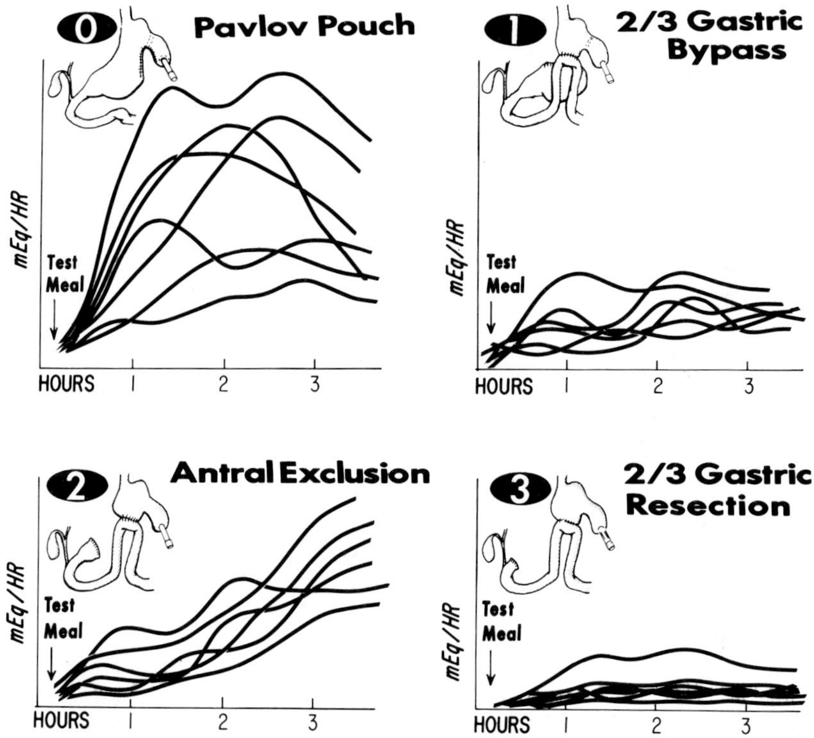

Figure 8-2. Shows a sequence of four operations, after each of which the gastric secretory response to a standard meal was determined. Bypass caused nearly as marked a suppression of gastric acid secretion as did resection.

Sixty-seven patients, weighing between 200 and 530 pounds, were operated upon between 1966 and 1970. There were 5 postoperative deaths, 3 from infections and 2 from pulmonary embolism. Two of the patients have developed signs of ulceration, but one of these responded to antacids and has remained well for over 2 years. The other patient had a resection of the excluded stomach and vagotomy.

One-third of the patients have lost more than 100 pounds; a third of the patients have lost between 50 and 100 pounds; and a third of the patients have lost less than 50 pounds. The average patients preoperatively weighed about 300 pounds and after a year weighed close to 200 pounds and have remained at approximately this weight for the years that they have been followed. Patients who lose a great deal of weight tend to remain at their lower weight. The greatest weight loss occurs in patients who are the heaviest to begin with. Men lose more weight than do women, and middle-aged patients have a better weight loss than the young or the elderly. Patients who have previously experienced myocardial infarction, angina, poliomyelitis, or some other disability which restricts their activity are less likely to lose weight at the desired rate.

Those patients who have mild diabetes require less medication, and many of them require no medication as they begin to lose weight. Elevated blood pressures are usually lowered. Some of the patients tend to retain fluids and require diuretics. The patients have not developed anemia or lowering of their plasma proteins or other signs of malnutrition. These patients level off at a normal weight or slightly above their ideal weight, and we have not been required to reconstitute the stomach because of excessive weight loss.

During the year 1971, we attempted to simplify the operation analogous to performance of a Billroth I. The stomach was partially divided, beginning at the lesser curvature and leaving a passageway along the greater curvature. This stoma was created small enough so that it felt a little tight around the surgeon's palpating index finger and was approximately 1.5 cm in diameter. This operation was referred to as a gastroplasty. A temporary suction gastrostomy of the Witzel type was placed in the upper pouch to keep it empty during the early period of convalescence, and another Witzel gastrostomy was placed in the lower segment of stomach to permit feeding of the patient during his convalescence. After we had performed 50 of these operations, a comparison was made between the weight loss in first 6 months in gastroplasty and gastric bypass, and it was found that the bypass patients were losing a greater amount of weight. The indications at that time were that longer term follow-up would probably exaggerate this difference, and since gastric bypass was a more effective procedure, we returned to the use of the earlier operation which included a gastroenterostomy (Fig. 8-1).

At the present time subtotal gastric bypass is being used for treatment of our grossly obese patients. We require that these patients be at least twice their ideal weight, as determined from the average weight for people with middle-sized frames (Table 8-1). No special diet and no special medications are required following this operation. These patients do not develop pernicious anemia. They do not have any fluid or electrolyte imbalance. There is no enlargement of the liver or other indication of increasing fatty metamorphosis. Some of the patients do tend to retain fluid and develop ankle edema which can be controlled with diuretics and

TABLE 8-1. AVERAGE WEIGHTS OF INSURED PERSONS HAVING MEDIUM-SIZED FRAMES IN THE UNITED STATES WITH LOWEST MORTALITY RATES.

Height ft in	(in shoes) cm	lb	kg
	MEN		
5-2	157.5	123.5	56.0
5-3	160.0	127	57.6
5-4	162.6	130	59.0
5-5	165.1	133	60.3
5-6	167.6	136.5	62.0
5-7	170.2	140.5	63.8
5-8	172.7	145	65.8
5-9	175.3	149	67.6
5-10	177.8	153	69.4
5-11	180.3	157.5	71.4
6-0	182.9	162	73.5
6-1	185.4	166.5	75.6
6-2	188.0	171	77.6
6-3	190.5	176	79.6
6-4	193	181	82.2
	WOMEN		
4-10	147.3	101.5	46
4-11	149.9	104	47.2
5-0	152.4	107	48.6
5-1	154.9	110	49.9
5-2	157.5	113	51.3
5-3	160.0	116	52.6
5-4	162.6	119.5	54.1
5-5	165.1	123	55.8
5-6	167.6	127.5	58.8
5-7	170.2	131.5	60.6
5-8	172.7	135.5	61.5
5-9	175.3	139.5	63.3
5-10	177.8	143.5	65.1
5-11	180.3	147.5	66.9
6-0	182.9	151.5	69.7

(From Metropolitan Life Insurance Company Statistical Bulletin 40. November-December, 1959)

does not result from hypoproteinemia. In those patients who lose 100 to 300 pounds, there usually is a need for removal of redundant skin from the lower abdomen and in some patients from the chest wall, upper arms, thighs, and elsewhere. The removal of redundant skin is not carried out until after the patient has reached a satisfactory weight reduction.

During the care of the first 45 extremely obese patients considered for gastric bypass, there were 5 sudden deaths. Two of these occurred preoperatively while patients were being prepared for operation with an overly zealous regimen of weight reduction. One of the patients died during induction of anesthesia. Two of the patients died postoperatively, one at 36 hours and the other at 10 days. Autopsies were performed in 4 of the patients. In one of the patients before operation and in the one at 36 hours after operation, massive pulmonary embolism was found. The patient who died 36 hours after operation from a massive pulmonary embolus had not received any glucose during that entire period of time. Following this, all operations for obesity were temporarily discontinued while an extensive search was made through the literature and while plans were made for investigation of the fatty acid levels in these patients. The results of this study support a suspicion that fatty acid elevation was precipitating intravascular thrombosis and in other ways contributing to the morbidity and mortality risk for these patients, as outlined earlier in Chapter 7. Presently, each of these obese patients receives an infusion of 5% glucose which is begun the night before operation and is continued at the rate of 2000 ml per day until such time as the patient is receiving sufficient nutrients by mouth to suppress serum fatty acid levels.

Those who have reported results of treating obese patients with intestinal bypass have also noted occasional occurrence of pulmonary embolism. During our experience with the last 134 patients who have been operated upon for extreme obesity we have not observed thromboembolic complications, and the convalescence has been smoother in other respects, particularly with regard to pulmonary function. It would seem logical that the extremely obese patient could tolerate a period of starvation after a major operation, but this does not appear to be true. Adequate nutrition should be maintained, so that lean body tissues are preserved but of probably greater importance, so that excessive mobilization of fat is prevented. Even in the dietary treatment of obesity, there is nothing to be gained by subjecting patients to complete starvation. Such starved overweights also lose lean body tissue and the loss of fat stores is not increased above that which can be obtained with a 1000-calorie diet.

REFERENCES

Aoki, V. S., Connor, W. E., and Wilson, W. R.: Effectiveness of cholestyramine in the treatment of hypercholesterolemia. Circulation *38* (Suppl. II) VI-34, 1968.

Bonbar, G. F., and Pisesky, W.: Severe and lethal complications following small intestinal short-circuiting operations for obesity. Arch. Surg. (Chicago) *94*:707 1967.

Buchwald, H.: Lowering of cholesterol absorption and blood levels by ileal exclusion: experimental basis and preliminary clinical report. Circulation *29*:713 1964.

Buchwald, H., Moore, R. B., Bertish, J., and Varco, R. L.: Effect of ileal bypass on cholesterol levels, atherosclerosis and growth in the infant rabbit. Ann. Surg. *175*:311, 1972.

Buchwald, H., Moore, R. B., Frantz, I. D., and Varco, R. L.: Cholesterol reduction by partial ileal bypass in a pediatric population. Surgery *68*:1101, 1970.

Buchwald, H., Moore, R. B., Lee, G. B., Frantz, I. D., Jr., and Varco, R. L.: Treatment of hypercholesterolemia: combined dietary, surgical, and bile salt-binding resin therapy. Arch. Surg. (Chicago) *97*:275, 1968.

Buchwald, H., and Varco, R. L.: A bypass operation for obese hyperlipidemic patients. Surgery *70*:62, 1971.

Carey, J. B.., Jr., Buchwald, H., and Varco, R. L: Intestinal absorption of bile salts in man and rabbits with ileal bypass. J. Clin. Invest. *44*:1033, 1965.

Carey, J. B., Jr., and Williams, G.: Relief of the pruritus of jaundice with a bile acid sequestering resin. J.A.M.A. *176*:432, 1961.

Dowling, R. H., Bell, G. D., and White, J.: Lithogenic bile in patients with ileal dysfunction. GUT *13*:415, 1972.

Dowling, R. H., Mack, E., and Small, D. M.: Effects of controlled interruption of the enterohepatic circulation of bile salts by biliary diversion and by ileal resection on bile salt secretion, synthesis and pool size in the Rhesus monkey. J. Clin. Invest. *49*:232, 1970.

Drenick, E. J., Simmons, F., and Murphy, J. F.: Hepatic morphology after treatment of obesity by fasting, diet and bowel bypass. New Eng. J. Med. *282*:829, 1970.

Gomes, M. M. R., Bernatz, P. E., Kottke, B. A., Juergens, J. L., and Titus, J. L.: Ileal bypass in treatment of hyperlipidemia: rationale and present status: subject review. Mayo Clin. Proc. *45*:229, 1970.

Hofmann, A. F., and Poley, J. R.: Cholestyramine treatment of diarrhea associated with ileal resection. New Eng. J. Med. *281*:397, 1969.

Kremen, A. J., Linner, J. H., and Nelson, C. H.: An experimental evaluation of the nutritional importance of proximal and distal small intestine. Ann. Surg. *140*:439, 1954.

Leren, P.: The effect of plasma cholesterol lowering diet in male survivors of myocardial infarction: a controlled clinical trial. Acta Med. Scand. *Suppl.* 466:1, 1966.

Lewis, L. A., Turnbull, R. B., and Page, I. H.: Effects of jejunocolic shunt on obesity, serum lipoproteins, lipids and electrolytes. Arch. Intern. Med. (Chicago) *117*:4, 1966.

Mason, E. E., and Ito, C.: Gastric bypass in obesity. Surg. Clin. N. Amer. *47*:1345, 1967.

Mason, E. E., and Ito, C.: Gastric bypass. Ann. Surg. *170*:329, 1969.

Morgan, A. P., and Moore, F. D.: Jejunoileostomy for extreme obesity: rationale, metabolic observations and results in a single case. Ann. Surg. *166*:75, 1967.

Moutafis, C. D., and Myant, N. B.: Increased hepatic synthesis of cholesterol after ileal bypass in monkeys. Clin. Sci. *34*:541, 1968.

Payne, J. H., DeWind, L. T., and Commons, R. R.: Metabolic observations in patients with jejunocolic shunts. Amer. J. Sug. *106*:273, 1963.

Richardson, J. D., and Griffen, W. O., Jr.: Ileocecal valve substitutes as bacteriologic barriers. Amer. J. Surg. *123*:149, 1972.

Salmon, P. A.: The results of small intestinal bypass operations for the treatment of obesity. Surg. Gynec. Obstet. *132*:965, 1971.

Scott, H. W., Sandstead, H. H., Brill, A. B., Burko, H., and Younger, R. K.: Experience with a new technic of intestinal bypass in the treatment of morbid obesity. Ann. Surg. *174*:560, 1971.

Sherman, C. D., May, A. G., Nye, W., and Waterhouse, C.: Clinical and metabolic studies following bowel bypassing for obesity. Ann. N.Y. Acad. Sci. *131*:614, 1965.

Shibata, H. R., MacKenzie, J. R., and Long, R. C.: Metabolic effects of controlled jejunocolic bypass. Arch. Surg. (Chicago) *95*:413, 1967.

Tennent, D. M.: Plasma cholesterol lowering action of bile acid binding polymers in experimental animals. J. Lipid Res. *1*:469, 1960.

Tilson, M.D., and Wright, H. K.: Adaptation of functioning and bypassed segments of ileum during compensatory hypertrophy of the gut. Surgery *67*:687, 1970.

Varco, R. L.: Intermittent external biliary drainage for relief of pruritus in certain chronic disorders of liver. Surgery *21*:43, 1947.

Wagensteen, O. H.: Personal communication.

Wood, P. D., Shioda, R., Estrich, D. L., and Splitter, S. D.: Effect of cholestyramine on composition of duodenal bile in obese human subjects. Metabolism *21*:107, 1972.

Wright, H. K., and Tilson, M. D.: The short gut syndrome. Curr. Prob. Surg., June 1971.

Chapter

9

Circulation and Shock

Shock is failure of the circulation so that vital organs are not supplied with sufficient oxygen and nutrients. Cells, organs, and life are in jeopardy. Normal circulation requires an adequate volume of blood, extracellular fluid, and total body water so that there is fluid to circulate. There must be pumping of the blood by the heart balanced by peripheral resistance so as to maintain blood pressure and allow for regulation of blood flow to those areas which need perfusion and away from those areas where metabolic activity is at a resting level. Normally, there is continual opening and closing of portions of the microvascular bed and adjustments rather analogous to the regulation of the flow of water in a city water system. In the summertime when many people open their faucets to water their lawns, the system may decompensate, and temporary emergency measures are required to assure that the most vital areas are provided with flow.

There must, of course, be an adequate mass of red blood cells to permit gas exchange, both in the lungs and in the tissues. The red cells need an adequate supply of 2,3-diphosphoglycerate so that they will release the oxygen where it is needed. There must be an adequate colloid osmotic pressure generated by albumin in the vascular space so as to preserve normal plasma volume. The lining membranes of the vascular bed must be competent to retain albumin. Cellular membranes depend for their integrity upon a normal metabolic activity so as to maintain the chemical distinction of cellular fluid as opposed to extracellular fluid.

Shock is a state of increasing entropy. *Entropy* means a state of uniformity and absence of energy-requiring gradients. Entropy implies a flowing towards uniformity. Health by contrast, is a state of "negentropy," which implies efficient use of energy to maintain not only flow, pressure gradients, and metabolism, but chemical gradients, with differences between cellular and extracellular fluid, and also differences in the subcellular particles so that mitrochondria with their elaborate enzyme systems are maintained distinct from lysosomes, endoplasmic reticulum, Golgi apparatus, nucleus, and the other parts of the microanatomy of the cell. Each part of the body is perfused so as to provide nourishment and remove waste products according to the needs of that tissue bed. In shock, these highly complex relationships between the pump and the resistances in various organs and the consequent regulated flow of fluid with substrates and waste products are disturbed. Shock comprises both a cause and a series of responses. Shock is dynamic with changing magnitudes of the various contributing factors so that there must be continued observation, re-evaluation, and appropriate modifications of treatment.

A variety of observations supply the data base for defining the presence and evolution of shock in a given patient. What begins as hemorrhagic shock may progress through any sequence of hypovolemic, cardiac, septic, or neurogenic shock. The initial history and physical findings allow formulation of an initial diagnosis which helps define the initial problem and treatment, but the most important unifying principle in the management of patients in shock is the recognition of the evolution of functional defects that may occur. Of equal importance to documentation of current abnormalities in function is the observation of response to treatment through continual monitoring of vital signs.

A great many statements have been made about the inadequacy of "low blood pressure" as a definition of shock, and yet, measurement of blood pressure remains one of our most valuable observations. It is true that the arterial blood pressure can be regulated so as to provide a normal reading up until the time of death through the appropriate infusion of norepinephrine. In selected patients, restoration of blood pressure by infusion of norepinephrine may coincide with restoration of normal tissue perfusion, and this treatment may contribute to recovery of the patient. Much more often the use of a powerful vasopressor, while it supports a normal blood pressure reading, contributes to a decrease in tissue perfusion and the hastening of death. Blood pressure is a valuable index but we need to think beyond single measurements of arterial blood pressure or central venous pressure. Even when cardiac output is measured along with blood gases and when a number of dimensions can be plotted or analyzed in complex ways so as to separate the various groups of patients with different types of circulatory failure, our hope is that these separations will identify different variations from normal circulation and will provide information about what really is the underlying problem that requires treatment. Modern data processing allows the analysis of large amounts of data in a formal mathematical way. Most of the time, the experienced physician is collecting and analyzing the data with the self-reproducing computer that is carried around on the upper end of his body. Treatment is formulated on the basis of a synthesis of data and some conclusion that the patient has an inadequate blood volume or that he has inadequate cardiac function or that peripheral resistance is inappropriate or that in some other way there is interference with perfusion of the tissues and exchange of oxygen.

RECOGNITION

Recognition of shock depends upon some index of suspicion that the patient has a condition which might produce shock. When a patient is vomiting large amounts of blood, the diagnosis of shock is scarcely even verbalized. The patient is immediately treated with fluids and early infusion of blood. His blood pressure, pulse, and urine output are monitored. If necessary, blood is given at several infusion sites, and as the blood pressure rises it is evident that the blood volume has been at least partially restored. If the blood pressure falls again, one concludes that bleeding has increased or resumed and that the patient needs additional blood. If the blood loss is less rapid, the blood pressure may remain normal but the pulse rate will vary inversely with the blood volume. The pulse rate may function as a very sensitive and accurate index of the adequacy of replacement, even though the blood pressure remains normal.

Shock follows hemorrhage less often when bleeding is obvious. When hemorrhage is obvious, the signs of circulatory insufficiency are used as indices of the severity of the blood loss and the adequacy of treatment. A low blood pressure, rapid pulse, and inadequate urine output in the face of rapid blood replacement are an indication of need for early intervention to secure a bleeding vessel. Under these circumstances not only is shock diagnosed early, it is treated immediately, vigorously, and appropriately.

By contrast, if a healthy-appearing and previously well person faints from obscure internal bleeding and is brought to the emergency room, there may be delay in arriving at a diagnosis of hemorrhage. The diagnostic sequence is one of first recognizing the signs and symptoms of shock and then raising the question as to whether there is internal bleeding which could explain the anxiousness, thirst, rapid pulse, low blood pressure, pale color, cool extremities, poor capillary refill, and decreased or absent urine formation.

There may be a history of a recent blow over the spleen or recent symptoms consistent with infectious mononucleosis which might have set the stage for spontaneous rupture of the spleen. Perhaps spontaneous rupture of a splenic artery aneurysm is the cause, and the suspicion as to the site of bleeding may come from shoulder pain, abdominal discomfort, or increasing abdominal girth. But the diagnosis is initially one of shock, and success in treatment depends upon early recognition of the signs and symptoms of shock even though there is no external evidence of blood loss.

Shock is even less likely to be recognized when bleeding is diffuse, slow, and hidden as in the patient with multiple fractures. The signs and symptoms may be overlooked initially because of the many injuries. Too often a head injury is blamed for low blood pressure and rapid pulse. Patients with multiple injuries and head trauma who develop shock are bleeding until proven otherwise. The diagnosis of irreversible shock must never be made in such a patient. Too many patients who have been diagnosed as having irreversible shock have been found at autopsy to have a large amount of blood in the peritoneal cavity or in the pleural space or about fractures of the femur and pelvis. If a patient has multiple injuries, bleeding from a ruptured spleen should be considered as a more likely cause than injury to the brain. If a patient has pelvic and vertebral fractures or a fractured femur, he may need four or five units of blood to replace the blood loss into the fracture sites and if the patient is still hypotensive after treatment with blood, re-examination of the chest and abdomen may reveal an accumulation of blood that was not present initially and which explains the continuing circulatory insufficiency.

Cardiac and septic shock are likely to occur in patients who are under care for some serious illness or have recently undergone a major operation. The recognition of shock in such patients may be delayed until the patient becomes anuric or until other changes occur in other organs which further complicate the picture. Acute renal failure is sometimes diagnosed without anyone having recognized that the circulation has at any time been inadequate. As with hemorrhage, there are other situations in which shock is anticipated and the signs and symptoms are actually looked for, such as in the patient who has a shaking chill during the change of a urethral catheter. Under such circumstances the physician cultures the blood and institutes frequent observation of pulse, blood pressure, and urine flow. He obtains a white blood cell count and differential blood cell count and monitors the temperature and gradually begins to gather the necessary data to substantiate a diagnosis of endotoxic shock.

If a patient is awake and has sudden severe chest pain along with signs and symptoms of circulatory insufficiency, the physician immediately suspects a myocardial infarction and obtains an electrocardiogram and begins to monitor serum enzyme levels and attempts to document a diagnosis of cardiogenic shock. However, the diagnosis of cardiogenic and septic shock is frequently not as quickly arrived at as is the case in a patient with shock from obvious external bleeding.

DATA COLLECTION AND ANALYSIS

The diagnosis and management of shock are dependent upon a sequence of collecting data from observation of the patient, analyzing this data in terms of the underlying problems such as deficient volume, inadequate cardiac output, abnormal vasomotion, and so forth. On the basis of this analysis, a treatment plan is followed and then the physician returns to the observations in order to find out if the treatment is appropriate and effective and also to be alert to the development of new problems which might require a change in treatment. There is a circular sequence of observing, analysis, treatment, and back to observation as is summarized in Figure 9-1.

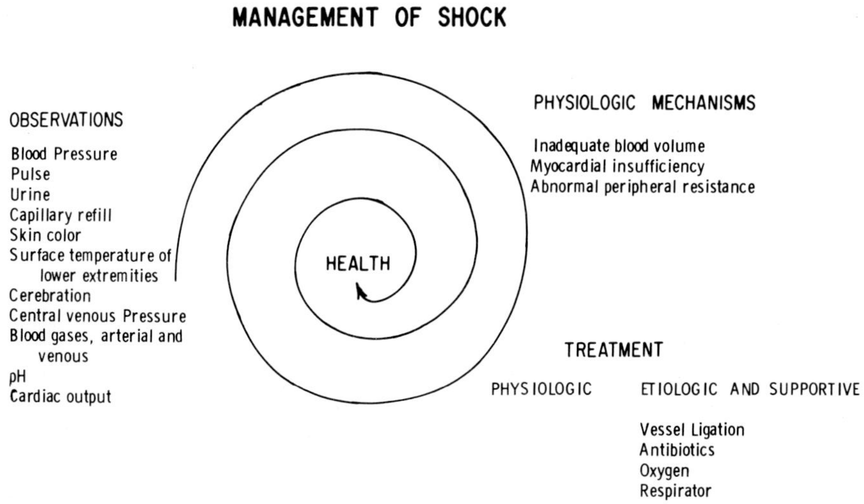

Figure 9-1. Emphasizes the need for continued observation, interpretation, and alteration of treatment until recovery. For physiologic treatment, see Figure 9-6.

The data which are collected consist always of certain commonly used parameters such as blood pressure, pulse, respiration, urine output, and other information which is easily obtained at the bedside without any special equipment. There are, in addition, more complex bits of information such as analysis of blood gases and determination of cardiac output by analysis of dye dilution curves. Finally, with the help of computations of varying complexity, parameters of ventricular function, vascular tone, peripheral shunting, and pulmonary shunting can be determined.

Arterial blood pressure, as measured in a noninvasive technique with the inflatable blood pressure cuff and listening with the stethoscope for Korotkoff's sounds, is the most frequently used and valuable bit of information for the recognition and treatment of shock. Like every other single parameter, it has its limitations. The sounds result from the sudden expansion of a relaxed artery below the site of compression of the inflated cuff. If the arm is large and obese and the cuff is small, the cuff pressure required to compress the artery may be considerably higher than the actual arterial blood pressure at any given stage of the determination. Whenever blood pressure is abnormal, one of the first considerations should be that the blood pressure cuff is not correctly applied.

There are situations in which accurate blood pressure readings cannot be obtained in spite of repeated readjustments of the blood pressure cuff. Inaccuracies are more likely if the blood pressure is low or if the pulse pressure is small. When the cardiac output is decreased, it may be necessary to use direct arterial blood pressure readings through a catheter inserted into the radial artery or some other artery. If the patient is critically ill and the accuracy of arterial blood pressure is critical to the care of the patient, an indwelling arterial catheter should be used.

There are hazards to the direct monitoring of blood pressure, especially in the elderly person or when circulation is impaired. If possible, the catheter should be inserted in a radial artery where it is evident that an ulnar artery is also present and in the nondominant extremity. Take the patient's supinated wrist and compress the radial and ulnar arteries. After all blood is drained from the hand lower it to a dependent position and release one artery and watch for flushing. Repeat and release the opposite artery. If the patient's circulation is sufficient, it should be possible to demonstrate that an adequate ulnar artery is present and could nourish the hand if the radial artery were irreparably damaged.

Cohn and Luria measured blood pressure at the bedside using both direct and indirect techniques in 50 patients with hypotension or clinical shock. They discussed 7 patients, mainly individuals with cardiac failure from acute infarction, but some with an element of bacterial endotoxic shock. The measurements revealed that the direct pressures determined by needle puncture of the femoral artery were significantly higher than the pressures obtained with the sphygmomanometer cuff. It was also observed that the blood pressure was being pushed to hypertensive levels with vasopressors at times because the arm band blood pressure was unreliably low, and under such circumstances improvement of the circulation resulted from discontinuing the use of vasopressors. It was Cohn and Luria's impression that the availability of direct arterial pressure measurements made a great difference in the management of shock in these patients, but the additional availability of other physiologic data, such as the determination of cardiac output and right atrial pressure, was also important.

Serial blood pressures, like measurement of any other parameter, are of more value than single blood pressures, and comparisons should be made with earlier blood pressures obtained when the patient was known to be well, if they are available. What seems to be a normal blood pressure may represent serious hypotension in a patient who has previously had very high blood pressure. The difference between the systolic and diastolic pressure, or pulse pressure, is related to the volume of output with each stroke of the heart. For any given cardiac output, pulse pressure is inversely related to the rate. The diastolic pressure is frequently maintained in shock by increasing peripheral resistance, and narrowing of pulse pressure is likely to be an indication of circulatory insufficiency.

Pulse rate in some patients under certain circumstances may be of greater value than blood pressure in monitoring the rate of blood loss and the adequacy of replacement. With increasing pulse rates, the pulse becomes more thready for any given cardiac output. If the pulse rate slows, the pulse will become more bounding and easier to feel, but this may not necessarily indicate an increased cardiac output.

Central venous pressure measurements require a catheter with the end in the superior vena cava. This can be placed from a percutaneous jugular approach or by way of the subclavian vein, or it can be provided by use of a longer catheter placed from the antecubital vein either by percutaneous puncture or through a cutdown in the arm. Such a catheter used for monitoring central venous pressure and for administration of medications and fluids should be removed as soon as the shock is corrected, since in the excitement of treating shock and with the repeated manipulations the chances of contamination are greatly increased.

Central venous pressure determinations are very valuable in assessing blood volume and cardiac function, but they also may be misleading. Central venous pressure is dependent upon the return of blood to the large veins, the vascular tone of these veins, and the competence of the heart in pumping blood that returns to the right side of the heart. Additional information can be obtained by changing the position of the patient with mild elevation of the head of the bed or mild elevation of the foot of the bed and observing the effects of the change in position upon not only central venous pressure but the blood pressure, pulse, and general appearance of the patient.

The temperature of the skin, especially that of the lower extremities, is a valuable index of the perfusion of tissues. The patient with inadequate circulation is likely to have increased sympathetic discharge with constriction of the vessels to the skin. The skin is cold or cool. In a cool room a patient with normal circulation has cool feet, but if the back of the hand is run along the skin of the leg and thigh and coolness is detected at the knee or above, this should suggest circulatory insufficiency.

Capillary refill is of additional help in evaluating the perfusion of peripheral vascular beds. The nailbeds of the fingers and toes are compressed and then released. The time required for the capillary bed to fill with pink blood is an index of adequacy of circulation. Peripheral veins can be used as a crude flowmeter if the patient is not markedly vasoconstricted. The extremity is elevated, emptying out all of the blood from the veins, and then when the veins are collapsed, the extremity is placed in a dependent position; the time required for filling of the veins is a measurement of the rate of arterial flow into the extremity, provided of course the patient has competent valves in the veins.

Arterial and venous blood gas analyses and pH determinations are available in most hospitals, particularly in intensive care facilities. A measurement of arterial Po_2 when the patient is breathing 100% oxygen at atmospheric pressure allows calculation of the gradient between the pulmonary alveoli and arterial blood and is an index of perfusion of the lungs. Arterial Pco_2 and pH allow determination of acid-base balance which is frequently disturbed in shock and may require correction for optimum response to other therapeutic measures. The mixed central venous Po_2 together with an arterial Po_2 allows calculation of the arterial-venous oxygen difference which is related to the peripheral utilization of oxygen. If oxygen consumption can be measured along with the arterial-venous oxygen difference, then cardiac output can be calculated.

The injection centrally of cardio-green dye followed by continuous determination of the appearance of this dye on the arterial side of the circulation also permits calculation of cardiac output. Such dye dilution curves contain information about the mixing of the dye in the blood and heart and its dispersion during flow through the lungs which provides information which has been used by Siegel (1972) in establishing both diagnosis and prognosis in patients with myocardial infarction.

Ventricular function curves based on Starling's law of the heart are shown in Figure 9-2. The normal ventricular stroke volume output is related to the amount of stretching of the myocardial fibers which in turn is related to the amount of blood returning to the heart. A crude impression of cardiac output can be obtained on the basis of capillary refill and urinary output. In occasional intensive care wards, it may be possible to obtain serial estimates of cardiac output on the basis of dye dilution curves. The other parameter, venous return, is estimated by measurements of central venous pressure. Regardless of the degree of sophistication of the monitoring, at least two sets of data are required in most instances; these are obtained before and after the rapid infusion of blood or fluids so as to increase central venous pressure.

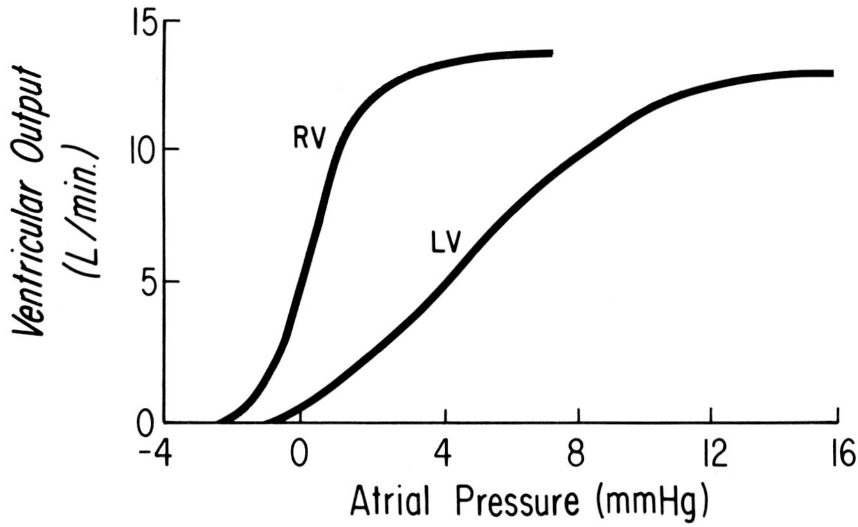

Figure 9-2. Starling function curves are shown for the two ventricles. When venous filling increases as indicated by increased atrial pressure, there is a lengthening of myocardial muscle fibers during diastole and an increase in cardiac output.

If the patient has evidence of excellent cardiac output and a low central venous pressure, it can be concluded that his cardiac function is satisfactory and probably the patient is not in shock. At the other end of the scale, if the central venous pressure is high and cardiac output seems to be inadequate, it may be deemed dangerous to test cardiac function with additional blood or fluid, since the ventricular function is already demonstrated to be inadequate. Lewin et al. have determined the ventricular function curves for elderly patients in an effort to predict operative mortality. Such studies may reveal diminished cardiac reserve in patients who are not in obvious congestive heart failure.

The fact that cardiac outputs cannot be determined or that a computer facility is not available for determining more complex relationships should not deter the surgeon from thinking in terms of ventricular function curves in his evaluation of a patient with circulatory insufficiency. When the blood volume is expanded, the question may come down to deciding whether this expansion of volume leads to an improvement in the sytemic blood pressure or a rise in central venous pressure. There should be some of both but the predominant rise of one or the other will separate those patients with excellent ventricular function and a deficient blood volume from other patients in whom the problem is one of borderline cardiac failure. The physician should decide whether there is an improvement in skin color and sensorium, capillary refill, and urinary output or, on the other hand, whether the expansion of blood volume is perhaps leading to an increase in pulmonary congestion. Of course if the determinations are available, cardiac outputs should be obtained along with arterial venous oxygen differences as an estimate of improvement in perfusion. Alveolar-arterial oxygen differences (while the patient is breathing 100% oxygen) are an index of improvement in pulmonary distribution of blood flow and gas exchange.

In the absence of actual measurement of cardiac output an experienced physician who has been watching the patient is in the best position to interpret central venous pressure measurements and changes in blood pressure and tissue perfusion after a rapid infusion of 200 ml of blood and to decide about the adequacy of the ventricular function. Central venous pressure is dependent upon the amount of blood returning to the right heart, the tone of the large veins, and the function of the right ventricle in overcoming pulmonary resistance as well as the relationships between right and left ventricular function.

Central venous pressure is normally between 4 and 8 cm of water, but values ranging between 2 and 15 cm of water are observed without necessarily signifying any need for a change in treatment. A central venous pressure below 2 cm of water indicates hypovolemia. A value above 15 suggests a venous return exceeding the capacity of the heart and represents either hypervolemia or cardiac failure or both. Wilson et al. found the infusion of 200 ml of saline during a period of 10 minutes to provide helpful information. If the central venous pressure rose more than 2 cm during the infusion and remained elevated for an additional 10 minutes following the infusion, this indicated myocardial failure. Excessive use of saline for such a test carries a danger in that it is lost rapidly from the vascular space into both pulmonary and systemic vascular beds and can produce pulmonary edema without having caused an elevation of central venous pressure. Blood or plasma may provide a more reliable and safer test of loading.

The effect of anesthetic agents, barbiturates, and norepinephrine and its antagonists should be considered for their influence on large vein tone. Peripheral resistance is a function of the muscular activity of the walls of the precapillary arterioles and can be measured by determining the blood pressure in relation to cardiac output. The potential vascular space in the body is much greater than the available blood volume. Blood pressure is sustained by the maintenance of an appropriate peripheral resistance in the various vascular beds. In the presence of blood loss shock and in other types of shock, blood flow through the coronary and cerebral vessels is maintained by virtue of increased venous tone and increased peripheral resistance in other vascular beds. A sudden faint as is observed in an occasional patient after a needle puncture is due to relaxation of peripheral resistance generally so that there is an inadequate amount of blood perfusing the cerebral vessels.

Peripheral resistance is regulated by the sympathetic nerves primarily and to a lesser degree by the circulating levels of catecholamines. Norepinephrine is the most frequently used drug in increasing venous tone and peripheral resistance. Norepinephrine acts on both beta and alpha receptors. The alpha receptors cause an increase in peripheral resistance. There are beta receptors which cause a mild vasodilatation, but the overall effect of the drug is to cause constriction of precapillary sphincters. Norepinephrine acts upon beta receptors in the heart to produce increased myocardial contraction: inotropic action. Alpha blocking agents are used with norepinephrine at times to prevent excessive constriction of precapillary sphincters when norepinephrine is given to stimulate improved myocardial contraction.

Shock implies an inadequate perfusion of tissues but it may come about because of an inappropriate distribution of blood flow so that tissues which need increased blood flow do not receive it. The concept of a peripheral shunt has been used to categorize this aspect of the problem. Whether arterial-venous shunts actually open up or whether the blood simply channels through portions of the capillary bed where little gas exchange occurs, leaving other large areas in deficit, is difficult to document in any particular instance or in any one part of the circulatory system. The concept need not be entirely one of a hydraulic abnormality but can also result from chemical changes which prevent the release of oxygen from hemoglobin during the transit of blood through the capillary bed.

Release of oxygen from hemoglobin is related to the concentration of inorganic phosphates, particularly 2,3-diphosphoglycerate, in the red blood cells. As is shown in Figure 9-3, such a deficiency shifts the oxygen dissociation curve to the left. This is referred to as a *chemical shunt* in that the blood passes through the tissues without giving up its oxygen. The result of chemical and hydraulic shunts is that the venous blood has a higher concentration of oxygen than is normal and the arterial-venous difference is narrow.

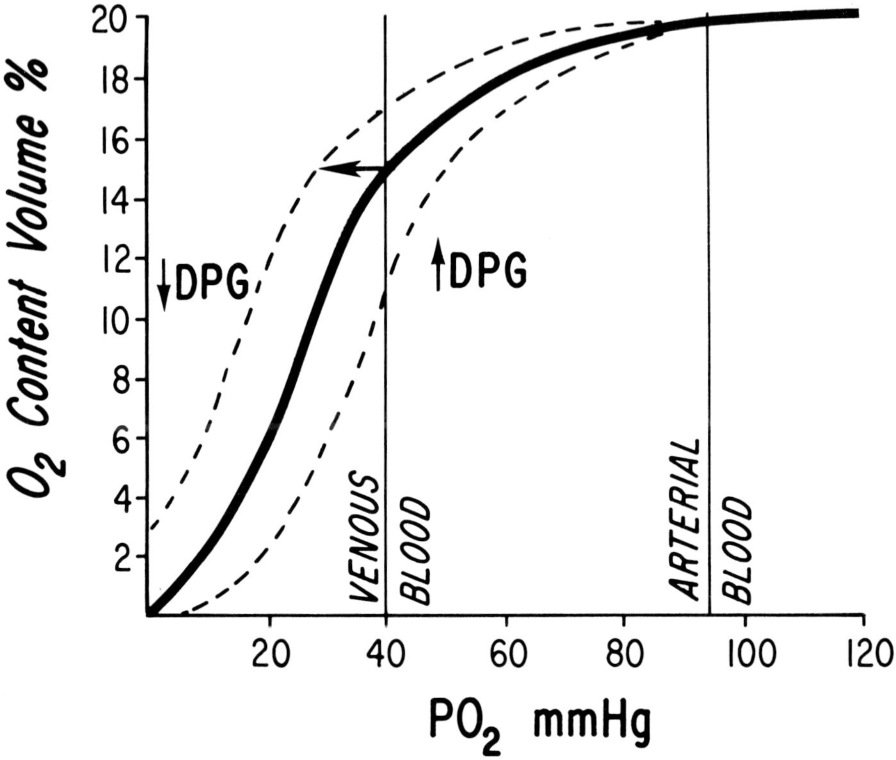

Figure 9-3. This illustrates how an increase in red blood cell 2,3-diphosphoglycerate causes a shift of the oxygen dissociation curve to the right so that more oxygen is released at any given Po_2. By contrast a deficiency of 2,3-DPG shifts the curve to the left, and less oxygen is released at the same Po_2.

Anoxic tissues shift to anaerobic metabolism with the production of lactic acid so that the venous return has a higher concentration of lactic acid (which is another measure of inadequate perfusion) and poor gas exchange in the capillary vascular bed. There is also an associated reduction in pH, evident first in tissue, then in venous blood, and finally in arterial blood. Patients in shock also are likely to develop shunts in the lung. As with the peripheral circulation, this may not represent a direct anatomical connection between an artery and a vein but is due to blood passing through a capillary bed in an area in the lung which is not aerated, with the consequence that the arterial blood is not saturated with oxygen. Pulmonary shunts are measured by administration of 100% oxygen to the patient and calculation of the difference between alveolar and arterial Po_2.

HEMORRHAGIC AND OTHER VOLUME DEFICIENCIES

The most common cause of shock is bleeding, and the most common cause of "irreversible shock" is found at autopsy to be unrecognized internal bleeding or bleeding in excess of what was thought possible on the basis of the ante-mortem history and physical and laboratory findings. A person, after donating 500 ml of blood, is soon able to walk away from the blood bank without significant symptoms. For a 60-kg lean person the estimated blood volume amounts to 4.8 liters so that such a donation represents about 10% of his blood volume. If 20 to 30% of the blood volume is lost, an otherwise healthy person will usually collapse. If the blood is lost slowly, however, there is considerable compensation during the blood loss, and the blood pressure and circulation are maintained.

The blood vascular space is made up of a high pressure or arterial space, which is relatively small in volume, and a low pressure system which is much larger in volume, containing 80 to 85% of the total blood in the body. This latter space is composed of the vena cava and other large veins and includes most of the blood within the chest. Gauer, Henry, and Behn found continual adaptation between blood volume and vascular capacity. The low-pressure, high-volume region is 11 to 200 times as distensible as the arterial tree, according to Gauer and Henry. When a patient with large varicose veins stands up, a significant portion of the blood volume pools in these dilated veins. This may be a problem in individuals who have been extremely obese and then lose several hundred pounds. It is a problem in patients who have had extensive sympathectomy, either surgically or by the administration of drugs. The tonic adaptation of the veins to the available blood in the low pressure system is important in maintaining venous return to the right side of the heart and sustaining an adequate cardiac output. The loss of venous tone can cause hypotensive episodes without any external blood loss. Contraction of central veins will sustain an adequate circulation in spite of a liter of blood loss.

Gauer and Henry found a gradual decrease in rate of firing of the arterial baroreceptors and a more rapid decline in the rate of firing from cardiac atrial receptors as blood was withdrawn slowly from experimental animals. There was a gradual increase in secretion of antidiuretic hormone and a more rapid rise in the release of aldosterone. The pulse rate increased rather steadily as more and more blood was removed. Finally when the blood loss approached 30% of the estimated normal blood volume, there was a marked and rapid rise in the tone of the capacity vessels. This did not occur until other compensatory mechanisms had been exhausted in these animals that were losing blood slowly.

The high pressure system also responds to blood loss. Parker et al. studied the canine gracilis muscle, isolated except for nerve and blood supply. The most striking change in peripheral resistance occurred with a slow loss of blood volume which was carried to 60% of the estimated normal volume. By contrast, if this much blood was lost suddenly, the increase in peripheral resistance was less marked, evanescent, and followed within 2 hours by death even in spite of reinfusion. The marked difference in response of the individual according to whether blood loss is rapid or slow is dependent upon the need for a certain amount of time for mobilization of defense mechanisms. There are, therefore, differences in hemorrhagic shock, according to the rate of the blood loss. Shock is always a composite of the etiologic mechanism and the body reactions. The result of rapid blood loss may be death of the individual within a few hours whereas the loss of an equal amount of blood over a longer period of time may allow the individual to survive the immediate episode but to develop other complications such as acute renal failure at a later stage in his illness.

Because shock is always a combination of stimulus and response, there are many variables involved. Early attempts to find a standard experimental shock model by removal of a specified volume of blood were unsuccessful. Wiggers and Werle used a specified level of lowered blood pressure for a given period of time, an approach which gave more predictable results. Their technique was refined further by Huizenga et al. and consisted of the following: (1) rapid removal of blood (55 ml/min) to lower the arterial blood pressure to 50 mm Hg where it was maintained for 90 minutes; (2) removal of additional blood slowly (4 to 5 ml/min) so as to lower the blood pressure to 30 mm Hg and use of that blood for small reinfusions so as to maintain the 30 mm Hg pressure for 15 to 30 minutes; and finally (3) all remaining removed blood was warmed, filtered, and reinfused. This model produced death in 76.5% of 21 control dogs and in 75% of a group of dogs treated with adrenal cortical extract. This has been one of the most commonly used experimental models in study of hemorrhagic shock.

Hemorrhage is followed by reformation of plasma volume from extracellular fluid (Fig. 9-4). This requires up to 48 hours after removal of 800 ml of blood from healthy young people and is followed by a slower replenishment of albumin and blood cells by increased production in the liver and bone marrow. Normally, 60% of the albumin in the body is outside of the vascular space, and much of this is located in the skin. The formation of tissue fluids occurs on the arterial side of the capillary bed because hydrostatic pressure exceeds colloid osmotic

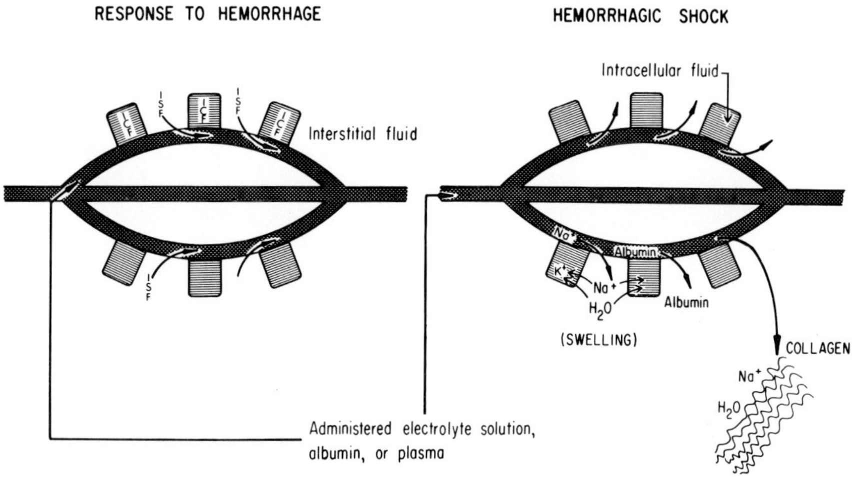

Figure 9-4. Contrasts the refilling of the vascular space from interstitial fluid after hemorrhage with the inactivation or sequestration of sodium, fluid, and albumin that occurs in hemorrhagic shock.

pressure. There is flow of extracellular fluid back into the vascular space on the venous side of the capillary bed where colloid osmotic pressure exceeds hydrostatic pressure. In addition there is fluid which moves as lymph from the extracellular fluid along lymphatics and back into the venous circulation through the larger lymphatic channels. The gradual movement of extracellular fluid with albumin to replenish plasma volume is probably due to a decrease in the formation of extracellular fluid as a result of a reduction in pressure on the arterial side of the capillary bed, either because of decreased cardiac output or because of contraction of the precapillary sphincters. At the same time, because of continued flow of lymph through the lymphatics, the net result is that interstitial fluid and albumin move into the vascular space.

The chronically ill and malnourished person may have all available albumin within the vascular space. Hemorrhage in such an individual is likely to be followed by a sustained loss of plasma volume, rising hematocrit, and clumping together of red blood cells to produce the sludging which has been demonstrated with microcinematography and dynamically described by Knisely et al.

Carey et al. studied young men brought to the hospital in Vietnam shortly after severe injuries in which an estimated 40% loss of blood volume had occurred. They were able to study these individuals with initial observations before any treatment and subsequently during and after treatment with saline. With these massive traumatic injuries and hemorrhagic shock, there was endogenous refilling of the plasma volume, initially at the rate of 1000 ml per hour. Dilution of red blood cells occurred, and there was dilution of plasma proteins, more so for globulin than for albumin since some albumin was mobilized and came into the vascular space. As evidence of poor tissue perfusion, the lactate levels, which are normally around 10 to 20 mg%, were 45 mg% at the time of admission, an average of 83 minutes following wounding. The lactate level was 65 mg% by the end of the operation and had returned to less than 20 mg% by the 18th hour postoperatively. By contrast, in those individuals who died, the serum lactate levels remained elevated.

The patients were given saline or lactated Ringer's as an initial fluid for resuscitation until blood had been cross-matched. Then blood was replaced, but additional saline solution was also used so that the total administration during the first four days after wounding amounted to some 12 liters of saline and 8 liters of blood. Comparisons between saline solution with 5% albumin and saline solution without albumin led to the conclusion that the saline solution was effective and that perhaps the patients receiving saline solution improved more rapidly than did those patients treated with added albumin. Later on at this hospital an attempt was made to reduce the volume of saline solution, and the result was that more blood was required. The chief concern about the use of saline solution for resuscitation is that the patients may develop pulmonary edema, but in these young men the incidence of pulmonary insufficiency did not seem to be related to the type of resuscitation fluid used. Moss produced hemorrhagic shock in the baboon and compared the effects of blood alone, saline solution with red blood cells, and saline solution with 5% albumin plus replacement of the red blood cells. He found no significant difference between the animals treated with saline solution and those treated with 5% albumin, insofar as the lung water content was concerned. Electron micrographs showed no edema in the lungs of the animals treated with saline solution.

The explanation for the requirement of large amounts of saline solution in the resuscitation of the patient with traumatic and severe hemorrhagic shock is the sequestration of sodium and water in collagen (Fig. 9-4). Grayson et al. depleted patients of sodium and studied their hematocrit, urinary excretion, pulse rate, and blood pressure and found certain similarities to the individual who has undergone recent hemmorrhage. Having hypothesized that perhaps damaged collagen was the source of the sequestration, they undertook to demonstrate this by placing the collagenous part of the tail of a rat beneath the rat's skin and then subjecting these rats to hemorrhagic shock. They were able to demonstrate that there was in fact an increased sodium and water uptake in the collagen. This type of experiment was repeated by Fulton, who also found uptake of sodium and water in collagen during shock just as had been proposed by Moyer's group. Fulton concluded that the quantity of sodium absorbed by the collagen was of an order of magnitude which could well explain the supposed irreversibility of the Wiggers type of hemorrhagic shock. According to this thesis there are close similarities between the patient with an excessive body surface burn and the individual with traumatic or hemorrhagic shock.

Many massive injuries are produced by the automobile, and we see patients with them fairly soon after injury. It would seem that the lessons learned from the care of massively injured individuals in Vietnam could be applied directly to certain of the civilian patients seen in our emergency rooms. Several liters of saline or lactated Ringer's solution should be given while obtaining cross-matched blood. Further resuscitation should then be governed by the blood pressure, central venous pressure, pulse rate, urinary output, level of consciousness, capillary refill, and warmth of skin. The infusion of blood and saline solution in proportions of approximately 2 parts to 3 parts should be used in whatever volumes are necessary to restore and sustain normal circulation and to maintain this circulation until appropriate measures can be taken to secure bleeding vessels and remove devitalized tissues.

If the patient turns out to be less seriously injured than initially supposed and responds to the saline solution alone, and his circulation remains adequate, it may not be necessary to give blood. Certainly caution should be used about the administration of large amounts of blood and saline solution to patients whose injuries are small or whose shock is mild. The thesis that shock and trauma, like a burn, can alter collagen and cause sequestration of sodium and water implies that these large amounts of resuscitation fluids are required to replace what has been lost to the functional blood and extracellular fluid volume. To give such infusions to patients who do not need them is likely to cause an overload and pulmonary edema.

There are those patients who, because of age, chronic illness, severe infection, or poor nutrition, may not respond in the way that has been described for the young, previously healthy individual. In such persons the use of albumin and plasma may be crucial, and the use of saline solution may need to be limited. Ideally, if a patient has a serum albumin of less than 3 gm% this should be corrected before a major operation. However, if the urgency of the situation requires an operation in the face of a low serum albumin concentration, then it would seem reasonable to incorporate human albumin in the resuscitation fluids.

CARDIOGENIC SHOCK

Following myocardial infarction there is a reduction in cardiac output and a rise in central venous pressure. In terms of Starling's cardiac function curves the patient is on a lower curve so that when central venous pressure increases, there is not a corresponding increase in cardiac output (Fig. 9-5). Improvement in the circulation requires improving the stroke volume output. This may not occur in spite of digitalis. Isoproterenol will probably cause an increase in heart rate and arrhythmias plus a decrease in peripheral resistance which further interferes with coronary perfusion. Norepinephrine may be of some help if it is given slowly in low doses so as not to excessively increase peripheral resistance. Norepinephrine and phentolamine given together will provide an inotropic effect without the deleterious effect of excessive increase in peripheral resistance.

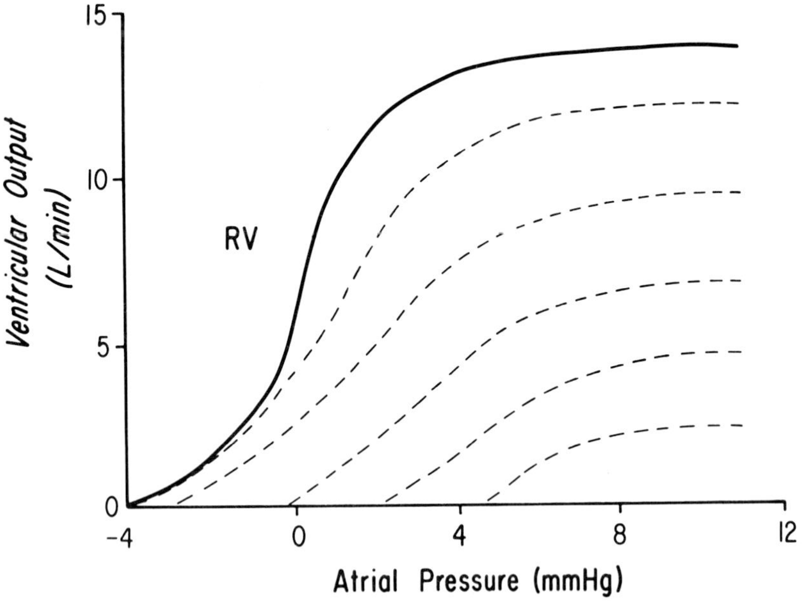

Figure 9-5. Illustrates a series of cardiac function curves and a basis for determining whether a patient needs an increase in venous filling pressure or a shift to a more efficient function curve. Does a trial expansion of blood volume cause an increase in atrial pressure or an improved cardiac output?

A cardiogenic component of shock sometimes appears in patients who have hypotension on the basis of hemorrhage or sepsis. This can be recognized by a rising central venous pressure without an increase in cardiac output when blood volume is expanded by a rapid infusion of several hundred ml of saline. Digitalis in such a situation is more likely to be helpful than in the patient who has had an acute myocardial infarction.

Cardiac insufficiency may result from increased peripheral resistance and may be complicated by the fact that there are two ventricles of the heart and that the left ventricle may fail before the right ventricle so that there is an increase in pulmonary pressure and pulmonary edema. Under such circumstances it may be impossible to give the patient needed blood or fluids until the peripheral resistance is reduced and a balance is re-established between the output of the left and right ventricles. Relaxation of the metarterioles with the use of phentolamine or Dibenzyline allows a better perfusion of the peripheral capillary beds and a shift of blood towards the systemic circulation and out of the pulmonary and central blood volume. This may cause the patient to remain or to become more hypotensive but now the patient can be given blood, plasma, or saline with restoration of a satisfactory blood pressure without causing pulmonary edema. Dibenzyline is a competive inhibitor of norepinephrine at the alpha receptors but is irreversible in its action. This is perhaps an advantage in that the effect is more permanent. On the other hand, phentolamine is also a competitive inhibitor of norepinephrine at the alpha receptors but is reversible and transient in its effect. If the predicted improvement is not observed, phentolamine can be stopped or the dosage of norepinephrine can be increased.

Surgical patients sometimes develop cardiogenic shock during or following major operations while there is on-going blood loss and replacement and when the patient is unable to report those symptoms which under other circumstances would center attention upon the heart. An electrocardiogram is of help in any patient in whom the circulation in inadequate and in whom there does not seem to be an appropriate blood loss or other cause for the shock. Hypotension occurring during anesthesia induction or following an episode of sudden operative blood loss and replacement may be antecedent to the development of cardiogenic shock which is actually due to myocardial infarction.

An infarct results in a decrease in stroke volume output because the infarcted muscle not only fails to contract but begins in time to develop paradoxic motion so that some of the energy which should be converted to kinetic energy and an outflow of blood is expended in useless ballooning (paradoxical motion) of the infarcted area. The remaining muscle may not sustain an adequate cardiac output. As stroke volume falls, the peripheral resistance usually increases. This helps to sustain coronary perfusion but increases the workload of a failing heart.

There has been some difference of opinion as to whether cardiogenic shock is usually accompanied by a decrease in cardiac output with an inadequate peripheral resistance or whether the dominant problem is either a decrease in cardiac output or a decrease in peripheral resistance. Whether expansion of blood volume should be used in the treatment would depend upon the predominant effects of the infarction upon these various parameters. Gammill et al. found a normal cardiac output in the majority of patients. An inverse relationship between stroke volume and peripheral resistance was observed in patients with lowered blood pressure. After four weeks the blood pressure and peripheral resistance were significantly decreased. Myocardial infarction may not be recognized until a patient with long-standing hypertension is found to have a normal blood pressure as in a preoperative physical examination. Venous pressure was observed by Gammill et al. to decrease during the time the patient was in the hospital. They concluded that cardiogenic shock was synonomous with cardiac failure.

On the other hand there may be instances of inadequate sympathetic stimulation even though peripheral resistance is normal and vasopressors are therefore indicated to maintain the blood pressure at a low normal level so as to assure an adequate coronary perfusion. Digitalis has not provided much help in the treatment of patients with acute infarction.

Gunnar et al. compared isoproterenol and norepinephrine infusions and were of the opinion that norepinephrine was the superior drug. The mean arterial blood pressure should be maintained at between 80 and 110 mm of mercury in a patient who has previously had a normal blood pressure. Somewhat higher levels might be needed in a patient who has been hypertensive. Urinary output as an index of renal blood flow is a practical bedside way of monitoring cardiac output in attempting to evaluate the effectiveness of various treatment regimens. Peripheral resistance should not be increased any more than is necessary to sustain a low normal urinary output which in turn suggests that the blood pressure is sufficient so as to sustain a satisfactory coronary perfusion.

For the most seriously infarcted muscle, it has been suggested that a balloon inserted into the aorta and pumped in relation to the cardiac cycle so as to improve cardiac output will take some load away from the injured heart and may be of sufficient temporary assistance to allow the myocardium to recover and subsequently to sustain life when a life would otherwise be lost. Kantrowitz et al. have reviewed some of the early attempts to assist the circulation with mechanical devices.

The usual patient with cardiogenic shock, which is said to occur in about 12% of patients with myocardial infarction, should be treated with a supine or slightly head elevated position but should not be placed in Trendelenburg's position since this interferes with respiration. Chest pain should be relieved with adequate intravenous injections of morphine or Dilaudid. Oxygen at 6 to 8 liters per minute should be given by nasal catheter. Intravenous saline solution with 5% glucose can be given in volumes up to 4 to 5 liters if necessary, provided the central venous pressure remains low. If the central venous pressure rises to 15 cm of water or above, then inotropic drugs should be tried with initial preference given to digitalis. Ouabain has the advantage of a rapid onset in action.

If the central venous pressure is high as a result of overzealous volume expansion and there is concern about, or evidence of, pulmonary edema, it may be helpful to perform a phlebotomy providing this can be accomplished without excessive lowering of the arterial blood pressure. Sinus bradycardia may add to the inefficiency of the heart and should be treated with atropine sulfate, 1 mg given intravenously. Ventricular tachycardia can be treated with lidocaine intravenously, 1 mg/kg as a single dose or 100 to 150 mg/hr given as a continuous intravenous infusion. Norepinephrine should be used with caution so as to maintain the systolic blood pressure at 30 or 40 mm Hg less than the normal level for that individual. It is said that norepinephrine given in small doses has primarily a beta stimulation effect. If norepinephrine is required in higher doses, it is desirable to add phentolamine to the mixture in order to prevent excessive peripheral vasoconstriction. Vasoconstriction increases the work of the heart. Also if a solution of norepinephrine extravasates into the extravascular tissues, the excessive local vasoconstriction will cause a slough of the overlying skin. This can be prevented by mixing phentolamine with the norepinephrine as first described by Zucker et al.

Lillehei et al. have used a combination of norepinephrine and phenoxybenazamine in the treatment of dogs with coronary shock and feel that this may have a place in the treatment of patients, although experience with patients is limited to those individuals who have undergone a cardiopulmonary bypass for more than 4 hours during open heart surgery. In these patients with weakened heart action, there is need for an increase in plasma catecholamines. The phenoxybenzamine is given 24 hours before the operation, and then the norepinephrine can be given at whatever rate is necessary to provide the necessary effect in elevating blood pressure. Lillehei noted that these patients continued to excrete urine at 1 cc/kg/hr during the actual cardiopulmonary bypass. At the end of the bypass the patient could be transfused until the blood pressure was satisfactory, and the patient appeared warm and pink with a wide pulse pressure and low central venous pressure. They noted that in some patients cardiac failure and shock developed 24 to 36 hours following the operation at a time when the effect of the phenoxybenzamine was wearing off. Such patients improved again when additional phenoxybenzamine was given.

It should be obvious in view of the many changes which occur during the management of shock that equally important with the various drugs and modalities of treatment is the close observation by professional intensive care nurses who have been trained in monitoring vital signs in these patients. They are also trained to handle defibrillation and administer resuscitation when necessary.

Patients with septic shock have shown a wide range of cardiac output. Some are classified as hypodynamic and others hyperdynamic. Apparently in some of these patients there is benefit from increasing cardiac output by expanding blood volume or by boosting the cardiac function to a more efficient curve. The primary defect in septic shock is probably not cardiac but interference with utilization of oxygen peripherally. Kho and Shoemaker observed that increasing the cardiac output by the administration of blood or dextran 40 increased oxygen consumption in traumatic and hemorrhagic shock but failed to increase oxygen consumption in septic shock. This would suggest that the defect in septic shock may be interference with gas exchange peripherally and that the need for an increased cardiac output is to compensate for this peripheral interference with gas exchange or utilization.

VASOMOTION

The response to prolonged blood loss is a progressive increase in peripheral resistance. Such a response helps to sustain blood pressure and continued perfusion of the cerebral and coronary arteries, even at the expense of blood flow through skin, kidneys, and other areas that are of less immediate importance to continued survival. If such peripheral vasospasm continues after blood volume and cardiac output have been restored, there may be injury to the kidney. The use of an alpha-blocking drug is therefore to be considered in restoring perfusion of the kidney when it is known that blood volume has been restored. The response to phentolamine or alpha-receptor blockade should be a widening of pulse pressure, improved skin color and warmth of skin, increased urine flow, and a sustained systolic blood pressure. If both systolic and diastolic pressure fall, the patient needs more blood or extracellular fluids or an increased plasma volume.

Whereas increased peripheral resistance is the usual pattern in shock, there are patients, particularly with septic shock, in whom the peripheral resistance is lower than normal. This is also a characteristic of patients with severe liver disease. There may be an increased requirement for blood flow in inflamed tissues or as a result of bacterial toxins where there is interference with oxygen release, possibly on the basis of an inadequate concentration of red blood cell 2,3-diphosphoglycerate. At the same time that peripheral resistance is decreased and oxygen delivery impaired, bacterial toxins may have a deleterious effect on the myocardium so that cardiac output is insufficiently increased to meet the larger peripheral circulatory demand. Improvement may therefore result from increasing venous return by expanding blood volume or extracellular fluid volume. Frequently, however, the administration of these fluids causes a rise in venous pressure because the heart is already functioning on the flat portion of an abnormal function curve. It may be possible to boost the heart to a more efficient function curve by the administration of digitalis. Isoproterenol has been used but has the disadvantage of causing peripheral vasodilatation.

It is attractive to classify septic shock as simply a problem in vasomotion, but it also involves other factors and, as in the other types of shock, there are times in the course of the treatment when a patient may need agonists and other times when antagonists are required. There are times when the patient may need inotropic support and other times when expansion of blood volume is more effective. Septic shock includes many possibilities, and it is necessary not only to evaluate each patient but to evaluate each patient repeatedly in the course of his illness.

Siegel (1968) published convincing evidence that patients with severe liver disease and patients with septic shock have a decrease in peripheral resistance and a failure to adequately increase cardiac output. Miller et al. have observed in addition that the red blood cell 2,3-diphosphoglycerate concentration is increased to above normal levels in patients with severe liver disease whereas others have found that 2,3-DPG is below normal concentration in the red blood cells of patients with septic shock.

The death or survival of patients with septic shock is in large part related to the underlying disease and whether the cause of the sepsis can be corrected. Abscesses must be drained, and antibiotics effective against the organisms causing the shock must be administered. Since the patient may succumb before sensitivity studies are completed, a broad-spectrum antibiotic should be selected and treatment begun as soon as the diagnosis is made.

TREATMENT AND PREVENTION OF COMPLICATIONS

Early and appropriate treatment is so intertwined with recognition and understanding of pathophysiology that it has been discussed in what has been presented (Fig. 9-6). Obviously if treatment is delayed and inappropriate, complications will develop or the patient will fail to respond. There are two major complications of shock that have received a great deal of attention: acute renal failure and respiratory distress syndrome. Acute renal failure has been under study for many years and is discussed in Chapter 10. Respiratory distress syndrome has become a subject of major attention recently, although it is not a new problem. There are those who would discuss respiratory distress syndrome as a complication of overzealous use of crystalloid solutions and, as noted in Chapter 3, when the syndrome is present it is aggravated by fluid overload.

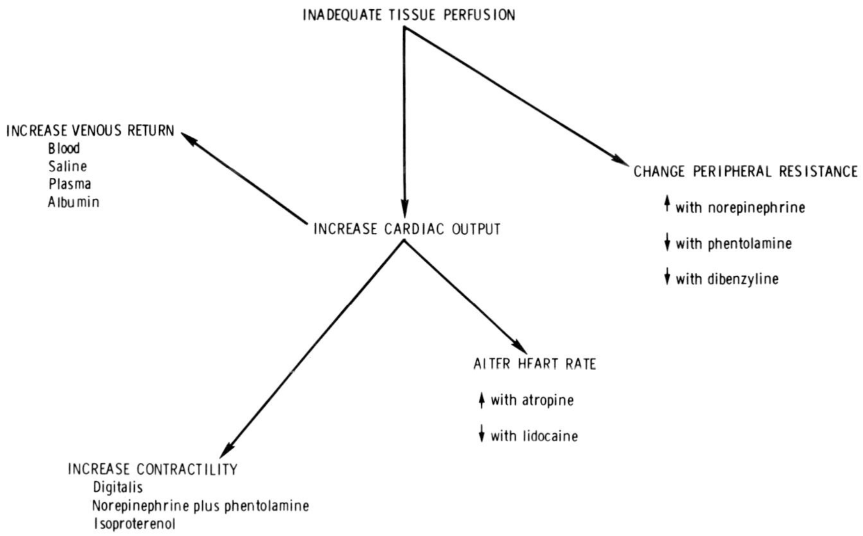

Figure 9-6. Treatment is based upon the type of physiologic disturbances that are present, as was indicated in Figure 9-1.

The mechanism of injury is only partially understood. For a detailed review of what is currently known, the historical review of Simeone and other papers published with it should be consulted. The lungs are injured during shock by the flow of blood through the lung. There is an increase in permeability of the endothelium such that the plasma proteins leak into the interstitial space. Blebs form separating the endothelium from the basement membrane, and these rupture exposing the basement membrane. Platelets adhere and thromboses occur. At the same time there is injury to the type II alveolar cells which produce surfactant. Use of excessive concentrations of oxygen adds to the injury of alveolar membranes. Particulate material from wounds and from inadequately filtered blood contributes to the plugging of the pulmonary vessels. Excessive intravenous fluid, especially if venous pressure is raised, contributes to the pulmonary edema though it is not the basic cause.

These changes are prevented by early and adequate resuscitation even when large volumes of saline are used as a part of the resuscitation. They are prevented or minimized by limiting the oxygen concentration to that which will provide an arterial Po_2 of 85 to 90 torr and by reducing the time when oxygen in excess of 40% is used. They are prevented by keeping the pressure in the pulmonary vessels at a normal level, by avoiding a too rapid administration of fluids and occasionally by reducing systemic peripheral vascular resistance. Patients with head injuries who develop cerebral edema have a rise in pulmonary pressure which may not be preventable unless the cerebral circulation is improved.

Shock produces changes in blood which reduce flow through small vessels. This has been studied from many viewpoints over the years but has come to attention again through the work of Swank, who has studied the effect upon flow through the brain and lung. Hemorrhage causes an increase in platelet adhesiveness, which in turn causes an increase in the pressure required to filter blood through a fine screen, screen filtration pressure (SFP). Platelet aggregates are filtered out in the lung and cause an increase in pulmonary artery pressure and impaired gas exchange. The treatment of shock requires blood transfusions, and stored blood also develops microaggregates which, if infused, add to the obstruction of pulmonary blood flow. Mosley and Doty demonstrated that filters which have been used in blood transfusion sets are not effective in removing all of such material, and if one filter is used for repeated transfusions more and more of the aggregated material escapes filtration. The use of Dacron wool filters designed by Swank for blood transfusions may reduce the incidence and severity of the acute respiratory syndrome in patients treated for shock.

The most effective treatment of the respiratory distress syndrome is the use of *continuous positive pressure breathing* (CPPB), as described by Petty and Ashbaugh. Such treatment requires that the patient have a normal blood volume and adequate venous return since the increased intrathoracic pressure impedes venous return. This is advantageous in fluid overload. The expansion of alveoli from CPPB corrects the atelectasis and may be needed for 4 to 5 days until regeneration of type II cells of Macklin again provides sufficient surfactant. Along with this if there is fluid overload, the use of diuretics will speed recovery of normal pulmonary function. If renal failure prevents the use of diuretics, then ultrafiltration by dialysis is another way to remove excess body fluid.

RECAPITULATION

Shock is a state of abnormal circulation brought about by one or more causes and influenced in time by a complex response. Optimum management requires early correction of the cause, careful monitoring of vital signs, and appropriate modifications in treatment to fit the current physiologic defect. With or without frequent direct measurements of cardiac output, central venous pressure, and blood gas determinations, the surgeon should think about his patient in terms of disturbed physiology. The main questions relate to whether replacement with blood and saline will restore cardiac output, central venous pressure, and peripheral perfusion. Myocardial infarction and sepsis both cause shock which is likely to be primarily due to abnormal myocardial function in the first instance and abnormal perfusion and peripheral exchange in the second. All manner of mixture of physiologic abnormalities may occur at some stage of shock in any patient, so that observation, analysis, and treatment must follow in an unending recurring cycle until the patient recovers.

Siegel (1972) presented a large amount of data in a manner that facilitates thinking about the physiologic derangements which exist in cardiogenic shock and during various stages of septic shock (Fig. 9-7). In this circular diagram eleven variables are shown as radii of a circle. A normal group is depicted as a circle and increases or decreases from normal are depicted in standard deviations from normal along each radius. Typical examples are shown of cardiac as contrasted with varying degrees of decompensation in septic shock. A patient with cardiogenic shock has a decrease in cardiac output and an increase in arterial-venous oxygen difference. The pump is weak, but peripheral utilization of oxygen remains as normal as the perfusion will allow. Venous P_{CO_2} and pH remain normal. In septic shock the example shows an initial increase in cardiac output, and even in the decompensated state cardiac output remains normal. In spite of a strong pump, there is a 2 standard-deviation decrease in arterial-venous oxygen difference until decompensation, suggesting that the tissues are not well perfused. However, when decompensation occurs, there is then an increase in oxygen extraction with a normal venous P_{O_2} but a washout of areas previously poorly perfused, with release of carbonic and lactic acid so that venous P_{CO_2} is 3 standard deviations above normal and venous pH is 4 standard deviations below normal.

How would such a diagram appear for a typical patient with hemorrhagic shock? Early in the course it would simulate cardiogenic shock, because the basic problem is that the heart does not receive enough blood to maintain an adequate cardiac

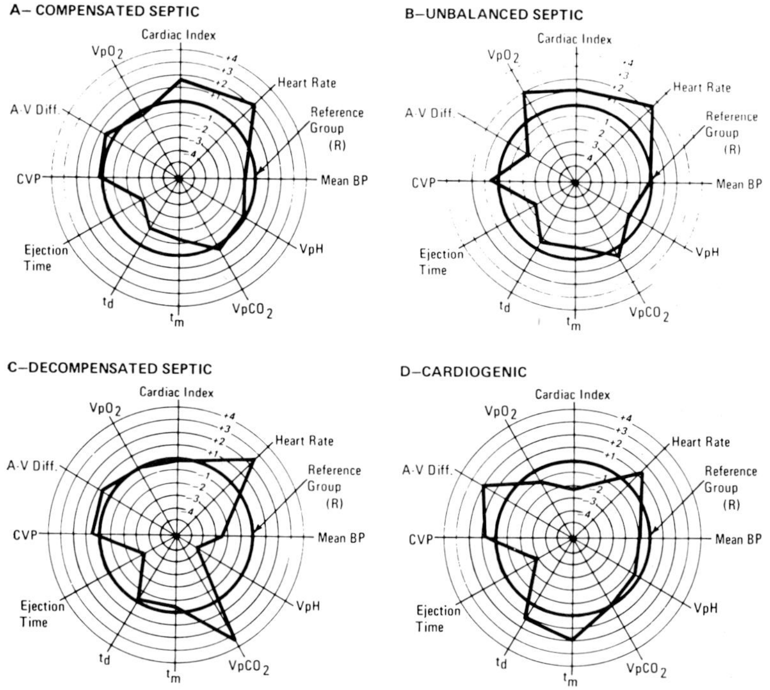

Figure 9-7. Patterns in multiple variables in three stages of septic shock contrasted with cardiogenic shock. (From Siegel, J. H., Farrell, E. J., Goldwyn, R. M., and Friedman, H. P.: The surgical implications of physiologic patterns in myocardial infarction shock. Surgery *72*:126, 1972.)

output. Later as peripheral tissues are injured, the distortion would probably simulate decompensated septic shock. These are the parameters in which a clinician should think even though he may not obtain the sophisticated and profuse amount of data available in some of these studies. Measurement of depicted variables permits use of computer analysis, but unavailability of such facilities does not detract from a logical approach to treatment of shock based upon physiologic principles.

REFERENCES

Carey, L. C., Lowery, B. D., and Cloutier, C. T.: Hemorrhagic shock. Curr. Prob. Surg. January, 1971.

Cohn, J. N., and Luria, M. H.: Studies in clinical shock and hypotension. J.A.M.A. *190*:891, 1964.

Fulton, R. L.: Absorption of sodium and water by collagen during hemorrhagic shock. Ann. Surg. *172*:861, 1970.

Gammill, J. F., Applegarth, J. J., Reed, C. E., Fernald, J. D., and Antenucci, A. J.: Hemodynamic changes following acute myocardial infarction using the dye injection method for cardiac output determination. Ann. Intern. Med. *43*:100, 1955.

Gauer, O. H., and Henry, J. P.: Circulatory basis of fluid volume control. Physiol. Rev. *43*:423, 1963.

Gauer, O. H., Henry, J. P., and Behn, C.: The regulation of extracellular fluid volume. Ann. Rev. Physiol. *32*:547, 1970.

Grayson, T. L., White, J. E., and Moyer, C. A.: Oxygen consumption: concentrations of inorganic ions in urine, serum and duodenal fluid, hematocrit, urinary excretion, pulse rates and blood pressure during duodenal depletion of sodium salts in normal and alcoholic man. Ann. Surg. *158*:840, 1963.

Gunnar, R. M., Loeb, H. S., Pietras, R. J., and Tobias, J. R.: Ineffectiveness of isoproterenol in shock due to acute myocardial infarction. J.A.M.A. *202*:1124, 1967.

Huizenga, K. A., Brofman, B. L., and Wiggers, C. J.: The ineffectiveness of adrenal cortex extracts in standardized hemorrhagic shock. J. Pharmacol. Exper. Therap. *78*:139, 1943.

Kantrowitz, A., Tjonneland, S., Freed, P. S., Phillips, S. J., Butner, A. N., and Sherman, J. L.: Clinical experience with intraaortic balloon pumping in cardiogenic shock. J.A.M.A. *203*:113, 1968.

Kho, L. K., and Shoemaker, W. C.: Evaluation of therapy in clinical shock by cardiorespiratory measurements. Surg. Gynec. Obstet. *127*:81, 1968.

Knisely, M. H., Eliot, T. S., and Block, E. H.: Sludged blood in traumatic shock. I. Microscopic observations of the precipitations and agglutination of blood flowing through vessels in crushed tissues. Arch. Surg. (Chicago) *51*:220, 1945.

Lewin, I., Lerner, A. G., Green, S. H., Del Guercio, L. R. M., and Siegel, J. H.: Physical class and physiologic status in the prediction of operative mortality in the aged sick. Ann. Surg. *174*:217, 1971.

Lillehei, R. C., Longerbeam, J. K., Bloch, J. H., and Manax, W. G.: The nature of irreversible shock. Ann. Surg. *160*:682, 1964.

Miller, L. D., Oski, F. A., Diaco, J. F., Siegerman, H. J., Gottlieb, A. J., Davidson, D., and Delivoria-Papadopoulos, M.: The affinity of hemoglobin for oxygen: its control and in vivo significance. Surgery *68*:187, 1970.

Mosley, R. V., and Doty, D. B.: Changes in the filtration characteristics of stored blood. Ann. Surg. *171*:329, 1970.

Moss, G. S.: An argument in favor of electrolyte solution for early resuscitation. Surg. Clin. N. Amer. *52*:3, 1972.

Parker, P. E., Dobbins, D. E., Weidner, W. J., Haddy, F. J., and Grega, G. J.: Effects of hemorrhagic, endotoxic and catecholamine shocks on canine gracilis muscle vasculature. Biol. Med. *138*:971, 1971.

Petty, T. L., and Ashbaugh, D. G.: The adult respiratory distress syndrome. Chest *60*:233, 1971.

Siegel, J. H., Farrell, E. J., Goldwyn, R. M., and Friedman, H. P.: The surgical implications of physiologic patterns in myocardial infarction shock. Surgery *72*:126, 1972.

Siegel, J. H., Greenspan, M., Cohn, J. D., and Del Guercio, L. R. M.: The prognostic implications of physiologic abnormalities in operation for portal hypertension. Surg. Gynec. Obstet. *126*:249, 1968.

Simeone, F. A.: Pulmonary complications of nonthoracic wounds: a historical perspective. J. Trauma *8*:625, 1968.

Swank, R. L.: Platelet aggregation: its role and cause in surgical shock. J. Trauma *8*:872, 1968.

Wiggers, C. J., and Werle, J. M.: Exploration of a method for standardizing hemorrhagic shock. Proc. Soc. Exp. Biol. Med. *49*:604, 1942.

Wilson, R. F.: Sarver, E., and Birks, R.: Central venous pressure and blood volume determinations in clinical shock. Surg. Gynec. Obstet. *132*:631, 1971.

Zucker, G., Eisinger, R. P., Flock, M. H., and Singer, M. M.: Treatment of shock and prevention of ischemic necrosis with levarterenol-phentolamine mixtures. Circulation *22*:935, 1960.

Chapter

10

Acute Renal Failure

PATHOPHYSIOLOGY OF ACUTE RENAL FAILURE

"Acute renal failure" can be defined as a sudden inability of the kidney to excrete the daily solute load. Renal failure might be classified as either prerenal, renal, or postrenal (Fig. 10-1). Prerenal failure is exemplified by poor circulation such as might occur in heart failure. Postrenal failure exists when the ureters are blocked. Renal failure represents a disease involving the nephron and can be divided into circulatory, toxic, and obstructive types. The circulatory insufficiency involves a decrease in glomerular filtration whereas the toxic form implies injury to the tubule. Obstructive changes causing renal failure might be illustrated by blockage of the lower parts of the nephron with casts of hemoglobin or with casts formed from urate crystals as in the patient with leukemia who is treated with an effective chemotherapeutic agent to the extent of releasing large quantities of uric acid (Fig. 10-2).

There are also various stages of classic acute renal failure: the situation immediately before injury or predisposing to the injury, the period during which the damage occurs, an oliguric period during which the urine volume is less than 500 ml per day, and a period of diuresis and recovery (Table 10-1). Oliguria lasts from a few days to as long as 3 weeks and is followed by the diuretic phase which lasts usually about as long as the oliguric phase and consists of a period when the volume of urine is excessive but the quality of the urine is not greatly different from the composition of plasma. It is only toward the end of the diuretic phase that the blood urea nitrogen begins to return toward a normal level. Finally the recovery or late stage extends for several months during which time there is gradual improvement in renal function usually with return to normal function. There may not be an oliguric phase if the osmolarity of the plasma is high as is commonly the case in the patient with an extensive body surface burn. Patients treated with osmotic diuretics may not develop an oliguric phase but may still develop

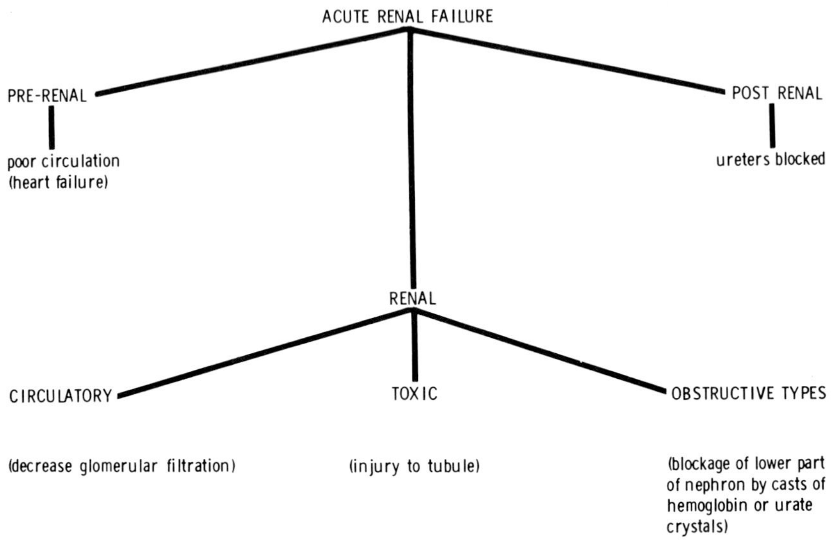

Figure 10-1. Calls attention to some of the considerations of differential diagnosis in acute renal failure.

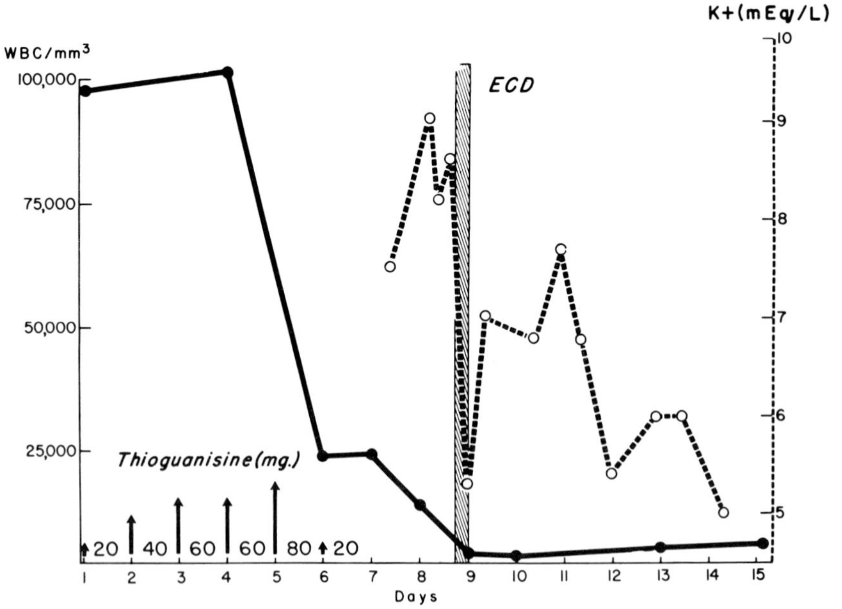

Figure 10-2. Shows the result of a too rapid lysis of abnormal lymphocytes in a 12-year-old boy treated with thioguanisine for leukemia. Uric acid precipitates temporarily obstructed the tubules so that acute renal failure coincided with a rapid rise in serum potassium. One treatment with hemodialysis prevented death from hyperkalemia and removed enough uric acid so that renal function returned. (From Hockmuth, R. E., Faber, L. C., and Mason, E. E.: Extracorporeal dialysis in renal failure. J. Iowa Med. Soc. 52:199, 1962.)

TABLE 10-1. STAGES OF CLASSIC RENAL FAILURE

	DISCOVERY	OLIGURIC	DIURETIC	RECOVERY
Duration	Extremely variable	Few days to 3 weeks	Equal to oliguric	Several months
Urine vol.	Usually decreasing	Below 500 ml/day	In excess of 1 liter/day	Normal
Characteristic	Conditions that cause: 1. Volume deficits: TBW, ECF, blood, plasma 2. Vasospasm a. Pitressin b. Epinephrine c. Norepinephrine 3. Toxicity a. Hemoglobin or myoglobin b. Antibiotic toxicity c. Iodinated contrast media d. Hypercalcemia 4. Obstruction a. Pigment b. Uric acid 5. Cirrhosis or jaundice 6. Localized Schwartzman reaction a. Sensitization by: 1) Bacterial products (or) 2) Pregnancy (or) 3) Cortisone (and then) b. Reaction to bacterial products	May be absent if: 1. High osmolality of plasma as in burn patients 2. Treatment with osmotic diuretics	1. Urine quality similar to plasma 2. BUN returns towards normal beginning after the first few days 3. Severity of diuresis is related to the degree of over hydration present when diuresis begins	1. Gradual improvement to normal in majority 2. Some patients do not recover normal renal clearance 3. A few patients remain azotemic

acute renal failure with an inability to excrete the daily solute load and with a rising blood urea nitrogen.

There are also variations in the severity of the morphologic lesions observed in patients dying at various stages of acute renal failure. There are many instances in which no morphologic injury can be found by light microscopy even though the functional disturbance is as severe as in other patients who have extensive histologic changes. There are patients in whom tubular lesions can be found, so-called tubulolysis (dissolution of cells lining the tubule) and tubulorrhexis (breaks in the basement membrane). The most severe lesions are renal cortical necrosis. Knowledge of these variations in the clinical course and the pathological changes of acute renal failure is the basis for understanding its development and the various forms of treatment designed to stop the development or to limit the extent of damage.

Dehydration is commonly present both in patients and in experimental situations where acute renal failure develops. It is more difficult to produce acute renal failure if the animal is well hydrated and undergoing a brisk diuresis. Depletion of extracellular fluid volume, loss of plasma volume, and dehydration seem to be a part of the clinical and experimental situation in which acute renal failure develops. Various agents which produce vasospasm also seem to be commonly present in the situations in which acute renal failure develops; among these are pitressin, bacterial toxins, epinephrine, and norepinephrine. In the pregnant animal or the cortisone-treated animal the introduction of Adrenalin may precipitate acute renal failure.

Patients who have bled and whose blood volume has not been restored when they are subjected to major operative trauma are more likely to develop renal failure. Patients with cirrhosis, especially those with ascites, and patients who are severely jaundiced are predisposed to renal failure; under these circumstances the term *hepatorenal syndrome* has been applied. Dawson has demonstrated a decrease in creatinine clearance following operations in patients who are jaundiced. Mason et al. found that patients who were jaundiced had a decreased concentration of urine sodium, increased urine potassium, and an elevated leucine aminopeptidase level in the urine similar to the pattern of nonjaundiced patients who are subjected to operative trauma. When the jaundiced patients were then subjected to an operation, they had a further increase in urinary leucine aminopeptidase (Fig. 10-3) and a further decrease in urinary sodium and increase in urinary potassium suggesting that the operative trauma and the jaundice were additive in their effects upon the kidney. The etiology of these changes is probably renal ischemia.

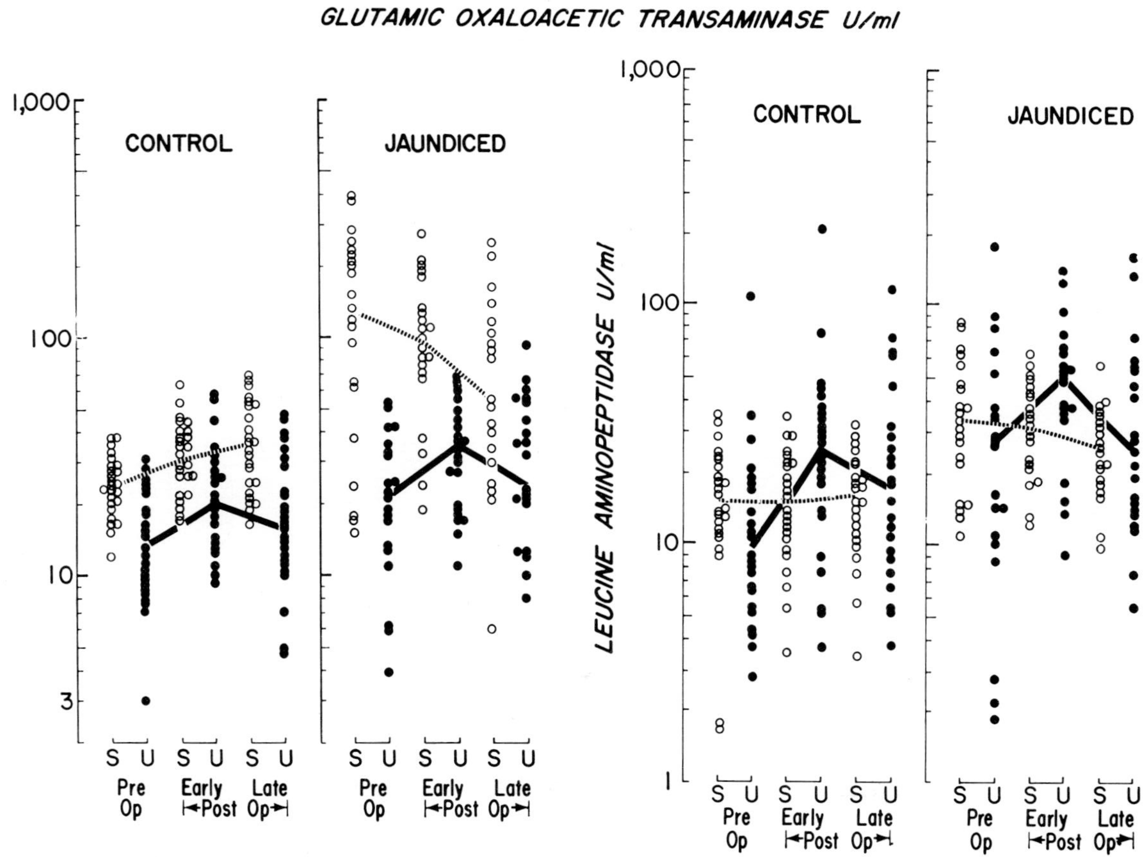

Figure 10-3. Shows the effects of operative trauma in jaundiced and nonjaundiced patients upon serum (S) and urine (U) glutamic oxaloacetic transaminase and leucine aminopeptidase. (From Mason, E. E., Chernigoy, G. A., Gulesserian, H. P., and Tectar, A. J.: Enzymuria in icteric surgical patients. Surg. Gynec. Obstet. *122:* 333, 1966.)

An ischemic episode is a common antecedent of acute renal failure. If the ischemia lasts for a sufficient length of time, there may be acute tubular necrosis, but acute renal failure can occur without tubular necrosis. The necrosis results from the ischemia, and the renal failure is also a consequence of impaired circulation rather than a consequence of the necrosis. Sheehan and Moore examined specimens from patients dying at varying times during the course of renal failure and came to the conclusion that there must have been a series of episodes of vasospasm with resumption of perfusion in between these episodes, but with progressive damage over time. Most of what we know about renal failure has been learned from observations made after the failure has developed.

Delay in treatment of the patient increases the incidence of acute renal failure. Among those with major wounds in the Korean War the incidence was 1 in 200 whereas during the Vietnam War it was 1 in 400. This was in spite of the fact that the ratio of wounded to killed was 3 to 1 in Korea and 6 to 1 in Vietnam. In other words more severly wounded men were reaching the hospital but the incidence of renal failure was less. The difference is probably related to 3½ hours between injury and hospitalization in the Korean War as compared with an average delay of only 40 minutes in Vietnam. The sequence of events from injury to acute renal failure can be interrupted by early restoration of circulation and treatment of injuries.

The kidneys normally receive about 20% of the cardiac output and have a blood flow in the range of 500 ml per hundred grams of kidney per minute. There is an obvious advantage in evolution for survival of the species by having a mechanism which can temporarily divert this volume of blood flow from the kidney to other organs such as the brain and heart. After renal failure is established the measured renal blood flow ranges between 60 and 260 ml per hundred grams of kidney per minute or in the range of 30% of normal renal blood flow. The glomerular filtration, however, is decreased to a greater extent than renal blood flow.

Any morphologic changes which are observed are now generally considered to represent the effects of ischemia and the effects of the cause of acute renal failure rather than being in themselves the cause. Oliver et al. dissected out individual nephrons in dilute hydrochloric acid and described the two main types of lesions observed: lysis of cells and breaks in the basement membrane. This disruption of the lining of the tubule was used as an explanation for oliguria. It was postulated that glomerular filtration continued, but there was massive passive diffusion of filtrate back through the tubule wall so that no urine reached the collecting system. This was an explanation for the period of oliguria. Then, as the cells began to grow out over the wall of the tubule and re-establish a complete lining, the period of diuresis began. As the tubules thickened and developed their subcellular structure and became capable of performing osmotic and chemical work, the diuretic phase ceased and normal renal function was re-established.

Such a theory did not explain the many instances commented upon by Brun and Munck in which there was an impressive contrast between the very limited structural change and the complete functional breakdown. Balint et al. measured oxygen consumption in the kidney and found that it was closely related to filtration rate and therefore to reabsorption of sodium. This indicated that the sodium which was filtered and then reabsorbed was reabsorbed by an active energy-consuming process and was not a passive flow as might occur through a disrupted tubular lining. In experimental animals given intramuscular glycerin, which causes hemolysis and loss of extracellular fluid into the site of injection, micropuncture studies indicated that glomerular filtration was decreased by 40%. This would result in a decreased amount of filtrate in the upper part of the nephron and would not support the theory of continued normal filtration and increased passive proximal tubule flow back into the blood.

Currently, one of the more attractive explanations for acute renal failure involves a temporary inappropriate overactivity of the juxtaglomerular apparatus. Normally this apparatus regulates renal blood flow at a constant rate in the face of variations in blood pressure from 80 to around 200 mm Hg. Renin is produced in the juxtaglomerular cells and converts angiotensin I into angiotensin II, which in turn causes a contraction of vascular smooth muscle. The highest concentration of renin in the kidney is in the afferent arterioles of glomeruli located in the cortex of the kidney. These glomeruli are responsible for the regulation of glomerular filtration. Glomeruli closer to the medulla of the kidney do not have a juxtaglomerular apparatus. The conditions which seem to predispose to acute renal failure are also the conditions in which an elevation of renin has been found. Acute renal failure patients also have plasma renin levels that are highest early after the onset and gradually decrease as the patient has an improvement in renal function. Dehydration, contraction of extracellular fluid volume, and hemorrhage all cause an elevation of plasma renin. Skillman et al. found that the release of aldosterone and consequent retention of sodium, which are so characteristic of hemorrhage and operative procedures, are mediated in large part by the renin-angiotensin-aldosterone system. The suggestion that renin might play an important part in the genesis of acute renal failure was made by Goormaghtigh who observed that "in no other pathological condition yet examined is the hypertrophy and granularity of the fibrillar constituent of the juxtaglomerular apparatus so marked." J. J. Brown et al. in 1970 reviewed the many observations which tend to support this hypothesis.

This theory would place the obstruction to nephron fluid flow in the arterioles just proximal to those glomeruli located in the cortex. This would explain why the milder lesions are found only in the cortex and why, in the most severe instances of acute renal failure, necrosis is located in the cortex. It would explain a decrease in tubular flow and how debris and pigment which happened to be circulating would be concentrated in the distal nephron as glomerular filtration decreased. The formation of casts, like the tubular lesions, would be a consequence of obstruction proximal to the glomerulus rather than a cause of renal failure. Hemorrhage causes a tenfold increase in antidiuretic hormone (ADH) levels, and an increase in tonicity of body fluids produced by infusing hypertonic saline interacts with hemorrhage to produce an even higher level of ADH according to Saito and Yoshida. ADH causes smooth muscle contraction in vessels. There is also a sympathetic nerve discharge after hemorrhage and these nerves end in the region of the afferent artery of cortical glomeruli which may add to the renal vasospasm.

Hollenberg et al. studied patients with acute renal failure in a variety of clinical situations by arteriography and found the cortex was poorly perfused. Xenon washout studies following intra-arterial injection showed an absence of the early fast component which is characteristic of flow in the cortex. Epinephrine will cause a similar decrease in glomerular filtration in the outer renal cortex. There are a number of mechanisms whereby such a change in distribution of renal blood flow might occur, and probably several of these contribute to the production of acute renal failure. Probably the elevation of renin and angiotensin in renal failure is more of a sign of renal cortical ischemia than a part of the cause of ischemia. Since the action of renin on angiotensin occurs in the lung, any effect of angiotensin upon renal blood flow would be part of a systemic effect and not a localized renal effect.

Such a theory does not exclude toxic and obstructive factors. Following a hemolytic transfusion reaction or following the release of myoglobin from a crushed extremity, the circulatory effects would be accompanied by the toxic effects of pigments concentrated in the tubule. As the glomerular filtration is resumed, there could well be obstruction in the lower nephron with dilatation of the convoluted tubule and flattening of the epithelium.

Rather than explaining renal failure on the basis of damage to a part of the nephron, it seems more likely that whole nephrons are temporarily or permanently defunctionalized and that any urine which is formed at any stage of the disease comes from nephrons which are still functional. If there are only a small number of these nephrons working, they would be subjected to an osmotic diuresis. This could explain the composition of the urine as being similar to plasma in some instances. There are patients with acute renal failure in whom the urine has a rather low concentration of sodium, suggesting efficient reabsorption of sodium in the tubules. This is rather characteristic of patients with extensive burns who develop renal failure.

RECOGNITION, DIAGNOSIS, AND PROGNOSIS

Acute renal failure is usually diagnosed when the urine volume decreases, the patient is unable to excrete his solute load, the blood urea nitrogen is rising, and the patient does not respond to treatment designed to improve the rate of urine formation and the efficiency of solute excretion. Knowledge of the circumstances in which acute renal failure occurs will lead to measures to prevent its occurrence or to early recognition of renal failure when it does appear. A decrease in urinary output is the most easily recognized indication of inadequate renal function and should cause a search for possible prerenal or postrenal cause. The circulation may be inadequate for perfusion of the kidneys. There may be obstruction to the urinary catheter or to ureters. A sudden complete cessation of urine in a patient whose urinary output has been normal should lead to a suspicion of some obstruction outside of the kidney such as embolism to the renal arteries, in which case the patient will usually have severe pain in the flank and abdomen, gross hematuria, and ileus.

High-dose intravenous pyelograms may be helpful even in the patient with oliguria or anuria. C. B. Brown et al. have used pyelograms plus tomography, taking repeated roentgenograms until they have seen a nephrogram or even a pyelogram. In spite of the formation of very little urine, given sufficient time enough of the contrast medium will reach the collecting system to allow visualization of the kidney and to provide valuable information as to the patency of the external collecting system as well as providing information about the size and contour of the kidneys.

Sometimes what appears to be acute renal failure in a patient with supposedly normal kidneys is actually failure superimposed upon chronic renal insufficiency and the kidneys are small, scarred, or atrophic. If large, smooth, nonobstructed kidneys are visualized and the cause of renal failure is not apparent, it may be desirable to perform a biopsy. A retrograde pyelogram could be performed, but this carries the added risk of infection in a situation in which antibiotics and high urinary flow rates cannot be efficiently used in the treatment of urinary tract infection.

Renal failure without decrease in urine volume is less easily detected and has given rise to a number of functional criteria to identify renal failure, such as a ratio of urine urea to plasma urea of less than ten or a decrease in creatinine clearance to less than 20 ml per minute. The urine sediment should be examined for casts. The concentration of sodium in the urine is not a very reliable indication of failure since the concentration of urinary sodium is related to sodium intake. A patient who is taking excessive amounts of sodium may have a urinary sodium as high as the plasma sodium concentration even with normal renal function.

The work of the kidneys is to excrete a daily load of solute, most of which is urea. This is normally accomplished simultaneously with a regulation of water excretion so that for any given solute load there is an inverse relationship between the concentration and volume of the urine. If a patient with decreasing urine volume does not have an increasing urine concentration, this should raise suspicion that the kidneys are failing. At any time that the blood urea nitrogen and creatinine are rising, this is an indication that the kidneys are not performing their task, and if the patient is adequately hydrated and there is no remaining extrarenal cause of azotemia, acute renal failure is likely. When the diagnosis is made early and there is no response to either expansion of extracellular fluid or hydration of the patient or administration of mannitol or furosemide, then this failure of response to treatment confirms the diagnosis and should lead to restriction of intake of fluids, protein, and potassium and the usual management of established acute renal failure.

The prognosis cannot be determined from the early course of acute renal failure. Alwall treated patients from all over Sweden who were brought to Lund with renal failure and was unable to predict which patients would recover. He did observe that in patients with a marked and progressive decrease in size of the renal outline, the prognosis was poor because of renal cortical necrosis. Hager et al. have selected patients from their experience who illustrate the broad spectrum of the disease. One patient with hepatorenal syndrome was anuric for 37 days and subsequently recovered completely. Another patient with acute renal failure whose biopsy showed minimal anatomic damage finally died of anuria 2 years after the initial onset. A patient with rising BUN and high urinary output does not necessarily have mild damage. A patient who has had an episode of renal failure and is recovering is not protected from a second episode, should circulatory insufficiency or some other insult supervene.

PREVENTION AND EARLY TREATMENT

Diuresis in a well-hydrated patient and in the experimental animal protects from renal failure during anesthesia and operative trauma and during episodes of myoglobinuria, hemoglobinuria, and release of various vasoactive substances known to predispose to renal failure. The diuresis should result from being well hydrated. In this way renin will be suppressed. A patient who has been allowed no fluids by mouth overnight should be given an intravenous infusion of lactated Ringer's in 5% glucose beginning before the anesthesia. Several liters of this solution can be administered during the early portion of a major operation provided the patient's circulatory reserve is normal as evidenced by a normal central venous pressure. Barry et al. observed that there was a decrease in renal plasma flow, glomerular filtration rate, and urine flow in patients anesthetized after having had a restriction in their fluid intake, whereas patients who were well hydrated had a decrease in renal blood flow only if the anesthetic agent had been administered at high concentrations. The only risk of the administration of salt-containing solutions during major operative procedures is the risk of fluid overload. If urinary ouptut decreases, and the patient seems to be retaining excessive amounts of fluid, then mannitol or furosemide should be given. The sequence of treatment is to provide adequate hydration and extracellular fluid volume and then to resort to diuretic agents, rather than to give diuretic agents to a patient who might be in need of expansion of his extracellular fluid or total body water.

It is true that the traumatized patient has increased levels of antidiuretic hormone and aldosterone and has difficulty in excreting salt and water, but with the diuretic agents now available it is more logical to keep the patient well hydrated and to give diuretic agents as needed than to withhold salt and fluids on the thesis that they are not well tolerated. We are in the habit of managing the fluid balance by replacing those fluids lost from nasogastric suction and other sites, but to look upon the kidneys as having some innate ability to govern their own function. In the context of anesthesia and major operative procedures, renal function also needs to be managed. During the early postoperative days the surgeon should take charge of water and salt balance, keep the patient well hydrated, and keep the flow of urine at a rate that will minimize the chance of renal failure. This will simplify management of the patient's fluid, electrolyte, and nutritional needs. It is much easier to order the necessary fluids, electrolytes, calories, and amino acids in a patient who has a high urinary output than in a patient who is oliguric. Normally the kidneys are balancing organs, and examination of the urine serves to indicate what the homeostatic mechanisms are designed to do to maintain a normal composition of body fluids, but in the early postoperative period and certainly after major trauma, the kidneys may need diuretic medication to maintain normal body composition and to preserve renal function.

There are instances when hydration cannot be established before anesthesia and trauma. The longer the period of oliguria before hydration and normal circulation is re-established, the more difficult it may be to restore renal function. The early use of lactated Ringer's in resuscitation from hemorrhage and trauma is the first step in establishing adequate urinary flow. As soon as circulation seems to be satisfactory, if urine flow is still inadequate, then the patient should be treated with mannitol.

It is difficult to find any good evidence that mannitol does, in fact, prevent renal failure in patients who are otherwise well hydrated and have normal circulation. Berne and Barbour reviewed patients with postoperative acute renal failure and in the 10 who developed oliguria in their hospital all had received lactated Ringer's and either furosemide, ethacrynic acid, or mannitol without an effective response. Brun and Munck in 1957 commented upon the frequent hydropic changes in the kidneys which they attributed to the frequent use of low molecular dextran, sucrose, and sulfate in attempts at re-establishing urine flow in patients developing acute renal failure. Acute renal failure is infrequent, and many patients with oliguria respond to diuretics. One seldom knows whether acute renal failure has been averted by diuretic administration. Dawson has shown that the fall in creatinine clearance which is noticed in jaundiced patients postoperatively can be prevented by administering mannitol during the operative and early postoperative period.

Review of the records of patients who have developed acute renal failure often suggests that preventive measures were not instituted early enough and were not accompanied by adequate replacement of extracellular fluid. In other patients with multiple injuries and abdominal operations where many units of blood are administered and in whom 3 or 4 liters of lactated Ringer's solution are administered in addition to the blood replacement and in some in whom mannitol is given, the renal function continues in a normal fashion or shows very mild insufficiency with mild and transient elevation of blood urea nitrogen. Although there is no definite proof that mannitol or furosemide has helped, it seems probable that they have been effective in some instances in preventing renal failure.

Montoreano and others gave furosemide to patients with elevated blood renin levels and observed a decrease in renin concentration. All patients with acute renal failure who have been examined have had a high concentration of renin in their blood early in the course of their disease. If a high volume of urine can be produced with a diuretic, this would seem to imply that flow through the kidney is being maintained. If there is a positive feedback in the renin-angiotensin regulation, the maintenance of high flow rates may serve to break this source of inappropriate spasm of the afferent arterioles. If there are any hemoglobin, myoglobin, or other potentially noxious materials passing through the kidney, they will be washed out in the larger urine volume.

Mannitol should be given in a dose of 12.5 to 25 gm over a period of a few hours; if an adequate response is obtained administration should be continued, using 5% mannitol, until the patient is able to sustain a urinary output of 1500 ml per day without the help of the mannitol. Some patients who fail to respond to mannitol will respond to furosemide. Initially the dose should be 40 to 80 mg intravenously; if a very brisk diuresis occurs, it may be necessary to replace some of the fluid and electrolyte that is lost. If the patient does not respond to these usual doses of furosemide, it is possible in some instances to obtain a response with a dose of 800 mg given intravenously over several hours. There have been instances where patients would respond to a combination of mannitol and furosemide when neither of these agents was effective alone. Whenever diuretics are given and a response of over 40 ml per hour of urine is obtained, the diuretics should be continued for several days as needed to maintain this flow rate of urine. The fluid and sodium loss in the urine may need replacement. If response does not occur, mannitol should be stopped after the first 25 gm. Continued use draws fluid from cells into the extracellular fluid and leads to intracellular dehydration and an extracellular fluid overload with dilution of extracellular fluid electrolytes and a fall in serum sodium concentration, not unlike the situation in some patients with high blood sugar levels in uncontrolled diabetes, as was discussed in Chapter 3.

The mechanism of action of mannitol is unsettled. Mannitol is distributed in the extracellular fluid and therefore causes an expansion of plasma volume which is a part of extracellular fluid. In the patient who is well hydrated, this may increase renal blood flow and glomerular filtration rate. Unless the mannitol reaches the tubule it will not improve the flow of fluids through the nephron, and it is difficult to see how mannitol would improve the situation in a patient with severe renal ischemia unless it also caused an increase in renal blood flow. To the extent that filtration occurs and mannitol reaches the tubule, it functions as an osmotic diuretic and maintains a larger amount of fluid in the tubular lumen and thereby dilutes any noxious substances which might otherwise injure the tubular epithelium or become concentrated and a cause of obstruction.

The action of furosemide is completely localized to the kidney and requires glomerular filtration. Furosemide inhibits sodium reabsoption in the proximal tubule and thereby increases the amount of filtrate which reaches the lower nephron and thereby increases urine volume. It would appear that the presence of a diuresis, however produced, in some way promotes better perfusion of the kidney. There is an inverse relationship between urine volume and plasma renin concentrations. The juxtaglomerular apparatus control of flow through the cortical glomeruli, by regulation of the size of the afferent arteriole, is an efficient means of regulating renal blood flow and glomerular filtration in the normal patient, but probably becomes inappropriately and excessively active under circumstances of markedly reduced renal blood flow and reduced urine formation. This sequence of events is as yet poorly understood, but clinical and experimental observations suggest that the sequence can be prevented by adequate hydration and preservation of normal circulation to the kidneys and that when the regulation becomes disturbed in the direction of acute renal failure it can be reversed if treatment is instituted early enough so that circulation and urinary volume are restored and maintained.

EMERGENCY TREATMENT OF ESTABLISHED RENAL FAILURE

Emergency treatment is not required so often now because patients are treated with peritoneal dialysis and hemodialysis before emergencies arise. In neglected patients, in patients with massive injuries where potassium is released in large amounts into the extracellular fluid, and in patients overloaded with fluids, emergency treatment may be required.

Serum potassium levels of 7 mEq/l or potassium levels that are rapidly rising signal the need for early institution of dialysis. Hemodialysis is more efficient than peritoneal dialysis. For those patients in whom the dialysis cannot be started immediately the intravenous administration of glucose and insulin will serve to drive potassium back into the cells temporarily. Calcium gluconate can be added to the infusion since calcium tends to counteract the effects of potassium on the heart. Sodium bicarbonate will correct any metabolic acidosis which is present and also will shift potassium back into the cell. Calcium and bicarbonate should not be mixed into the same infusion fluid. An electrocardiographic monitor should be used since the toxic effects of potassium are related to disturbances in the electrical activity of the heart. Exchange resins are effective in preventing hyperkalemia but should not be relied upon for its emergency treatment, since the rapidity and predictability of their action are insufficient for such an emergency. Sodium polystyrene sulfonate, a potassium-chelating resin, can be given by mouth or by enema and may provide some help even though neither route can be depended upon for a rapid action. Dialysis should be started as soon as possible. Very shortly after its institution the abnormal electrocardiogram will show improvement.

The patient who is overloaded with fluids and anuric or oliguric needs ultrafiltration with a dialysate containing higher than the usual concentration of glucose or with the artificial kidney arranged so that the blood is under pressure as it passes through the coils. Digitalis is indicated if there is specific evidence of cardiac failure but it should be kept in mind that there is an antagonism between digitalis and potassium; therefore if digitalis is used, care should be taken not to dialyze potassium from the patient to the extent of producing a subnormal concentration of serum potassium. Such a circumstance would potentiate the digitalis toxicity.

The pulmonary edema can be controlled in part by intubation of the patient and continuous positive pressure breathing while total body water is being reduced through ultrafiltration by the artificial kidney. There may be some delay in improvement of the roentgenographic picture of the lungs and positive pressure breathing may be required for a somewhat longer time than the period of ultrafiltration. The patient should be weighed repeatedly during this treatment and his body weight used to determine how much fluid to remove. A patient should lose about 500 gm a day during an illness in which food intake is not possible and while increased catabolism from trauma or other illness is present. Knowing the patient's previous weight, his present expected weight can be calculated. The excess is usually an increase in total body water and dilution in total body solute. The decrease in sodium concentration will correspond to the increase in total body water as calculated from observed as compared with expected body weight.

MANAGEMENT OF ESTABLISHED RENAL FAILURE

Once renal failure is established, fluid and electrolyte restrictions are required. The patient should be weighed daily and his body weight allowed to decrease at least 0.5 kg/day. The diet should be restricted to 1200 calories with 20 gm of protein and a low potassium and salt intake. Fluid and electrolyte administration should follow the usual plan of administering metabolic fluids, replacing abnormal losses, and correcting any abnormalities that exist. The patient is not losing urine so metabolic fluids consist only of fluid lost from evaporation from the skin and lungs. Since the patient is mobilizing fat stores and converting fat to water and CO_2, the needs for insensible loss are actually less than would be anticipated, and the average patient will need only about 500 ml of water per day.

As waste products accumulate the metabolic acidosis is manifest by a decrease in CO_2 concentration. If the patient has an ileus or is losing fluids from his stomach and if this loss is acid and contains an excessive concentration of chloride, the resultant hypochloremic alkalosis will compensate nicely for the accumulating metabolic uremic acidosis, and the CO_2 concentration will then be preserved at a near normal level. There is no necessity to treat hypochloremia *per se* since it is better to compensate for the accumulation of unmeasured anions by a decrease in chloride concentration than by a decrease in CO_2. Kayexalate can be given by mouth. It tends to remove some sodium bicarbonate as well as potassium so that it may be necessary to dilute the Kayexalate in sodium bicarbonate solution. It is usually necessary to give the patient a laxative to get rid of the Kayexalate. Magnesium salts probably should not be used because of the possible absorption of magnesium. Sorbital or some such orally administered osmotic agent will serve to remove fluid and thereby decrease the tendency to water overload. Kayexalate can be given by enema but is not as effective as if it is given by mouth. Since most of these patients are receiving frequent treatment with dialysis, there is also a danger now that low serum potassium levels will be produced by overenergetic treatment to reduce elevated potassium levels. This can be particularly hazardous if the patient is receiving digitalis. If the patient is losing potassium by some other route, such as loss of gastrointestinal fluids, it may be necessary to actually administer potassium but this can be governed by frequent serum potassium determinations.

Dialysis should be undertaken early and carried out frequently in order to prevent high levels of serum potassium, water overload, infections (particularly pneumonia), and gastrointestinal bleeding. A Scribner type of arterial-venous shunt or some modification of this should be established. In patients who have an intact peritoneal cavity and in whom the rate of tissue breakdown is reasonably low, peritoneal dialysis can be used. Peritoneal dialysis is less efficient than hemodialysis and will require 12 hours to accomplish what could be performed with hemodialysis in 6 to 8 hours.

CRUSH SYNDROME

According to Brun this was a familiar syndrome described in textbooks of the 1880 to 1890 era. It was rediscovered by the German physicians during World War I in soldiers who were crushed after shelling of their trenches. During the Battle of Britain in 1940 and 1941 there were many patients who were removed from bombed buildings and brought into a center established for the treatment of crush injuries in London. Four of these patients were described by Bywaters and Beall. The syndrome is not common but is of importance because of the misleadingly healthy appearance of the patient early in its inception and the 36- to 48-hour progression of renal failure, intoxication, and death if the condition is not recognized and adequately treated. It is a combination of acute renal failure and massive release of cellular materials, including potassium, with early death from potassium intoxication.

The patient is released from the crushing situation and may have few apparent injuries. He is likely not to have any fractures and to have good pulses in his extremities. The injury causes a combination of crushing damage to muscle followed by ischemic renal injury. There is progressive swelling and induration of the crushed extremities. Initially the patient passes urine in normal amounts, but the urine quickly becomes reddish or smoky in appearance from the passage of myoglobin. Vasoactive materials are thought to be released from the crushed tissues causing vasospasm. In the kidneys perhaps this is accentuated by increased concentrations of antidiuretic hormone, catecholamines, sympathetic discharge, release of renin, and activation of angiotensin. Plasma and fluid are lost into the injured extremities with reduction of circulating blood volume and increasing hematocrit, with decreased cardiac output and especially restricted renal perfusion. Glomerular filtration decreases, and the high concentration of myoglobin precipitates in the tubules, forming casts. The renal failure runs the usual stages of oliguria and diuresis, providing the patient survives that long.

It may be possible to prevent renal failure by early treatment with fluids and diuretics. A fairly satisfactory volume of urine under normal circumstances may be inadequate, however, to relieve the patient of his tremendous load of pigments and waste products so that stimulated diuresis with mannitol or furosemide (or both if necessary), supported by adequate replacement with intravenous saline, is most likely to be effective in preventing renal failure.

The secret of success in treatment of these patients once renal failure is established (urine at a rate of less than 500 ml per day in spite of treatment) is early prophylactic and continuous or frequent intermittent dialysis. Hemodialysis is required because of its greater efficiency, and there are some instances in which it is necessary to use both peritoneal dialysis and frequent hemodialysis. If hemodialysis is carried out for 6 or 8 hours and the chemistries seem to be satisfactory, within a few hours after stopping dialysis the serum potassium level may rise to near lethal levels. The frequent energetic treatment with dialysis must be continued for several days until the crushed muscles have released potassium and other material from damaged cells, and this material has been removed from the body. Subsequent dialysis can be carried out at less frequent intervals until such time as renal function returns to normal.

TRIAGE

One of the most frustrating problems in management of patients with renal failure relates to prognosis. There is often no way to determine whether a seriously ill patient will recover provided he is maintained with proper management or whether he has irreversible renal injury. If the kidneys are small by roentgenography or if they become small within a week or 10 days, then chronic renal disease or renal cortical necrosis is likely, and renal biopsy should be considered. A part of the problem arises from the frequency of azotemia in patients who are dying from serious illness or extensive trauma involving multiple organs or after complex and prolonged operations. Physicians will agree that the dying patient whose problem is basically related to other than renal damage should not be subjected to dialysis. Sometimes one cannot be sure of the relative importance of systemic disease and renal failure, and dialysis must be instituted and continued as required until recovery or until failure of some other organ settles the issue.

REFERENCES

Alwall, N.: Die aktive Therapie der Niereninsuffizienz. I. Ergebnisse von 700 Behandlungen mit der Kunstlichen Niere (Dialyse, Ultrafiltration) Während der Jahre 1946-1957, Sowie Mobilisierung, Tracheotomie, Respirations behandlung usw. und röntgenologische Kontrolle des Flussigkeitsgleichgewichts.

Balint, P., Chatel, R., Fekete, A., and Forgacs, I.: Haemodynamics and oxygen consumption of the kidney in post-ischaemic renal failure. Clin. Sci. *26*:471, 1964.

Barry, K. G., Mazze, R. I., and Schwartz, F. D.: Prevention of surgical oliguria and renal hemodynamic suppression by sustained hydration. New Eng. J. Med. *270*:1371, 1964.

Berne, T. V., and Barbour, B. H.: Acute renal failure in general surgical patients. Arch. Surg. (Chicago) *102*:594, 1971.

Brown, C. B., Glancy, J. J., Fry, I., and Cattell, W. R.: High-dose excretion urography in oliguric renal failure. Lancet *2*:952, 1970.

Brown, J. J., Gleadle, R. I., Lawson, D. H., Lever, A. F., Linton, A. L., MacAdam, R. F., Prentice, E., Robertson, J. I. S., and Tree, M.: Renin and acute renal failure; studies in man. Brit. Med. J. *1*:253, 1970.

Brun, C.: *Acute Anuria: A Study Based on Renal Function Tests and Aspiration Biopsy of the Kidney.* Copenhagen: Munksgaard, 1954.

Brun, C., and Munck, O.: Lesions of the kidney in acute renal failure following shock. Lancet *1*:603, 1957.

Bywaters, E. G. L., and Beall, D.: Crush injuries with impairment of renal function. Brit. Med. J. *1*:427, 1941.

Dawson, J. L.: Postoperative renal function in obstructive jaundice: effect of a mannitol diuresis. Brit. Med. J. *1*:82, 1965.

Goormaghtigh, N.: Vascular and circulatory changes in renal cortex in anuric crush syndrome. Proc. Soc. Exp. Biol. Med. *59*:393, 1945.

Hager, E. B., Hampers, C. L., Bailey, G. L., and Merrill, J. P.: Acute renal insufficiency: the spectrum. Ann. Surg. *168*:224, 1968.

Hockmuth, R. E., Faber, L. C., and Mason, E. E.: Extracorporeal dialysis in renal failure. J. Iowa Med. Soc. *52*:199, 1962.

Hollengerg, N. K., Epstein, M., Rosen, J. M., Basch, R. I., Oken, D. E., and Merrill, J. P.: Acute renal failure in man: evidence for preferential renal cortical ischemia. Medicine *47*:455, 1968.

Mason, E. E., Chernigoy, F. A., Gulesserian, H. P., and Tector, A. J.: Enzymuria in icteric surgical patients. Surg. Gynec. Obstet. *122*:333, 1966.

Mason, E. E., and Chernigoy, F. A.: Postoperative loss of heat-labile kidney leucine aminopeptidase. Surg. Gynec. Obstet. *128*:806, 1969.

Montoreano, R., Mouzet, M. T., Cunarro, J., and Ruiz-Guinazu, A.: Prevention of the initial oliguria of acute renal failure by the administration of furosemide. Postgrad. Med. J. *47*:7, 1971.

Oliver, J., MacDowell, M., and Tracy, A.: The pathogenesis of acute renal failure associated with traumatic and toxic injury, renal ischemia, nephrotoxic damage and the ischemuric episode. J. Clin. Invest. *30*:1307, 1951.

Saito, T., and Yoshida, S.: Levels of antidiuretic hormone in plasma after hemorrhage and infusion of hypertonic saline in dogs. Endocrinology. *88*:1511, 1971.

Sheehan, H. L., and Moore, H. C.: *Renal Cortical Necrosis and the Kidney of Concealed Accidental Hemorrhage.* Springfield, Ill.: Charles C. Thomas, 1953.

Skillman, J. J., Lauler, D. P., Hickler, R. B., Lyons, J. H., Olson, J. E., Ball, M. R., and Moore, F. D.: Hemorrhage in normal man: effect on renin, cortisol, aldosterone, and urine composition. Ann. Surg. *166*:865, 1967.

Chapter

11

Calcium and Phosphorus Metabolism

CALCIUM

Calcium is absorbed from the intestine, excreted in the urine, and deposited in bone, all under the influence of parathyroid hormone. The only well-known stimulus to the secretion of parathyroid hormone is a decrease in concentration of ionized calcium. The ions of calcium and phosphate are in equilibrium with bone minerals. An increase in the concentration of ionized calcium causes supersaturation in the region of osteoblasts and causes deposition of calcium and phosphate in bone. A decrease in concentration of calcium causes a shift of minerals from bone into the body fluids. If the product of ionized calcium and phosphate is high enough, precipitation occurs in soft tissues.

The degree of ionization of calcium and phosphate is dependent upon the hydrogen ion concentration of body fluids. Acidosis tends to increase the ionization and the capacity of body fluids for these salts, whereas a decrease in concentration of hydrogen ion (i.e., alkalosis) will cause more deposition of minerals in bone and, under some circumstances, in soft tissues. Krull and others, for example, made use of local transient acidosis to develop a test for hyperparathyroidism, in which they occluded the circulation in a patient's arm and had him rhythmically clench his fist for 10 minutes; then they measured the concentration of calcium in venous blood from that arm. In the presence of the osteolytic changes in bone in hyperparathyroidism there was an increase in the concentration of calcium, whereas in control patients there was no change in the concentration of calcium in the venous blood.

Almost half of the blood calcium is carried by adsorption to albumin. In uremic patients there are other substances which complex with the calcium and further reduce the proportion of free ionized calcium. Calcium is still reported as milligrams/100 ml in many hospitals. Since the molecular weight of calcium is

40, a blood level of 10 mg/100 ml would be the same as 5.0 mEq/l or 2.5 mM/l. Different laboratories use these different units for reporting results. A level of 8.5 in mEq/l would be alarmingly high but would actually be a low concentration if the scale of measurement intended was mg/100 ml. Since these patients are frequently referred from one physician or hospital to another with their recorded calcium values, it is essential that the appropriate unit designation be recognized.

For a 70-kg person with an extracellular fluid of 14 liters, there are roughly 70 mEq of calcium in extracellular fluid, whereas there are 35,000 mEq of calcium in bone. Only a fraction of bone calcium is rapidly exchangeable, and the release of calcium is dependent upon osteoclastic activity which is stimulated by parathormone. Jowsey has measured areas of bone resorption and areas of bone formation in biopsies of bone and finds that resorption is more markedly altered than bone formation when there is excessive function of the parathyroids.

PHOSPHATE

Large stores of phosphate are deposited in bone, but phosphate is also present in soft tissue. High-energy phosphate bonds are formed as phosphocreatine and as adenosine triphosphate. The energy is derived from the metabolism of carbohydrates in the citric acid cycle as well as from fats and amino acids. The affinity of hemoglobin for oxygen is decreased by increased levels of 2,3-diphosphoglycerate in the red blood cell in circumstances when tissue oxygen supply might otherwise be inadequate. Inorganic phosphate in blood is derived from cellular metabolism, from absorption by the intestine, and from resorption of bone and is excreted in the urine and stool.

In the presence of renal insufficiency the serum phosphate levels rise. There is an inverse relationship between ionized calcium and ionized phosphate. A rise in concentration of plasma phosphate leads indirectly to the stimulation of secretion of parathyroid hormone by way of the associated decrease in concentration of ionized plasma calcium. Phosphate is excreted as disodium phosphate which may then be converted to monosodium dihydrogen phosphate through the trapping of hydrogen in the lumen of the renal tubule, thus facilitating the excretion of excess acid and preservation of body bicarbonate. Wills has suggested that the evolution of parathormone may have been directed toward a control of cellular hydrogen ion concentration as mediated through inorganic phosphate. Barzel and Jowsey have found that the formation and release of bone salts are also influenced by alkalosis and acidosis and may be vital in survival of such events.

Barzel has studied the relationships of parathyroid hormone, blood phosphorus, and acid-base metabolism and has arrived at the generally held opinion that these are mechanisms for regulation of calcium balance, in contradistinction to the suggestion of Wills that parathormone evolved as a means for regulating acid-base balance. The question is not settled. A fall in ionized blood calcium occurs in alkalosis, and this stimulates secretion of parathormone which causes an increase in the body acid load. This in turn speeds bone resorption. The bone calcium restores the concentration of calcium in extracellular fluid, and the excess acid load and phosphate are excreted by the kidneys. In data from Barzel on a wide range of serum parathyroid hormone levels, regression analysis revealed that 65% of the variation in blood phosphorus could be predicted on the basis of observed changes in arterial pH, arterial P_{CO_2}, CO_2 content, and blood calcium. Probably the vector derived from these independent variables is the level of ionized calcium which in turn governs parathyroid hormone production. Wills and McGowan observed that in hypercalcemia caused by hyperparathyroidism there was an elevation of plasma chloride concentration and a metabolic acidosis, whereas in hypercalcemia due to other causes there were alkalosis and hypochloremia.

The product of calcium and phosphate is of equal importance to the consideration of the concentration of either one of these ions alone, because of the deposition of calcium in soft tissues and consequent soft-tissue injury when the product is high. This can occur in either hyper- or hypoparathyroidism. It is occasionally seen in chronic renal disease. Soft-tissue calcification is a potential hazard in the administration of phosphate for the treatment of toxic hypercalcemia. Alkalosis adds to the risk of "metastatic" calcification of soft tissues as is illustrated by the milk-alkali syndrome. McMillan and Freeman produced acute changes in patients by the administration of 1½ quarts of milk a day and an absorbable antacid, calcium carbonate. In the course of one week of such treatment, there was a rise in the concentrations of calcium, phosphorus, carbon dioxide, and creatinine in the serum. By contrast when aluminum hydroxide was substituted as the antacid, these abnormalities were reversed. Repeated or prolonged treatment with milk and absorbable alkali leads to soft-tissue deposition of calcium, damage to the renal tubules, and, if continued long enough, chronic renal failure.

PARATHYROID HORMONE AND CALCITONIN

Parathyroid hormone has been characterized to the extent that Aurbach (2nd ref.) has synthesized a peptide with amino acids 1 to 34 from the amino terminus. This peptide has approximately

25% of the activity of native hormone when activation of cyclic AMP is used as the index. The stimulus to the formation and secretion of parathyroid hormone and also the hyperplasia of the parathyroid tissues is a lowering of ionized calcium in the blood perfusing the parathyroids.

Parathyroid hormone is synergistic in its action with vitamin D. The three chief sites of action are kidney, bone, and intestine. Parathyroid hormone inhibits the reabsorption of phosphate by the cells lining the renal tubules so that increased amounts of phosphate are lost in the urine. Parathyroid hormone also stimulates the tubular reabsorption of calcium. This may not be apparent from urinary calcium measurement because of the increased filtration of calcium consequent to the elevated serum calcium concentration. The usual effect of increased levels of parathyroid hormone is an increase in the calcium in the urine. If for some reason the serum calcium level does not rise, then the decrease in urinary calcium as a result of the action of parathormone on the renal tubule may become evident. Osteoclastic activity is stimulated by parathyroid hormone with increased movement of calcium and phosphate into the body fluids. Intestinal absorption of calcium is also stimulated. The results of action at these three sites are a rise in serum calcium and a fall in serum phosphorus. These various actions were described in detail by Albright and Reifenstein.

Thyrocalcitonin discovered by Copp in 1961 counteracts the effects of parathyroid hormone on the osteoclasts and as a result has a hypocalcemic effect. Thyrocalcitonin is a polypeptide of 3700 molecular weight according to Rittel et al., and it has been measured in plasma by an immunologic method developed by Deftos et al. Hypercalcemia stimulates secretion of thyrocalcitonin.

Embryologically the third and fourth branchial pouches form parathyroid glands, and the fourth pouch provides the ultimobranchial body which gives rise to the calcitonin-producing cells which migrate into the thyroid and are called the C-cells or parafollicular cells. The thyroid arises in the midline from the foramen cecum at the base of the tongue. The thyroid gland descends in the neck and in most individuals divides and moves dorsally to the sides of the trachea. The parathyroid glands, arising from the fourth branchial pouches, remain posterior to the thyroid near the trachea and slightly cephalad to the transverse process of the sixth cervical vertebra (carotid tubercle). Parathyroids III, which arise from the third branchial pouches in conjunction with the thymus, descend in the neck to the lower part of the thyroid and frequently are located dorsal to the recurrent laryngeal nerve and near the inferior thyroid artery, but they may descend with the paired thymus into the superior mediastinum.

CYCLIC AMP

Aurbach (1st ref.) and others have reviewed the action of 3′, 5′-cyclic adenosine monophosphate in mediating the action of parathyroid hormone in kidney and bone. Parathyroid hormone activates adenyl cyclase in renal cortical tubules with a resultant increase in the cellular concentration of c-AMP. Some of the increased c-AMP appears in the urine. Elevation of urine c-AMP concentration, like elevation of urine phosphorus, can be used as an index of parathormone activity. Adenvl cyclase activity in bone is also increased by parathyroid hormone with resultant increase in c-AMP. Parathormone causes increased absorption of bone whereas calcitonin inhibits reabsorption and yet c-AMP is the second messenger for both hormones. It has been suggested that separate cell types are probably involved in these opposing actions of c-AMP in bone.

HYPERPARATHYROIDISM

Excessive secretion of parathyroid hormone may be produced by a neoplasm. This is usually an adenoma and very rarely a carcinoma. Parathyroid carcinoma is less frequent than parathyroid hormone-secreting cancers of lung, kidney, and other organs. Until recently most hyperparathyroidism was thought to be due to adenomas but now with more patients being operated upon in an asymptomatic stage of disease, more and more of the patients seem to have chief-cell hyperplasia and there are all degrees and combinations of adenoma and hyperplasia. In the earlier reports clear-cell hyperplasia was described but this now is a rare type of hyperplasia. There are also areas of clear-cell change in glands that are mainly composed of chief-cell hyperplasia as depicted by Hume.

When the stimulus is unknown hyperplasia is termed *primary*. If the cause of the hyperplasia is a chronic decrease in concentration of ionized calcium, then it is termed *secondary hyperplasia*. Parathyroid-like peptides are secreted by some malignant neoplasms of nonparathyroid tissue. This has been observed most often in oat-cell carcinoma of the lung and renal carcinoma, but other malignancies can be involved. Katz et al. reported hypercalcemia in two patients with breast cancer in whom bone metastases could not be demonstrated and in whom removal of a parathyroid adenoma in one and an adenomatous nodular hyperplastic gland in the other patient restored serum calcium levels to normal.

Bronsky has outlined a classification of parathyroid disease on the basis of our current knowledge of the etiology and pathogenesis. The most common cause of excessive secretion of parathyroid hormone is probably still the chief-cell adenoma. Pathologists have difficulty at times in deciding whether parathyroid specimens submitted represent adenomata or hyperplasia, and it has now become evident that there can be mixtures of the two and that the final conclusion as to the diagnosis may require examination of all of the parathyroid glands. At least snippet biopsy samples of normal-appearing parathyroids should be sectioned as suggested by Cope (1941). The final diagnosis may not be apparent for many years and is dependent upon prolonged observation of the patient's parathyroid function.

With electron microscopy it has been possible, according to Haff and Ballinger, to demonstrate that patients with grossly normal-appearing glands and with normal-appearing histologic sections by light microscopy may still have hyperplasia of the endoplasmic reticulum and Golgi apparatus, indicating that the glands are overactive and that the parathyroid cells are probably manufacturing excessive amounts of parathyroid hormone. Such findings support the recommendation for removal of seven-eighths of the parathyroid tissue when a distinct adenoma is not found and when all four parathyroid glands appear to be of approximately the same size, but this will be discussed later.

DIAGNOSIS OF HYPERCALCEMIA

Gordon and Roof have called attention to three steps in the diagnosis of hypercalcemia. The first step is to become suspicious that hypercalcemia might be present. Once the suspicion is raised, then it is necessary to establish that hypercalcemia is in fact present. Finally, the cause of the hypercalcemia must be determined. The diagnosis is made on the basis of symptoms arising from the kidney, musculoskeletal system, gastrointestinal tract, and central nervous system. These will become evident in what follows, but an overview of the entire subject is shown in Figure 11-1.

In 1925, when Mandl performed the first operation for the removal of a parathyroid adenoma, the patient had the extensive bone changes which are referred to as osteitis fibrosa cystica. These changes are the result of prolonged osteoclastic activity and lead to bowing of the legs and other obvious changes in the bone which would automatically raise a suspicion of hyperparathyroidism. Such extensive disease is seldom seen now. The first such patient operated upon in the United States was seen at Massachusetts General Hospital in 1926 and was very similar to

HYPERPARATHYROIDISM

1. Presenting Symptoms

"Stones, Bones, Groans and Psychic Moans"

↑ PTH PRODUCTION

KIDNEY	MUSCULOSKELETAL	GI	CNS

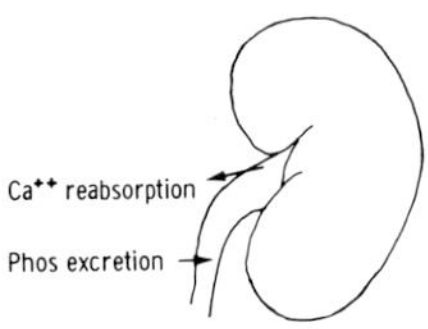

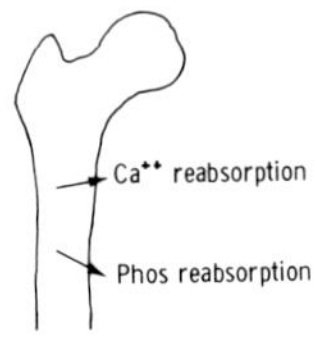

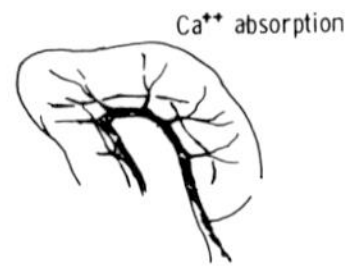

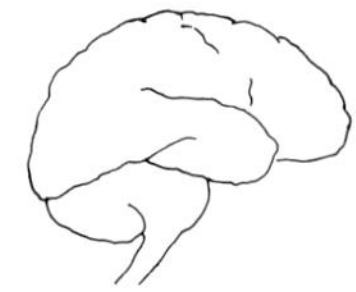

KIDNEY

Stones
- Renal colic
- UT infection
- Necrosis
  - Renin
  - Blood Pressure

ADH antagonized by Ca
- Polyuria
- Polydipsia
- Nocturia

MUSCULOSKELETAL

Bone Pain
Backache
Joint Pain
Weakness
Relaxation of ligament and joints
Unsteady Gait

GI

Abdominal Pain
Constipation
Diarrhea
Anorexia
Nausea
Vomit
Ileus
Pancreatitis
Duodenal Ulcers

CNS

Symptoms from mild to severe hypercalcemia
- Anxiety
- Depression
- Confusion
  - Suicide
  - Stupor
  - Hysteria
- Personality Change
- Seclusion
- Distraction
- Dullness
- Irritability
- Interest Loss
- Blurred Vision
- Hearing Loss
- Paralysis
- Coma

2. Hypercalcemia: calcium, phosphorus, albumin, and total protein determinations

3. Differental Diagnosis

POSSIBLE CAUSES	DIFFERENT TESTS	SERUM CALCIUM	SERUM PHOSPHATE	ALKALINE PHOSPHATASE	URINE CALCIUM
Vitamin D intoxication	History	↑	↑	↓ or N	↑
Immobilization	History	↑	↑ or N	N	↑
Milk Alkali	History and removal of absorbable alkali	↑	N	N	↓ or N
Osteomalacia	History	↓ or N	↓	↑	↓
Hyperthyroidism	T_3 & T_4 uptake	↑	N	↑ or N	↑
Parathormone Secreting Cancer		↑	↓ or N	N	↑ or N
Kidney	IV Pyelography				
Lung	Roentgenograms				
Bone Destructive Metastisis	Roentgenograms & Bone Biopsy	↑	N	↑ or N	↑
Prostatic Carcinoma					
Breast Carcinoma					
Multiple Myeloma	Plasma, Bence - Jones Protein	↑	N	N	↑ or N
Sarcoid	Plasma Roentgenograms Bone Biopsy	↑	↓ or N	↑ or N	↑
4. Hyperparathyroidism		↑	↓	↑ or N	↑

Parathormone Immunoassay
Roentgenograms - Hand and Skull
24 hour Urinary Calcium
Tubular Reabsorption of Phosphorus
Calcium Infusion
Dent Test - cortisone suppression of Calcium with bone metastasis
Serum Chloride elevation

Mandl's patient. The first patient operated upon for hyperparathyroidism at the University of Iowa Hospitals in Iowa City by Frank Peterson in 1929 was also a patient with severe bone disease. Lee et al. reported a patient with severe bone disease secondary to hyperparathyroidism who developed osteogenic sarcoma. There is no question that prolonged and severe hyperparathyroidism can be morbid if allowed to persist. Such advanced changes are seldom observed now.

The physicians at Massachusetts General Hospital were intensively interested in calcium metabolism and hyperparathyroidism and quickly came to realize that many such patients formed renal stones as the chief manifestation of hyperparathyroidism. In other hospitals around the country physicians with interest in parathyroid disease wondered why they did not see as many patients with renal stones and hyperparathyroidism as were seen in Boston. An example of this was the experience of Keating who, after a year's study at Massachusetts General Hospital, returned to the Mayo Clinic and in the course of the succeeding year discovered more patients with hyperparathyroidism than had been detected in the history of the Mayo Clinic up until that time. Renal stones have raised the question of hyperparathyroidism in more patients than any other manifestation of the disease, at least until the introduction of mechanized analytic screening of serum from people having routine or unrelated physical examinations.

Cope and others in 1957 described a relationship between hyperparathyroidism and pancreatitis. Analysis of serum calcium and phosphorus levels in patients with pancreatitis has led to the discovery of additional instances that otherwise might have been overlooked. Pancreatitis, through its formation of areas of fat necrosis and precipitation of calcium as calcium soaps in the necrotic fat, tends to cause a decrease in concentration of serum calcium which may obscure the fact that the patient has had an abnormally high serum calcium level as a part of hyperparathyroidism. It has also been suggested that there may be instances where the expected lowering of serum calcium in a patient with pancreatitis might be obscured by the basic underlying tendency toward hypercalcemia resulting from hyperparathyroidism. Paloyan, Lawrence, et al. have found pancreatic alpha cell hyperplasia and elevated levels of plasma glucagon in patients with chronic relapsing pancreatitis. Glucagon produced in alpha cells is said to stimulate release of calcitonin from the thyroid. The chronic lowering of serum calcium resulting from calcitonin could cause hyperplasia of the parathyroids which might eventually become autonomous, according to the observations of Avioli et al. Shieber has summarized these relationships.

Turchi and others reached the conclusion that in terms of the cause of pancreatitis, hyperparathyroidism ranked immediately behind alcohol, biliary tract disease, and trauma. They found 26 patients reported in the literature and added 4 additional instances of pancreatitis and hyperparathyroidism. Probably there is more than one mechanism for an occasional occurrence of pancreatitis and hyperparathyroidism in the same patient. It is possible, of course, that the pancreatitis could result from deposition of calcium and phosphate complexes in the pancreatic parenchyma with damage to the gland in the same way that the kidney is damaged. Disruption of ductules could cause pancreatic juice to mix with interstitial fluids and activation of the pro-enzymes could lead to the autocatalytic process which we recognize as pancreatitis. Cope, Culver, and others were under the impression that the calcinosis and lithiasis gave rise to the pancreatitis. Perhaps the pancreatitis gives rise to elevation of serum glucagon in some patients and in other patients the hyperparathyroidism is primary and leads to calcification and pancreatitis. Removal of the overactive parathyroid tissue seems to cause an amelioration of the chronic relapsing pancreatitis which adds further interest to this "chicken-egg" question of sequence.

In the earlier reviews of series of patients with hyperparathyroidism, there were occasional patients who also had duodenal ulcer. It gradually became evident that there must be some relationship between the two conditions, so that now there is a commendable tendency to obtain serum calcium and phosphorus levels in patients with symptoms of duodenal ulcer. This has added to the increasing number of diagnoses of hyperparathyroidism. There is apparently a synergism between calcium and gastrin in stimulating secretion of hydrochloric acid. Some of the patients who have duodenal ulcer and hyperparathyroidism are suffering from multiple glandular adenomas including gastrin-secreting adenomas of the pancreas. These patients succumb to their duodenal ulcer disease unless a total gastric resection is performed. A larger proportion of the patients with combined acid peptic disease and hyperparathyroidism do not have adenomatous hyperplasia of gastrin-secreting cells and are relieved of the ulcer diathesis after removal of the offending parathyroid tissue. In both situations the condition may be familial. Examination of other members of the family is indicated and will often lead to the diagnosis of additional patients with hyperparathyroidism.

Wilder et al. reviewed 52 patients with peptic ulcer and primary hyperparathyroidism. Where patients with peptic ulcer disease were studied for the possibility of hyperparathyroidism, the latter disease was found in 4 instances giving an incidence of slightly greater than 1%. The ulcer was duodenal in 41 patients, gastric in 9, and located in both areas in 2 patients. Half of the patients were in the fifth decade of life. The majority of patients had symptoms over a period of at least ten years. In 28 of the patients the ulcer disease was active at the time of the parathyroid operation, and in 23 of these patients the ulcer symptoms improved following removal of parathyroid tissue. If all of the hyperplastic and overactive parathyroid tissue is not removed or if the patient has a gastrin-secreting adenoma of the pancreas, then persistent or recurrent ulcer symptoms will require further diagnostic and therapeutic effort.

A woman with both a pancreatic adenoma and hyperparathyroidism was treated at the University of Iowa Hospitals with subtotal parathyroidectomy. This caused temporary relief, but ulcer pain soon returned and a total gastric resection was performed. She had a sister who had previously been operated upon in our hospital for an insulin-secreting adenoma of the pancreas. When this sister was re-examined it was discovered that she also had hyperparathyroidism. There were seven other siblings. A brother had passed renal stones. Another brother had had a parathyroid adenoma removed. A sister had passed renal stones and had two adenomas removed from her neck. A brother was examined and found to have hyperparathyroidism and underwent a subtotal parathyroidectomy. His 8-year-old son had passed a kidney stone and was found to have a high serum calcium and a low serum phosphorus. He subsequently developed Cushing's disease. The grandfather of this boy was found to have died of renal infection and to have passed kidney stones on numerous occasions between 1940 and 1947. He also had taken antacids over the years for symptoms which probably were due to a duodenal ulcer, although this diagnosis was never actually made. This man died at age 53 from his renal disease. It appears, therefore, that in this family at least three generations are involved, and it is likely that as more relatives are examined, more instances of hyperparathyroidism will be uncovered.

Kaplan et al. have suggested another possible basis for the interrelationship between hyperparathyroidism and gastrin-secreting pancreatic tumors. Secretion of gastric acid produces a metabolic alkalosis. Kaplan demonstrated that infusion of sodium bicarbonate caused a decrease in ionized calcium followed by a rise in serum parathormone. Eventually such stimulation would possibly result in sufficient hyperplasia of the parathyroids so that periods of hypercalcemia might result. Increasing concentrations of calcium increase the secretion of acid in response to gastrin so that once hyperplasia and hypersecretion of parathormone were established, acid peptic disease would be even more likely.

Ellison and Wilson reviewed the experience with gastrin-secreting adenomas of the pancreas in 260 registered cases and found associated endocrine disease in 55 or 21% of patients. They were starting with patients with known gastrin-secreting adenomas of the pancreas and looking into the incidence of involvement of other endocrine glands. They found parathyroid adenoma to be present more often than disease of any other endocrine gland. Only 8 patients had multiple glandular disease or Wermer's syndrome.

In the past the vast majority of patients with hyperparathyroidism have had signs and symptoms of renal stones which gave rise to the suspicion of possible parathyroid disease. In a review of the Massachusetts General Hospital experience published by Cope in 1966, out of 343 patients there were 195 with renal stones, 80 with bone disease, 27 with peptic ulcer, and 9 with pancreatitis. The diagnosis of hyperparathyroidism jumped by an order of magnitude when it was recognized that this could be a cause of renal stones and when the medical profession made a conscious effort to find these patients. "What you see is what you get." We are at the present time in the midst of another quantum jump in the incidence of diagnosis of hyperparathyroidism as a result of the routine chemical screening of large numbers of clinical patients. The incidence figures at the present time vary between 1 in 850 and 1 in 2000 patients screened. Operations on the parathyroids are becoming more common than operations on the thyroid (Fig. 11-2).

SIGNS AND SYMPTOMS OF HYPERCALCEMIA

The suspicion of hypercalcemia in the past has usually been raised by the presence of those signs and symptoms which are frequently seen in people with high serum calcium levels. These symptoms can be understood and remembered in terms of the various organ systems which are influenced, namely the gastrointestinal tract, kidneys, musculoskeletal system, and the central nervous system. The symptoms are not specific and may not be explained for years unless the disease is considered.

The effects of hypercalcemia on the gastrointestinal tract give rise to abdominal pain, constipation, diarrhea, anorexia, nausea, vomiting, and ileus. High serum calcium levels affect the kidneys in various ways. Calcium antagonizes the action of antidiuretic hormone in the distal tubule so that the patient has polyuria, polydipsia, and nocturia. The formation of stones gives rise to renal colic, and the presence of stones and the necrosis of tissue from renal calcinosis predispose to infection so that the patient may have signs and symptoms of urinary tract infection. Renal damage may also give rise to an increase in the production of renin and consequent elevation of blood pressure. Hypercalcemia causes increased peripheral resistance by direct action on blood vessels according to Frohlich et al. Shackney and

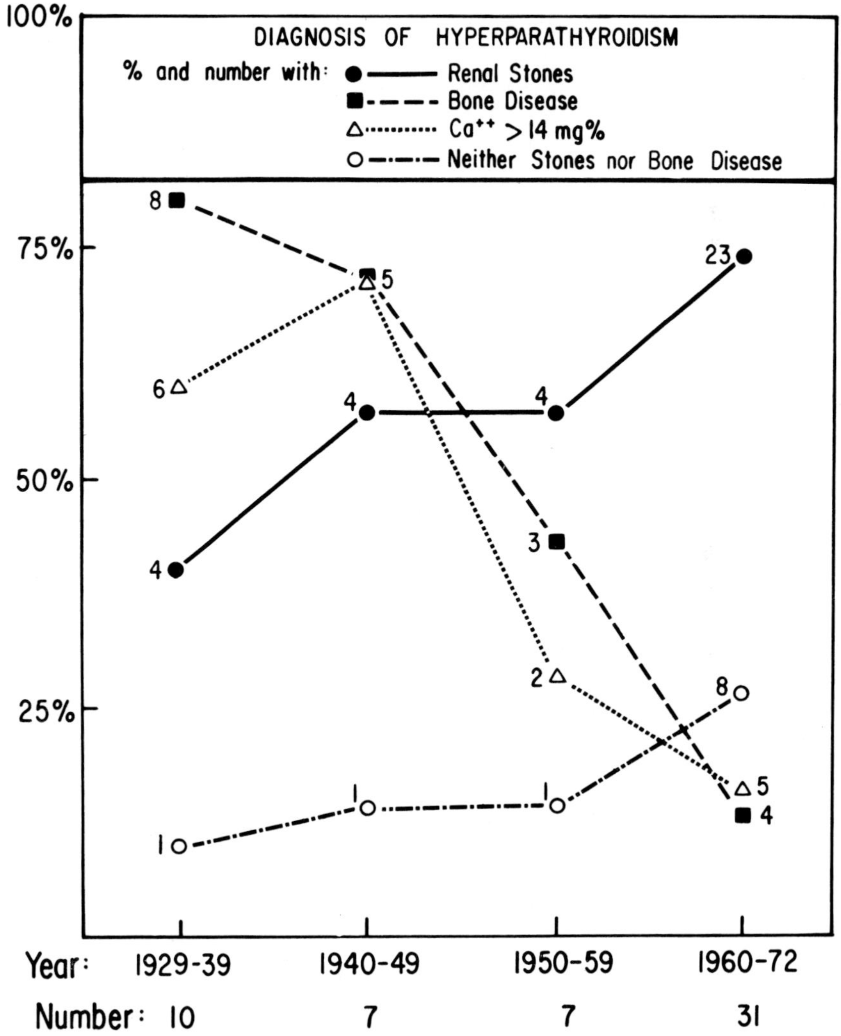

Figure 11-2. Shows the number of patients cared for at University of Iowa Hospitals and the percentage in each decade with different manifestations of the disease. The absolute number of cases is shown by each symbol in each decade. Notice the steady increase in renal stones and recent increase in patients with neither stone nor bone disease. There will be a sharp increase in the latter in the present decade due to automated serum analyses. (Prepared by John Hoines)

Hasson have even found evidence that renal cortical necrosis may occur in hyperparathyroidism, in part because of the special sensitivity of renal vessels to hypercalcemia.

Symptoms arising from the effects of high calcium levels on the musculoskeletal system include bone pain, especially at night and especially if the serum calcium level is extremely high. Patients complain of backache, joint pain, and weakness. There is a relaxation of the ligaments and joints so that the patient has an unsteady gait somewhat analogous to the relaxation of the pelvic girdle in pregnancy. A patient may be able to perform feats of limberness such as placing both feet behind one's head. The average patient will not have discovered this ability, and the physician may need to explain why he is conducting such an unusual physical examination. Be careful; the bones are susceptible to fracture in some of these patients.

The central nervous system effects of hypercalcemia are related to the degree of hypercalcemia and with progressive rise in serum calcium levels there may well be a progression of symptoms from mild anxiety and depression, through confusion, threats of suicide, changes in personality, seclusion, distraction, dullness, irritability, loss of interest, blurred vision, hearing loss, paralyses, and, with extremely high levels of serum calcium, hysteria, stupor, and coma. Tetany is not a symptom of hypercalcemia, but there have been instances, such as that reported by Friderichsen and Rosendal, where a newborn infant developed tetany, and this led to the diagnosis of hyperparathyroidism in the mother. High serum calcium levels in the mother apparently provided sufficient levels of calcium in the fetus so that the infant's parathyroid tissue was inadequate in its function and for a brief period of time after birth the infant was hypocalcemic. One instance of permanent hypoparathyroidism in an infant has been reported. Parathyroid hormone does not pass through the placental barrier so that osteitis fibrosa cystica and other changes which might be expected in the infant with increased maternal levels of parathyroid hormone are not observed. Osteitis has been reported in a newborn infant whose mother was deficient in parathormone. This was secondary hyperplasia of the infant's parathyroid due to chronic hypocalcemia.

ESTABLISHING THAT HYPERCALCEMIA IS PRESENT

Reliable calcium and phosphorus analyses are essential to the diagnosis of hypercalcemia. Hypercalcemia may be intermittent. A tendency towards hypercalcemia can be masked by malabsorption or by a high phosphorus intake. The presence of pancreatitis or renal failure and a low concentration of serum proteins may also obscure the diagnosis. Various nomograms have been proposed for the estimation of ionized calcium. A nomogram published by Chamberlin et al. takes into consideration both the globulin and albumin fraction of plasma proteins (Fig. 11-3). With their nomogram an estimated serum ionized calcium above 6.6 mg/100 ml indicates an elevation consistent with a diagnosis of hyperparathyroidism. In the presence of low serum proteins and also with acidosis, a total serum calcium of 10 mg/100 ml may be significantly elevated. The ionized calcium controls normal parathyroid function and hypercalcemia exists only when a diffusible or ionized calcium concentration is above normal.

Keating has published data relating calcium and phosphorus levels to age and sex in 756 healthy persons and in 260 patients

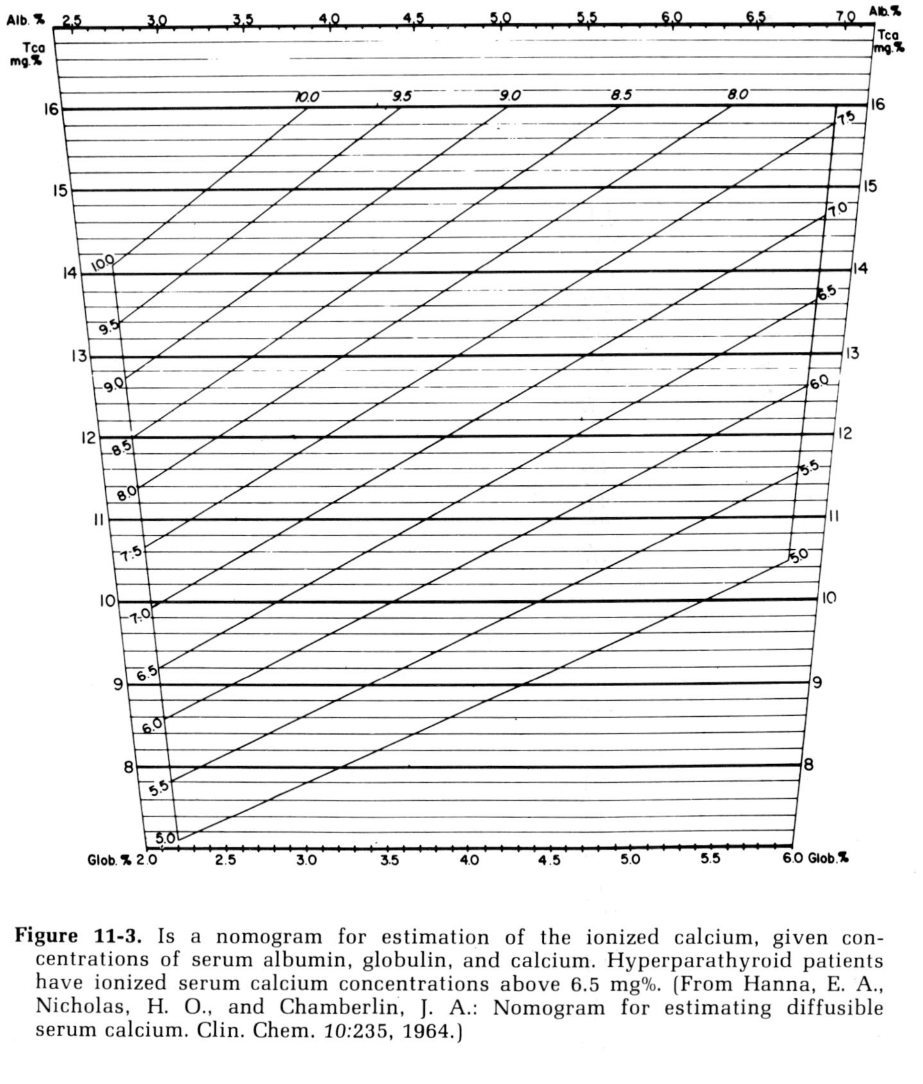

Figure 11-3. Is a nomogram for estimation of the ionized calcium, given concentrations of serum albumin, globulin, and calcium. Hyperparathyroid patients have ionized serum calcium concentrations above 6.5 mg%. (From Hanna, E. A., Nicholas, H. O., and Chamberlin, J. A.: Nomogram for estimating diffusible serum calcium. Clin. Chem. *10*:235, 1964.)

with hyperparathyroidism. There is a gradual decline in normal serum calcium concentration with age in men but not in women. Almost all patients with hyperparathyroidism fell above the 95% confidence limits for normal calcium in this collection of data. Shieber et al. described a few patients with hypercalciuria and hyperparathyroidism, as demonstrated by elevated serum parathyroid hormone levels, but with serum calcium levels in a normal range. Keating's data for serum phosphorus demonstrate that a lowering usually occurs in hyperparathyroidism and is of help in diagnosis, but the serum phosphorus levels are often within the 95% confidence limits for normal people. An elevated serum calcium concentration is the most reliable bit of information to obtain in establishing the diagnosis of hyperparathyroidism.

A high phosphorus diet can result in a rise in serum phosphorus, a lowering of serum calcium, and a decrease in urinary calcium so that the diagnosis of hyperparathyroidism may be overlooked. If hypercalcemia is suspected, but not found, the diet should be looked into, and all milk and milk products eliminated for at least three days before repeating serum analyses. The number of determinations of serum calcium and phosphorus required to establish hypercalcemia will depend upon the degree of elevation of the serum calcium, the reliability of the laboratory, and the number of other signs, symptoms, and laboratory abnormalities which contribute to the diagnosis. In situations where the major weight of the laboratory contribution is based on mildly abnormal serum calcium and phosphorus levels, it may be necessary to obtain half a dozen elevated serum calciums over a period of some weeks or months in order to be certain that a persistent and significant hypercalcemia does in fact exist. A tentative diagnosis of hypercalcemia should be retained over a period of 6 to 12 months before it is discarded. Repeated normal serum calcium and phosphorus levels are needed to allow one to discard the diagnosis if several elevated serum calcium levels have been reported at some other stage of the study. There often is variation in serum calcium and phosphorus levels. If the patient's values are borderline abnormal, an excellent laboratory becomes absolutely essential. An unreliable laboratory can be the cause of great expense and confusion and may lead physicians to such a feeling of hopelessness in the diagnosis of milder degrees of hyperparathyroidism that bona fide disease will be missed.

FINDING AND PROVING THE CAUSE

Once the presence of hypercalcemia has been established and the possibility of hyperparathyroidism comes into question, there are a number of other diseases that should be looked for and, insofar as possible, ruled out before subjecting the patient to an exploration of parathyroid tissue. The surgeon who operates on a patient for hyperparathyroidism may be obligated to spend a number of hours searching for the parathyroid bodies and he should therefore be convinced that the patient has hypercalcemia, that the cause is overactivity of parathyroids, and that other causes of hypercalcemia have been ruled out. If all parathyroid bodies are not identified at the time of a first operation, the consequent scar tissue will make any subsequent exploration much more difficult.

Excessive intake of vitamin D, sarcoid, immobilization (particularly of children or of patients with Paget's disease), and hyperthyroidism can all result in high serum calcium levels. Parathyroid hormone-producing cancers have already been mentioned; these are most commonly carcinoma of the lung and kidney. Other malignancies can cause hypercalcemia, simply by increasing the rate of bone destruction; included in this category are multiple myeloma, prostatic carcinoma, breast carcinoma, or any other malignancies with extensive bone metastases. Chronic renal disease, the milk-alkali syndrome, or osteomalacia may be present alone or together with hyperparathyroidism to further confuse the interpretation of laboratory data. In chronic renal disease, as excretion of phosphorus is decreased and serum phosphorus levels rise, the serum calcium tends to fall. A patient with hyperparathyroidism may have symptoms of duodenal ulcer which he treats with milk and calcium carbonate or other absorbable alkalis. A patient with milk-alkali syndrome and normal parathyroids should, when placed on aluminum hydroxide antacids and with elimination of milk and absorbable alkalis for a time, have a return of serum calcium and phosphorus levels to normal as the alkalosis is corrected. If hypercalcemia and low serum phosphorus levels persist, then it may well be that the patient also has hyperparathyroidism and that the suspected milk-alkali syndrome was superimposed.

Patients with prolonged vitamin D insufficiency may develop osteomalacia and low serum calcium levels with consequent stimulation of the parathyroid glands until these glands become hyperplastic and a secondary type of hyperparathyroidism exists. On the other hand, primary hyperparathyroidism may lead to osteomalacia, in the presence of vitamin D insufficiency. By contrast, in a patient with hyperparathyroidism who has a normal or excessive vitamin D intake, the response is more likely to be osteitis fibrosa cystica.

A plasma protein electrophoresis pattern will serve to rule out multiple myeloma and Boeck's sarcoid. Roentgenograms of the lung and intravenous pyelography will help to rule out primary carcinomas of the lung and kidney as well as metastatic neoplasm. Serum alkaline phosphatase may be elevated if the patient with hyperparathyroidism has significant bone disease. In the case of carcinoma of the prostate, the serum acid phosphatase may be diagnostic. Roentgenograms of the skeleton may reveal metastatic bone disease, osteomalacia, or osteitis fibrosa cystica. In hyperparathyroidism the outer ends of the clavicles are often decalcified. X-rays of the hand may show disintegration of the distal phalanges with disappearance of the phalangeal tuft and subperiosteal erosion, particularly of the middle phalanges. The lamina dura may be missing. In about half of the patients with roentgenographic evidence of bone changes, the changes are diffuse decalcification. The skull may give a ground glass appearance. Occasionally punched out areas are seen where masses of hyperplastic osteoclastic tissue have completely destroyed bone. Bone biopsy may on occasion be needed to rule out malignancy. Excessive osteoclastic activity of hyperparathyroidism is also evident in a bone biopsy. Diffuse multiple myeloma may be confused with osteomalacia if it is not considered and ruled out.

Because of the action of parathyroid hormone on the kidneys, special attention must be given to renal function. Creatinine clearance, when reduced to 30% of normal or less, should suggest the possibility of secondary hyperparathyroidism. On the other hand, a patient with long-standing hyperparathyroidism may have sufficient impairment of renal function to reduce the creatinine clearance to this level. In the presence of renal insufficiency, special tests of renal phosphate excretion are of little use in the differential diagnosis between hyperparathyroidism and primary renal disease. If the renal function is adequate, then a determination of phosphate excretion is helpful, and the simplest test is a serum phosphorus level. If a patient has established hypercalcemia and repeated serum phosphorus levels that are below normal, this may be sufficient evidence that the tubules are failing to reabsorb phosphorus under the stimulation of excessive parathyroid hormone. There are a number of conditions which should be considered, however, in which serum phosphorus levels may be abnormally low. Prime examples are dietary deficiency, alcoholism, and malabsorption. Antacids which bind phosphorus interfere with the absorption of phosphorus and could result in a low serum level. Patients with a vitamin D-resistant rickets and patients with the hypophosphatemic glycosuric osteomalacia or Fanconi syndrome, as well as patients with idiopathic hypercalciuria, may have low serum phosphorus levels. The latter condition may be due to hyperparathyroidism and require serum parathormone analysis. Hypophosphatemic osteomalacia was observed by Salassa et al. in 2 adult patients with small benign sclerosing hemangiomas. Removal of the tumors caused a dramatic restoration of normal serum phosphate levels, relief of symptoms, and recalcification of bone. These patients did not have elevation of the serum calcium concentration and the serum parathyroid hormone immunoreactive assay was negative before and normal after removal of the tumor in the second patient.

Parathyroid hormone inhibits tubular reabsorption of phosphate and Avioli, Gordon et al., and Krementz et al. have reviewed the use of this as a test for hyperparathyroidism. If tubular reabsorption of phosphorus is to be determined, the test should be performed before the administration of cortisone. Abnormalities of phosphate reabsorption are demonstrated most frequently when the patient has a high phosphate intake, as with a diet containing approximately 1.5 gm of phosphorus and with administration of an additional 1.5 gm of phosphate as sodium phosphate in divided doses by mouth each day. The tubular reabsorption of phosphate is usually less than 60% in patients with hyperparathyroidism. The normal reabsorption is 85 to 90%. If the serum phosphorus level is 1.5 mg/100 ml, then an 80% reabsorption is abnormally low. Serum phosphorus level and phosphorus intake should be known, and the investigator should have experience in the conduct and interpretation of the test if tubular reabsorption of phosphorus is to be of use in diagnosis.

A modification of the above test is sometimes used in which an intravenous infusion of calcium serves to raise the concentration of serum calcium, thereby reduce the output of parathyroid hormone, and consequently remove the inhibitory effect of parathyroid hormone on tubular reabsorption of phosphorus. Normally responsive parathyroids would cause urinary phosphorus to decrease following the infusion of calcium. This test is more likely to be of use in the diagnosis of hyperparathyroidism when serum calciums are near the normal range. Having established the diagnosis of hyperparathyroidism, the calcium infusion test might be expected to distinguish between primary and secondary hyperparathyroidism and between adenoma and hyperplasia. In other words, the test should help to determine if parathyroid function is responsive to changing levels of serum calcium or if the parathyroid secretion is autonomous as in an adenoma. Actually patients with primary hyperparathyroidism due to a single adenoma do not show a decrease in concentration of serum parathormone when calcium is infused, whereas patients with hyperplasia demonstrate a lowering of serum parathormone levels according to Reiss. However, change in urine phosphorus excretion following calcium infusion is not a very helpful diagnostic test in hyperparathyroidism.

Urine calcium is often measured in these patients. Hypercalciuria is present in hyperparathyroidism because of the high serum calcium levels even though the actual effect of parathyroid hormone on the kidney is to increase tubular reabsorption of calcium. Early in the course of hyperparathyroidism before the serum calcium has risen much above normal, the urine calcium excretion may be abnormally low. Later in the course of the disease, as there is a decrease in glomerular filtration rate, the urinary calcium excretion may again be low. The normal urinary calcium is less than 100 mg per day. With normal glomerular filtration and high serum calcium levels more than 250 mg of calcium will be excreted in the urine per day. Such a patient will have a serum calcium above the normal range, and a serum phosphorus below the normal range, and the hypercalciuria does not add anything to the evidence for probable parathyroid overactivity. Keating considered that a 24-hour urinary calcium in excess of 500 mg suggested sarcoid or malignancy rather than hyperparathyroidism.

A urinary calcium of 150 to 200 mg/day is suggestive of hyperparathyroidism, and between 200 and 500 mg/day of urinary calcium is usually indicative of hyperparathyroidism. The test is not sufficiently reliable, however, to justify the expense of hospitalization and maintenance of the patient on a 125-mg calcium diet for three days if there are other indices of hyperparathyroidism. In 1958 Henneman defined a condition of idiopathic hypercalciuria which may be a form of hyperparathyroidism. Shieber et al. in 1971 reported ten such patients with urinary calcium of more than 250 mg/24 hours while the patient was receiving a diet containing 800 mg calcium per day and with normal serum calcium concentrations, normal or low serum phosphorus levels, and tubular reabsorption of phosphate levels below 75%. These patients who had suffered from renal colic were relieved of symptoms, had an elevation of serum phosphorus, a slight drop in serum calcium, and a rise in tubular reabsorption of phosphorus after removal of 3.5 parathyroid glands. In four patients on whom serum parathyroid hormone assay was performed, the levels were above normal before and normal after operation. In six patients on whom electron microscopy was performed the glands were hyperfunctional. The high urine calcium excretion was an important indication of hyperparathyroidism in these patients.

The administration of 50 mg of hydrocortisone every 8 hours for 10 days, as described by Dent, will cause suppression of serum calcium levels in many of the conditions that cause hypercalcemia other than hyperparathyroidism. Of course, if the patient has a neoplasm which is producing parathyroid hormone, suppression might not occur. This test is not completely reliable, and it requires a number of days for its effect in some patients. If the patient has a high serum calcium level and there is any urgency about controlling the hypercalcemia, the test probably should not be attempted.

Immunoassay of parathyroid hormone as used by Berson and Yalow, Reiss and Canterbury, and Arnaud et al. would seem to be the most specific way of diagnosing hyperparathyroidism. It still is necessary to measure serum calcium, however, since patients with secondary hyperparathyroidism have very high serum parathyroid hormone levels but low concentrations of serum calcium. The highest levels of parathyroid hormone in serum have been found in patients with chronic uremia. If hypercalcemia is due to some other cause like metastatic bone disease, the serum parathyroid hormone concentration will be suppressed. The combination of serum calcium and parathormone level becomes diagnostic when both are elevated as shown by Arnaud et al.

Mild elevation of parathyroid hormone has been observed in patients with carcinoma of the lung. The serum parathyroid hormone levels in adenoma and hyperplasia of the parathyroid are somewhat higher than with nonparathyroid, parathormone-secreting neoplasms and generally somewhat lower than in patients with chronic renal insufficiency. Autonomy of the parathyroids can be determined by the infusion of calcium intravenously and simultaneous measurement of serum calcium and parathyroid hormone. Reiss has observed that parathyroid glands that are hyperplastic still are under the influence of serum calcium levels. Reiss has also been able to determine the side of the neck where an adenoma is located by measuring serum parathyroid hormone levels before and after compression of one side of the neck. Ackerman and Winder have had help in localizing hyperparathyroid tissue to one side of the neck in two patients by sampling venous blood at multiple sites and having Berson and Yalow analyze the samples for parathormone.

Serum parathyroid hormone levels should be of value in the long-term follow-up of patients where there is any question about the possible persistence of hyperplastic parathyroid tissue. Our patient, who was operated upon in 1929 and again in 1943 with supposed adenomas removed each time and who died of renal failure 17 years after his first adenoma was removed, would certainly have benefited if he could have had serum parathyroid hormone analyses early in the course of his disease and if he could have had the additional overactive parathyroid tissue removed before irreversible renal damage. The complexity of the problem was illustrated by a patient followed by Seldin and Castleman 18 years after the removal of a parathyroid adenoma. They had looked at and biopsied the other parathyroids and thought they ruled out hyperplasia, but the patient may have had sufficient renal disease so that with progressive renal insufficiency he finally developed secondary parathyroid hyperplasia. On the other hand, perhaps this was adenomatous hyperplasia from the beginning. The final diagnostic tests need to be performed over a period of years following extirpation of parathyroid adenomas and hyperplastic tissue, since the pathologist frequently cannot distinguish between adenoma and hyperplasia.

The vicissitudes of diagnosis and management have been discussed by Cope (1961) in a review of 47 patients. Thirty patients were explored for suspected hyperparathyroidism, but abnormal parathyroid tissue was not found. Seventeen patients were operated upon for other reasons. The latter experience led to the diagnosis of pseudohyperparathyroidism, vitamin D-resistant rickets, the milk-alkali syndrome, and idiopathic hypercalciuria with formation of renal stones. Cope, Barnes et al. mentioned the confusion that may arise between hyperparathyroidism and sarcoid. Sarcoid can infiltrate the bones of the hands and feet and provide x-ray changes which are most difficult to distinguish from those of hyperparathyroidism. The patients with sarcoid are disproportionately ill for the mild elevation of serum calcium. This is one situation in which bone biopsy could be helpful. There is at least one report of a patient with both sarcoid and hyperparathyroidism, and recently I was surprised to find nontuberculous granuloma in cervical lymph nodes removed during exploration and removal of a parathyroid adenoma from a patient with severe diabetes and chronic renal insufficiency.

Fraser and co-workers have used discriminant analysis to find linear combinations of commonly obtained laboratory data which, when properly weighted, would give maximum separation of different groups of patients. Two functions were developed and nomograms provided for their rapid determination. These two functions were then plotted on Cartesian coordinates. The first discriminant was influenced most by inorganic phosphate and urea and separated patients in the horizontal axis on the basis of renal function. The second discriminant separated patients vertically, primarily on the basis of alkaline phosphatase, and identified patients with bone disease as a separate group. In developing the discriminants some 87 patients were used from a retrospective study. In a prospective study the analysis was then evaluated, and in 90.4% of patients the authors were able to assign, by this analytic approach, the same diagnosis that had been reached by the physicians through their more detailed clinical study. Where problem cases arise, both approaches have pitfalls because they are basically similar, but the discriminant equation is an objective way to tie data together in formulating a diagnosis, providing the laboratory methods and circumstances are unchanged between the development of the equation from a retrospective study and the prospective application.

TREATMENT

The susceptibility of the kidney to calcification was demonstrated by Carone by giving parathyroid extract to dogs so as to maintain serum calcium levels between 13 and 18.8 mg/100 ml for 24 hours. This produced a severe impairment of renal concentrating ability, a decrease in glomerular filtration rate, and an elevation of blood urea nitrogen. The nephrons were then dissected out in dilute hydrochloric acid, and it was observed that there were lesions in the ascending limb of Henle, distal convolution and the collecting system with patchy degeneration of the epithelium, calcification, necrosis, and obstructing casts. Such observations and the knowledge that occasional patients with hyperparathyroidism develop progressive renal disease which may be lethal long after parathyroidectomy would seem to argue for treatment of hyperparathyroidism, even when it is asymptomatic, if the serum calcium levels are consistently above 11.5 mg/100 ml. A 19-year-old man was operated upon for severe osteitis fibrosa cystica by Frank Peterson at the University of Iowa Hospitals in 1929, and a parathyroid adenoma was removed. The patient had another adenoma removed in 1943 because of recurrent hypercalcemia and finally died in 1946 from uremia which was a consequence of renal damage from prolonged hypercalcemia. This patient was reported by Boyd et al. and was one of the earliest instances of removal of an adenoma. The subsequent course demonstrated the dangers of prolonged hypercalcemia and also raised the question of whether adenomas are simple, multiple, or a part of adenomatous hyperplasia. We are still searching for answers to these questions.

Indications for exploration of the neck vary in urgency from patients whose mild asymptomatic hypercalcemia is found during screening laboratory tests to patients whose hypercalcemia is so severe as to threaten life. The big question today is what to do with patients who have mild hypercalcemia without signs or symptoms of bone, renal, or other organ system abnormality. Hyperparathyroidism is like an iceberg which was first noticed in 1926 and has progressively risen in the waters of medical practice. We see now that it is a common disease. How can we select those patients for operative treatment who are destined to develop severe bone and renal disease? Probably patients with serum calcium levels between normal and 11.0 mg/100 ml should be followed for a few years if this is the only manifestation of parathyroid overactivity. Purnell et al. are following 171 patients, and after 30 months only 13.8% had required operative treatment. The reasons for operating upon 21 of these patients rather than continuing observation were listed: appearance of metabolically active stone disease in 5, decreasing renal function in 5, increasing serum calcium in 4, roentgenologic change in 2, psychologic problems in 2, and reconsideration of the original classification into the provisional group in 3. These last 3 actually had serum calciums between 11.0 and 11.5 mg/100 ml, and the authors felt that on this basis alone they should have been operated upon earlier instead of followed. The expense and inconvenience of prolonged and repeated studies are another reason for advising operation in some patients.

Hodgkinson et al. followed 12 patients with serum calciums which were less than 11.5 mg/100 ml, and over a period of 5 years only one patient was finally advised to have an operation. The others had no rise in serum calcium levels and no evidence of bone or renal disease. They suggested that postmenopausal osteoporosis might increase the indication for operation. In a group of 57 patients treated between 1929 and 1972 at the University of Iowa, the median age for 35 women was 51 years as compared with a median age of 38 in the 22 men. Senile osteoporosis may be an incorrect diagnosis in some patients and another area where our increasing awareness of hyperparathyroidism could improve medical care. At the present time patients without signs or symptoms of active renal or bone disease and with serum calcium levels that remain below 11.0 or 11.5 mg/100 ml (the exact cut-off level is still arbitrary) represent a relatively large group, who could be operated upon or followed, or randomized into a prospective cooperative study. The latter approach in some of the centers would eventually provide some basis for recommending a plan of management. It is unlikely that parathyroid crisis would develop in such a group of patients who were being followed every 3 months.

PARATHYROID CRISIS

At the other end of the scale from patients with asymptomatic and mild hypercalcemia are the patients with toxic levels of serum calcium. Fortunately the condition is infrequent and should be even less frequent as we learn to recognize and treat hyperparathyroidism during its early and milder stages. The recognition of parathyroid crisis is more common now than the recognition of thyroid crisis, analogous to the increasing importance of hyperparathyroidism and the decreasing requirement for surgical treatment of thyroid disease. In 1926 Collup produced death in dogs by administration of parathyroid extract according to Payne and Fitchett, who in 1965 reviewed 70 instances of parathyroid crisis reported in the medical literature. This is a true emergency, and the diagnosis is made when the serum calcium rises above 15 mg/100 ml (7.5 mEq/l; 3.75 mM/l). In the presence of hypoproteinemia or acidosis, a lower total serum calcium level may still be toxic. Some writers have listed the critical level for serum calcium at 17 mg/100 ml. A rapid rise in serum calcium concentration is also important as well as rapid change in the patient's general condition, with increasing symptoms of abdominal pain, anorexia, nausea, confusion, and loss of memory. Just as all of the signs and symptoms of hypercalcemia are exaggerated in parathyroid crisis, so are the complications more frequent. More of the patients have pancreatitis and symptoms of ulcer disease. Because high calcium levels interfere with renal concentration, a renal type of diabetes insipidus is present, and the patient is dehydrated.

It is important to rule out high doses of vitamin D as the cause and to obtain x-rays which might reveal metastatic malignancy or provide confirmation of hyperparathyroidism from changes in the bones of the hands, the clavicles, and skull. However, a delay in diagnosis for the sake of carrying out a wide variety of elaborate special laboratory tests is not justified. Deterioration in a patient's condition may accelerate with the development of high fever and rising blood urea nitrogen, or the patient may die suddenly. Since the recognition of this condition and the realization of the need for an early search for the offending parathyroid tissue, the most common cause of death in parathyroid crisis has been a failure to find the adenoma at the time of operation. A patient may have symptoms for some time, and the hypercalcemic crisis may be precipitated by the treatment of abdominal symptoms with milk and absorbable antacids. Crisis may come on suddenly. This suggests necrosis of a parathyroid adenoma with release of larger amounts of parathyroid hormone. A fairly large adenoma is usually present, and usually such patients have had a long history of symptoms but their symptoms have not been recognized as being due to hypercalcemia.

Boquist et al. described a patient whose admission was for acute cholecystitis. Because of mental confusion, vomiting, and weakness in the right arm and leg, a search was made for some lesion in the central nervous system. Echoencephalography and examination of the eye grounds revealed no abnormality. The serum calcium was 15.4 mg/100 ml and the phosphorus 2.1 mg/100 ml. A 3-cm diameter adenoma of the parathyroid was removed from behind the left lower pole of the thyroid. Later a cholecystectomy was performed, and the diagnosis of cholecystitis was confirmed. The patient remained in serious condition and finally died. The simultaneous presence of two conditions, both of which are of an urgent nature, could be coincidental. Recently Selle et al. studied all of their patients who had been treated for hyperparathyroidism and found a high incidence of gallstones. A patient who is asymptomatic and maintaining hydration might become symptomatic when some other condition prevents an adequate water intake. In patients who vomit and are unable to take fluid by mouth, dehydration, hypokalemia, and alkalosis may add to the fluid and electrolyte imbalance.

PREOPERATIVE TREATMENT OF CRISIS

The initial emphasis in preparing a patient with parathyroid crisis for operation should be on rehydration and expansion of the extracellular fluid in order to correct existing deficits but also to prepare the way for diuresis and an increased rate of calcium excretion. Sodium and calcium are both reabsorbed from the proximal convoluted tubule and from the ascending limb of Henle's loop. Suki and others have reviewed and compared the various treatments available for hypercalcemia and have outlined a treatment with large doses of furosemide, close monitoring of urine volume and electrolytes, and accurate replacement, except for calcium. Eight patients with initial serum calcium levels between 12.3 and 18.4 mg/100 ml were treated. In three patients the serum calcium was returned to near normal. In one patient the levels were reduced from an initial 18.4 to a final 14.6 mg/100 ml, and in another patient from an initial 18.0 to a final 14.8 mg/100 ml. From 0.7 to 2.7 gm of calcium were lost in the urine. There was considerable loss of magnesium. The mean furosemide dose level was 1240 mg given in amounts of 80 to 100 mg every one or two hours. The urine volumes were monitored hourly. A solution of four parts 0.9% saline and one part 5% glucose with the addition of 20 mEq/l of potassium chloride was infused at a rate equal to the rate of urine loss. Frequent measurements of body weight are of assistance whenever such large volumes of fluid are exchanged. They found that the amount of calcium excreted greatly exceeded the calcium theoretically present in extracellular fluid which would be consistent with ongoing release of calcium from the bones. In the presence of severe bone disease it may not be possible to reduce the serum calcium even by a diuresis of 20 liters a day. In such a patient we used phosphate infusion followed by an emergency operation.

The most immediate danger of hypercalcemia is probably its effect upon myocardial contractility and nerve conduction. There is also the danger of calcification of soft tissues if the product of serum calcium and phosphorus is excessive. A treatment which lowers the serum calcium by causing increased excretion in the urine would seem to be ideal for the immediate emergency situation. Any safe and effective method for correction of extreme hypercalcemia would seem to make the surgeon's position easier. Smith et al. in 1963 and Henley in 1964 reviewed the published cases from 1939 when Hanes first described parathyroid crisis, and they found that 25 of 38 patients had died. They concluded that hyperparathyroid crisis was a genuine surgical emergency, and that fever and a rising blood urea nitrogen added to the urgency rather than contraindicating an operation. Coffey et al. in 1965 reported two patients who died before operation and again emphasized that parathyroid crisis requires an emergency operation. The surgeon not only was forced into an emergency exploration but was made aware of the fatal outcome should he fail to find the offending adenoma. In 1966 Boyle and Mason reported such an unsuccessful exploration in a patient who died soon after the operation and in whom a mediastinal adenoma was quite evident at autopsy.

The possibility of an emergency treatment for hypercalcemic crisis which would allow for a scheduled operation was greeted with enthusiasm in 1966. Goldsmith and Ingbar in 1966 presented a series of patients whose hypercalcemia was corrected by treatment with phosphate. There may be a relative deficit of phosphate as a result of loss through the kidney under the stimulation of excessive levels of parathyroid hormone. Albright et al. in 1932 classified hyperparathyroidism as producing an anomalous saturation with very high serum calcium levels and abnormally low serum phosphorus levels so that the serum phosphorus capacity was unfulfilled. Albright (1932) observed that the administration of phosphate caused an increase in the threshold for calcium in the kidney and a decrease in calcium excretion. He warned of the danger of converting an anomalous saturation to supersaturation in that, if the serum phosphorus level rose in excess of a fall of serum calcium concentration, then deposits of calcium phosphate could be expected in the lung, stomach, kidney, thyroid, and other areas, similar to the situation in poisoning with excessive doses of vitamin D. He also warned of the danger of calcium phosphate stones in the renal collecting system, since phosphate excretion increases tremendously when additional phosphate is given either orally or intravenously.

Eisenberg has studied the effect of intravenous phosphate on serum strontium and calcium, and his data suggest that calcium phosphate must be deposited in areas other than bone, because of the rapidity with which it disappears from the blood and the rapidity with which the strontium tag reappears following such treatment. Probably, as the saturation of body fluids for calcium and phosphorus is increased, calcium phosphate is deposited in soft tissues and is then taken up by histiocytes. This has certain dangers, but may be a lesser evil than a high serum calcium, provided the renal output is high. It would appear that the treatment of hypercalcemia with phosphate is probably safe if the serum phosphorus levels are low, and if in the course of treatment the calcium decreases enough so that the product of calcium and phosphorus does not rise greatly above normal. Herbert et al. have recently confirmed the hypothesis of Albright, however, that the fall in calcium concentration bears a linear relationship to the product of the concentrations of calcium and phosphorus, suggesting that any effect obtained by phosphate infusion must result in precipitation in either bone or soft tissues. There is real danger in the use of phosphate infusions. Kahil et al. and Breidahl et al. have recommended phosphate infusion. Breuer and LeBauer have emphasized caution in its use. All who have had experience with it including Goldsmith and Ingbar have recommended that the *initial* dose be limited to 50 millimoles, although 100 millimoles over each 8-hour period may be required. In a patient who has some renal insufficiency and where the serum phosphorus level is normal or even slightly high, at a time when the serum calcium level is high, phosphate infusion is contraindicated. Another danger of intravenous phosphate is in its very effectiveness. There have been reports of hypocalcemia.

Intravenous isotonic sodium sulfate given at the rate of 200 ml/hr will cause a marked increase in urinary calcium and lowering of serum calcium. Sulfate is nonreabsorbable in the tubule and complexes with calcium so that the latter ion is removed, in contrast to phosphate, which actually decreases urinary calcium. Sulfate might therefore be safer for use over a longer period of time. Chakmakjian and Bethune found sodium sulfate to be effective in lowering elevated serum calcium in all of the 13 patients they studied.

Thyrocalcitonin might become a preferred drug management of toxic hypercalcemia in selected patients. Pak et al. used this approach. West et al. prepared a rapid test with a single injection, followed by a more prolonged infusion in those patients who showed a lowering of serum calcium in response to the rapid dose. Thyrocalcitonin inhibits bone resorption and should be most effective in patients whose hypercalcemia is caused by active bone disease. Haddad and Avioli found an additive effect of thyrocalcitonin and phosphate in counteracting the hypercalcemic effect of parathyroid hormone in rats, suggesting that perhaps a combination of these two methods would be of use in patients whose dangerously high serum calcium is associated with a very low serum phosphorus level. As with the use of phosphate alone, the management would require very close monitoring and cautious use of these agents. The metabolic clearance rate of porcine calcitonin is high, according to Riggs et al., so that the effect of a test dose should not be prolonged.

Brown and Kennedy found that mithramycin would lower serum calcium levels in normal people as well as in patients with hypercalcemia from bone metastases. Slayton et al. and Elias et al. have been successful in controlling toxic levels of hypercalcemia with a few doses of mithramycin, 25 mg/kg body weight given as bolus intravenous injections once a day. This is a lower dose than is required for cancer chemotherapy, but it is effective in hyperparathyroidism. Kennedy et al. found that mithramycin inhibits bone resorption in animals.

None of the measures used for the emergency treatment of hypercalcemia solves the underlying problem, and early operation is still a most important part of the treatment of parathyroid crisis. Continued use of intravenous phosphates for control of hypercalcemia may lead to extensive soft-tissue calcification and renal failure and may, therefore, cease to be either an effective or a safe emergency treatment. It is desirable to restore the serum calcium level to normal but at the same time to have the patient properly hydrated and in good balance as far as the other electrolytes are concerned when the operation is undertaken.

OPERATIVE MANAGEMENT OF CRISIS

Usually the cause of toxic hyperparathyroidism is a large adenoma, and most of these are found in the neck. If they are in the superior mediastinum, they will usually be in relation to the thymus, and there is often a large vascular pedicle extending down from the inferior thyroid artery to the adenoma. If the adenoma and the other parathyroid glands cannot be found, one and then the other lobe of the thyroid should be removed and sliced into multiple sections. If after removing the thyroid and all of the tissue between the carotid sheaths and the trachea, the adenoma still has not been found, then the mediastinum should be opened with a sternal splitting incision and an extensive search made. This is in contrast to the usual sequence in non-toxic patients in whom a cervical exploration is carried out on one day, and if the responsible parathyroids are not found, then a mediastinal exploration is carried out later as a separate operation. In an operation performed for parathyroid crisis the patient will probably die if the adenoma is not found, and delay of mediastinal exploration is not justified. Actually there are only about 5% of instances where the parathyroid adenoma cannot be found from the cervical approach.

There have been instances in which infarction of the parathyroid adenoma has caused crisis and subsequent early regression of symptoms and signs of hyperparathyroidism because of massive infarction of the gland. There have been instances reported where an adenoma was successfully removed, but the patient did not recover. In most cases the prognosis is directly related to the success of the exploration. If the adenoma is found and removed, the patient will be cured. If the adenoma is not found, the patient will die.

OPERATIVE PROCEDURE

Cope has described the operative approach to hyperparathyroidism on the basis of the embryology, and his description, published in 1941, should be consulted by any surgeon who is planning to perform these operations. Usually the four parathyroid glands are symmetrically placed along the posterior borders of the thyroid lobes. The uppermost parathyroids which embryologically arise from the fourth branchial pouch are to be found above the level of the inferior thyroid artery and usually slightly above the point at which the recurrent laryngeal nerve disappears into the larynx. The lowermost parathyroids which emerge from the third branchial pouch and which descend in the neck with the thymus are usually located slightly below the inferior thyroid artery and near and behind the recurrent laryngeal nerves. They may be located somewhat more caudad at the upper end of the thymus in juxtaposition to or even incorporated into the capsule or substance of the thymus. Over the years, it has become evident that many of these patients have adenomatous hyperplasia rather than single adenomas. It is therefore important to search for and identify all four parathyroid bodies.

If any of the glands is more than 5 mm in diameter, it probably is abnormal and should be removed. If a large adenoma is found and the other glands appear normal, then probably only the adenoma should be removed. Apparently, in some instances, there is a diffuse adenomatous hyperplasia even though only one gland is markedly increased in size. The parathyroid glands which are left behind should be marked by placing a metal clip close by, but placed so as not to interfere with the blood supply of the gland. If none of the glands is markedly enlarged, then three and a half glands should be removed. In the effort to cure the patient of hyperparathyroidism the patient should not be made deficient in parathyroid tissue. A major portion of a normal parathyroid must always be preserved with adequate blood supply. It should be biopsied and identified by frozen section. This conscious act will prevent eventual hypoparathyroidism if the last remaining parathyroid is finally identified and found to be an adenoma. Do not remove three normal-sized and grossly normal-appearing glands on the thesis that they may be hyperplastic, when a fourth gland cannot be found. The gland to be preserved should be biopsied before any other glands are removed so as to be as certain as possible of the viability and identity of this most important single gland. Prior to the concern about hyperplasia and more frequent subtotal parathyroidectomy this was less often a problem. Now we must prevent the creation of hypoparathyroidism which would be an unfortunate trade for hyperparathyroidism, especially if the latter is asymptomatic.

Cope observed a relationship between calcium levels and size of the parathyroid adenoma. If the calcium level is mildly elevated, between 11 and 12 mg/100 ml, any adenoma found is likely to be small, especially now with the increased number of asymptomatic patients found by screening. It is quite possible that the problem will be adenomatous hyperplasia. It may even be hyperplasia of a sort which is identifiable only by electron microscopy. If the blood calcium level is 14 mg/100 ml or higher, it can be anticipated that an adenoma weighing over 5.0 gm will be found. The possibility of hyperplasia of remaining parathyroids is not ruled out, however, by finding a large adenoma. At least biopsy should be performed on all of the parathyroid tissue found, and any parathyroid glands which appear to be enlarged should be removed.

The preoperative localization of parathyroids by some chemical compound in which radioactive materials are incorporated would greatly facilitate the diagnosis and treatment of these patients. At the moment there is no compound which is adequate to the challenge. Radioactive selenium in selenomethionine has been used, but the concentration in parathyroid tissue is not high enough so that the parathyroid tissue can be easily identified as separate from surrounding tissues. For intraoperative identification of parathyroid tissue, toluidine blue has been used. So far efforts to tag toluidine blue with radioactive iodine in order to provide a means of preoperative external scanning have not worked out. Apparently the addition of the iodine to the toluidine blue changes properties of the latter so that it no longer localizes in parathyroid tissue. Klopper and Moe observed in 1964 that toluidine blue stained the parathyroid and pancreas. Hurvitz et al. in 1967 reported its use in experiments in animals and in patients. Owens et al. in 1968 have also found this of use in patients. We have found it to be of help. The parathyroids are stained a darker blue than the thyroid and other tissues.

The dose is 5 to 10 mg/kg of body weight. It is made up as a 1% solution in saline and should be allowed to sit over night, because of the low solubility. It is then filtered and autoclaved at 105° C for 10 minutes. The material is added to 300 ml of normal saline and infused over a period of one hour at approximately 80 drops per minute, during which time the patient's electrocardiogram is observed for prolongation of the PQ interval, elevation of the ST segment, or inversion of T-waves. The toxicity of the material is such that higher doses should not be used. Direct injection into the arterial circulation of the parathyroids has been attempted in order to try to obtain more intense staining and to obviate some of the systemic effects. The result of this has been transient recurrent nerve paralysis. Yeager and Krementz have demonstrated a decrease in nerve conduction from toluidine blue. Postoperatively patients with toluidine blue injections have a bluish tinge to the skin which may be alarming to the nursing staff if they are not warned. The bluish discoloration will leave more quickly if the patient is given mannitol and additional fluids to promote a diuresis.

Carcinoma of the parathyroid is rare. Holmes found 50 instances reported in the literature as of 1969. A fibrous inflammatory reaction around the enlarged gland with adherence to surrounding structures should rouse suspicion of carcinoma.

POSTOPERATIVE CARE

Patients with bone disease, especially those with a markedly elevated alkaline phosphatase, may have a rapid return of calcium and phosphorus to bone with resultant tetany during the postoperative period. Mild hypocalcemia requires no immediate treatment. Calcium gluconate can be given intravenously to relieve the symptoms, but in order that repeated injections not be required it is preferable to add 50 ml of 10% calcium gluconate to a liter of isotonic saline and to infuse this at whatever rate is necessary to relieve the tetany. Such an infusion may need to be continued for a number of days.

Where the bone disease is extensive and it appears that prolonged treatment may be required, the patient should be managed in the same way that a patient with permanent hypoparathyroidism is managed, with high doses of vitamin D. This will be required only temporarily until parathyroid function returns to normal and until the bones have been partially recalcified. The patient should learn to perform the urinary Sulkowitch test and report back at any time that newsprint cannot be read through the test tube containing the mixture of equal parts of urine and Sulkowitch reagent. The Sulkowitch test is not reliable for detection of a low serum calcium, but it is helpful in avoiding vitamin D toxicity. In addition to the Sulkowitch test, the patient should have periodic serum calcium and phosphorus determinations. Very few patients require vitamin D, even though they may have tetany in the early days following removal of an adenoma. Long-term follow-up is indicated because of the possibility of abnormal function in remaining parathyroid tissue.

There has been an increasing need for something other than change in serum calcium and phosphorus levels to use as an index of the success or failure of operation. This is because the glands are often hyperplastic and a definite single large adenoma is not found. There are also some patients with normocalcemic hyperparathyroidism whose problem is one of repeated passage of stones. Goldsmith, Gall, et al. have used urinary phosphorus excretion and find that if the postoperative value per day decreases to less than 150 mg or to less than 20% of the preoperative level then one can be fairly sure that the cause of hyperparathyroidism has been found and corrected. This does not assure us that there will never be a recurrence of hyperparathyroidism and long-term follow-up is still indicated.

Recurrent hypercalcemia in a patient with carcinoma of the parathyroid has been successfully treated with 10-day courses of calcitonin. The effect has lasted considerably longer than the treatment. Knill-Jones et al. restored calcium levels to normal by hepatectomy and liver transplant for a parathormone-producing hepatoma. In most instances parathormone-producing neoplasmas are difficult or impossible to eradicate. It is possible that a patient with hypernephroma or with a localized carcinoma of the lung might be successfully treated by excision of the parathormone-secreting neoplasm.

SECONDARY AND TERTIARY HYPERPARATHYROIDISM

There are estimated to be around 22,000 new patients with chronic renal disease diagnosed each year, and there are increasing numbers of chronic dialysis programs in medical centers and for treatment of these patients in their homes. Buck and Robertson estimate that 80% of patients on a chronic dialysis program have spontaneous renal osteodystrophy from hypocalcemia and secondary hyperplasia of parathyroids. Patients with chronic renal disease have impairment of metabolism of vitamin D in the intestine and in other tissues so that the bones tend to develop osteomalacia initially. Later, under the stimulation of increased levels of parathyroid hormone, the typical lesions of osteitis fibrosa cystica appear. Soft-tissue calcification occurs and because of calcium crystals in skin, some patients are incapacitated by pruritus. If a successful kidney transplant can be provided, these changes are usually reversed, but if the chronic dialysis program is to be continued longer than 6 months, these patients need subtotal or total parathyroidectomy. Eilert et al. reviewed an experience with 75 patients maintained by chronic dialysis. Four patients were subjected to subtotal parathyroidectomy. Good results were obtained in three. In one patient small-vessel calcification led to multiple amputations and death. When the product of serum calcium and phosphorus begins to rise, parathyroidectomy should be considered before extensive soft-tissue and small-vessel calcification has occurred.

Following parathyroidectomy these patients can be regulated with high doses of vitamin D. Soft-tissue calcification will be reversed and pruritus relieved. Some of these patients appear to have parathyroid adenomas, but this is really adenomatous hyperplasia and at least three and a half glands should be removed and the remaining tissue localized with a metal clip for possible later removal. The similarity of a simple greatly enlarged parathyroid in secondary hyperparathyroidism to parathyroid adenoma deserves further study and should help us to understand the relationship of adenoma and hyperplasia in primary hyperparathyroidism.

Patients with chronic renal disease who have undergone prolonged dialysis and have developed secondary hyperparathyroidism may not have excessively high serum calcium levels until after they have undergone renal transplantation because the serum calcium levels are suppressed by the high serum phosphorus concentrations. As the new kidney functions and excretes phosphorus and as the serum phosphorus level falls, hypercalcemia becomes evident. As the serum phosphorus falls, high levels of calcium appear in the urine. The lowering of serum phosphorus in these patients is exaggerated by the fact that the patients are also being treated with steroids and, in order to prevent steroid-induced ulcers, they are frequently given aluminum hydroxide, which interferes with the absorption of phosphorus from the intestine. The classical chemical changes of hyperparathyroidism usually show up within a month to six weeks after renal transplantation. This is a situation in which total body phosphorus is probably depleted and in which administration of sodium phosphate can be used to correct the phosphorus deficit and to lower the serum calcium levels without the usual danger of soft-tissue calcification. The hyperplastic parathyroids gradually return to normal function. In an experience of 175 patients undergoing kidney transplantation at the University of Colorado, only one patient required parathyroidectomy for posttransplant hyperparathyroidism.

Wilson, Hampers, et al. reviewed their experience with 800 patients with chronic renal disease including 237 who received renal transplants. Twenty-eight patients required subtotal parathyroidectomy. Eight of these were operated upon before hemodialysis, 18 during hemodialysis, and only 2 after renal transplantation. Marchioro in the following discussion of Wilson's paper compared his experience with the above and found that of 59 patients with renal transplants 18 had persistent hypercalcemia but most of these returned to normal serum calcium levels within 6 months. In 7 patients persistent hypercalcemia (one as long as 2 years) and elevated parathormone levels led to subtotal parathyroidectomy which was performed at least 8 months after the transplantation. The frequency of hypercalcemia requiring parathyroidectomy in chronic uremia is related to the duration of hypocalcemic stimulation of parathyroid hyperplasia.

Buckle found two patients with long-standing renal disease, secondary bone disease, and metastatic soft-tissue calcification in whom the serum calcium concentration had gradually risen to a normal level in spite of elevation of serum phosphate. Serum immunoreactive parathyroid hormone was elevated and remained elevated in spite of calcium infusion and further elevation of serum calcium concentration. This is a specific way of separating out those patients in whom the parathyroid glands have become autonomous in function and in whom parathyroidectomy would appear to be indicated.

LIFETIME DISEASE OF PARATHYROIDS

An early return of normal serum calcium and phosphorus levels does not assure that the disease has been eradicated. Utley and Black observed that the final diagnosis requires the longest possible follow-up, and after such follow-up some of the patients initially classified as having adenoma are reclassified as having hyperplasia because of subsequent recrudescence of hypercalcemia. Johnson and Conn have noted that untreated patients may have prolonged periods of freedom from hypercalcemia only to become hypercalcemic again and therefore the diagnosis of hyperparathyroidism should not be easily discarded. Raisz has observed that, in those asymptomatic patients with borderline abnormalities of serum calcium and phosphorus, we need to know more about the hazards as well as the advantages of the "wait-and-manipulate" approach. Hellstrom has emphasized the need for long follow-up. There are potentially irreversible changes that may develop in blood vessels with resultant hypertension and in the kidneys with late renal failure, if abnormal serum calcium levels are allowed to persist for many years. Wilson, Bernhard, et al., in a review of acute parathyroid intoxication, mentioned the possibility of myocardial lesions due to lack of phosphorus diffusion and the possibility of brain damage from inability to metabolize glucose in the absence of phosphorus. There are bits of evidence that hyperparathyroidism has widespread injurious effects. Many patients who have had parathyroid overactivity (as well as those with deficient function) should be followed for a lifetime.

Unfortunately, few of these patients have been followed closely enough or long enough to know the frequency of chronic recurrent disease or the extent of progressive damage which might occur in the kidneys and other organs. Ohlsson found no evidence of progressive renal disease in 73 patients in whom inulin clearance was performed preoperatively and again more than two years postoperatively. This lack of progression of renal disease was observed even in patients whose inulin clearance was significantly reduced preoperatively. From this study it appears that the progression of renal disease is stopped once the patient becomes normocalcemic. On the other hand untreated or recurrent hyperparathyroidism will gradually destroy the kidneys and needs to be recognized and treated before renal function is impaired. In a recent review of patients operated upon at the University of Iowa it was observed that one-third had persistent hypercalcemia (Fig. 11-4).

HYPOPARATHYROIDISM

Hypoparathyroidism is divisible into primary and secondary types. Surgeons are concerned with secondary hypoparathyroidism which may be a complication of thyroidectomy or parathyroidectomy. Primary hypoparathyroidism is divisible into idiopathic and pseudohypoparathyroidism. Idiopathic hypoparathyroidism is a true deficiency of parathyroid hormone production. There has been one report of permanent hypoparathyroidism in an infant born to a mother who had hyperparathyroidism. According to Ludwig, 19 of the 20 infants reported in the literature as having been born to mothers with hyperparathyroidism have had only temporary, if any, sign of parathyroid insufficiency.

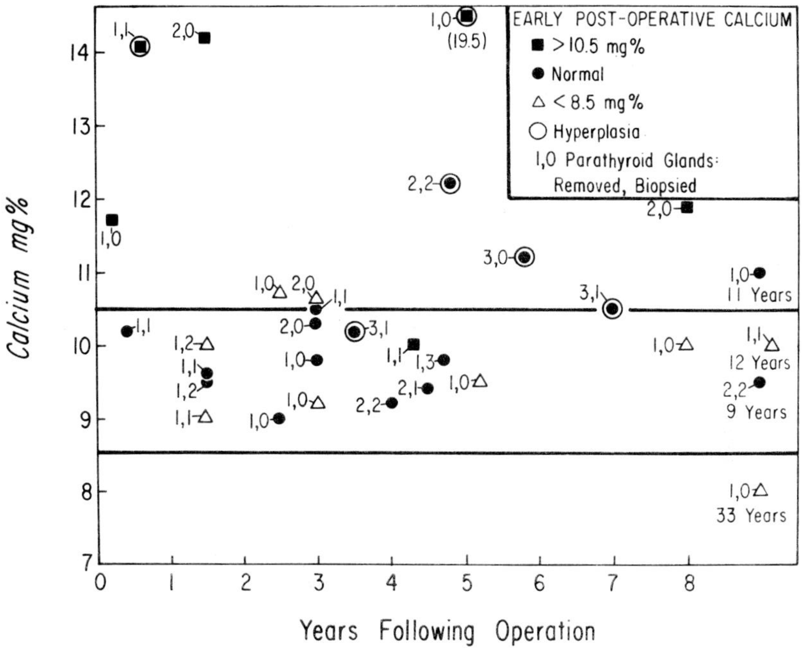

Figure 11-4. Shows the serum calcium levels of 31 patients reviewed in 1972 at the University of Iowa. Ten patients have hypercalcemia. Of these 5 had normal or low serum calcium levels in the immediate postoperative period. Four of the 10 had a diagnosis of hyperplasia, and none of the 10 with hypercalcemia had 3.5 glands removed. It is apparent that we have not been sufficiently aggressive in the surgical treatment of hyperparathyroidism. It is also evident that an early fall in serum calcium concentration does not obviate the need for prolonged follow-up. Hypercalcemia is more likely to persist in patients with hyperplasia and in patients whose early postoperative calcium concentrations are elevated. (Prepared by John Hoines)

Pseudohypoparathyroidism is a failure of end organ response to parathyroid hormone. There is a condition which is called "pseudopseudohypoparathyroidism" in which there really is no parathyroid disease at all but the patient has a high forehead and hands with short metacarpals of the third and fourth rays so that the fingers are all the same length. Such patients are short in stature and in general have the physical appearance of patients with pseudohypoparathyroidism, but the serum calcium and phosphorus concentrations are normal.

Postoperative hypoparathyroidism was observed in about 3% of patients having thyroidectomy for thyrotoxicosis, according to a review by Buckwalter and others, who reported 50 patients observed in the University of Iowa Hospitals between 1927 and 1955. With the increasing use of radioactive iodine for the treatment of hyperthyroidism, the occurrence of postthyroidectomy hypoparathyroidism has been seen less commonly. When it does occur, it is following thyroidectomy for cancer of the thyroid. With the current recognition of the need for 7/8 parathyroidectomy in patients with hyperplasia of the parathyroids it is likely that insufficiency will follow more frequently as a complication of parathyroidectomy.

The onset of signs and symptoms of hypocalcemia is most frequently within 48 hours of operation, and most of the patients who develop symptoms have them within the first week. There are some patients, however, whose deficiency is apparently borderline and who have no symptoms but do have an abnormally low serum calcium level. Some of these patients are finally recognized as having parathyroid insufficiency only after they develop complications, sometimes many years after thyroidectomy. The signs and symptoms observed in a review of 50 patients studied at the University of Iowa over some 28 years are shown in Table 11-1. Chvostek's sign was observed the most frequently but is not always present. In some patients with normal serum ionized calcium levels the sign can be elicited, so that it is not completely reliable. Nevertheless, for a given patient, Chvostek's sign is of help in that it tends to become more pronounced as the serum calcium level falls and less evident or absent when the serum calcium level is normal. The sign is elicited by tapping over the facial nerve and observing a quick contraction of the orbicularis oris or other facial muscles. Tingling of the hands and feet and about the mouth is a frequent complaint. Unfortunately, there are a significant number of patients who have no symptoms and yet whose serum calcium level is so low that over the years they will develop cataracts or other late complications as listed in Table 11-2. The occurrence of convulsions and mental deterioration has led to the diagnosis of brain tumor and, in some instances, patients have undergone operations to attempt to find such tumors. There have even been reports of obtaining brain biopsies with a needle with the operator observing that the feel of the needle during the biopsy was as though there were a tumor in the suspected area, and yet no tumor was found. This is referred to as "pseudotumor cerebri."

The management of postoperative hypoparathyroidism must take into consideration the possibility of a temporary insufficiency especially in the patient who has had a large adenoma removed and in whom it is thought that the hypocalcemia is probably due to the avid deposition of calcium and phosphate in the depleted bones. When the surgeon is quite certain that several parathyroid glands remain and have good blood supply, the patient should be treated with intravenous calcium gluconate which can be given slowly by syringe until symptoms are relieved, or as much as

TABLE 11-1. SYMPTOMS AND SIGNS OBSERVED IN HYPOPARATHYROIDISM AT UNIVERSITY OF IOWA

	Number of Patients
Chvostek's sign	33
Tingling	30
Muscle cramps	29
Carpal spasm	23
Trousseau's sign	21
Pedal spasm	20
Numbness	14
Paresthesias	9
Stiffness	8
Disorientation	6
Twitching	6
Convulsions	5
Ringing in ears	4
Hyperventilation	3
Erb's sign	3
Laryngospasm	2
Dysphagia	2
Anxiousness	2

From Buckwalter, et al.

TABLE 11-2. LATE COMPLICATIONS OF HYPOPARATHYROIDISM OBSERVED AT UNIVERSITY OF IOWA

	Number of Patients
Cataract	10
Convulsions	7
Mental deterioration	3
Psychosis	2
Cardiac insufficiency	1
Death	1

50 ml of the 10% calcium gluconate can be placed in a liter of intravenous fluid and given slowly but at a rate adequate to relieve symptoms. If after several days the patient is continuing to require intravenous calcium, vitamin D_2 should be started; the dose is several orders of magnitude higher than would be used for its vitamin effects in a patient with normal parathyroid function. Fifty thousand units a day are required, and in some patients the dosage must be higher than this.

The action of vitamin D_2 is delayed, and the patient should receive 50,000 units a day for several weeks before deciding that the dosage should be increased. Failure to understand this has led to increasing the dosage after a few days to 100,000 units or even higher and then gradually, as the serum calcium level rises up through normal range and into toxic levels, the physician is forced to stop all medication and may need to wait then for additional weeks before he can again attempt to regulate the medication at a proper level. This positive feedback problem is compounded by the production of increased sensitivity to vitamin D after vitamin D poisoning as described by Leeson and Fourman. If the patient has symptoms while waiting for the initial dosage of 50,000 units of vitamin D_2 a day to become effective, intravenous calcium gluconate should be given rather than an increase in dose of vitamin D.

The parathormone like effect of vitamin D_2 is mostly to stimulate and increase the intestinal absorption of calcium, and it has minimal effect upon the inhibition of phosphorus reabsorption in the renal tubule. As a result, the patients have a rise in their serum calcium but the serum phosphorus remains high. It was thought at one time that in order to counteract this, the patient should receive a low phosphorus diet by eliminating milk and milk products from the diet. Since milk is the prime source of calcium, giving a low phosphorus diet also meant a low calcium diet, and it was necessary to supplement the diet with calcium lactate or some other calcium salt by mouth. In the majority of patients, if the vitamin D_2 dosage is sufficient to raise the serum calcium level well into the normal range, the serum phosphorus will fall to a level only slightly above normal. It is not usually necessary to restrict the diet in any way or to provide extra calcium by mouth.

Dihydrotachysterol (AT-10) was popular at one time since it seemed to have somewhat more effect in lowering serum phosphorus than did vitamin D_2. Because the AT-10 was impure and not dependable in its effect and also because the cost was considerably higher for AT-10 than for vitamin D_2, it has not been used very frequently in the treatment of hypoparathyroidism until recently. Now a crystalline preparation of AT-10 is available and is effective; it still is expensive and probably does not have any advantage over vitamin D_2 when D_2 is given in adequate dosage.

The danger of vitamin D_2 is in overtreatment. This is especially true if the patient has a return of parathyroid function. In a patient with normal parathyroid function, 50,000 units of vitamin D_2 are extremely toxic and will cause a rise in serum calcium and, if allowed to continue, will cause calcification of all of those areas where there is a secretion of acid and an equal and opposite alkaline pH in the secreting cells. Patients develop calcification in the lungs, kidneys, stomach, and sometimes in other soft tissues, and death is likely to result from renal failure. In order to prevent toxicity, every patient with hypoparathyroidism should be given instructions in the performance of the Sulkowitch test, which should carried out daily, preferably on the first urine passed in the morning. The test is simple to perform and requires mixing an equal amount of urine and Sulkowitch reagent, shaking the test tube and looking at the precipitate which forms in relation to the amount of calcium present. Normally, the urine will be clear or mildly cloudy, but it will be possible to read newsprint through the solution. If at any time the precipitate is so heavy that the patient cannot read newsprint through the test tube, he should return to his physician for a repeat of the serum calcium and phosphorus determination and for instructions in temporary discontinuation of the vitamin D_2. The Sulkowitch test is not a sufficiently accurate test to regulate the serum calcium level but it is of benefit in warning the patient that his serum calcium levels may be dangerously high.

Patients should have serum calcium and phosphorus determinations every few months initially and several times a year subsequently for the rest of their lives, if they do have permanent hypoparathyroidism. If it is necessary to increase the dose of vitamin D_2 to 100,000 units a day or even higher levels, then it is especially important to repeat serum calcium and phosphorus levels, since over a period of months at these higher dosage levels the serum calcium may gradually rise to a toxic level. Once a patient has received sufficient vitamin D_2 to develop a serum calcium of about 11 mg%, it is likely that he will for a time be more sensitive to the effects of vitamin D_2. This makes regulation difficult and may mislead the physician into thinking that the patient actually had a temporary hypoparathyroidism and that he does not need further treatment or observation. Whenever it is felt that the hypoparathyroidism is temporary and that medication should be discontinued, the patient should be followed for several years with repeated serum calcium and phosphorus determinations to make certain that there is not a recurrence of parathyroid insufficiency.

In the patient who is started on vitamin D_2, the serum phosphorus concentration can be of great assistance in indicating whether the patient's parathyroid function is returning. Vitamin D_2 will not alone reduce serum phosphorus to the level that is observed when parathyroid hormone is active. The patient who has a normal serum calcium level and continuing insufficiency of parathyroid function will have a high normal or even above normal level of serum phosphorus. On the other hand, if the parathyroids are beginning to function again, the serum phosphorus will fall to a normal or low level; in such circumstance the vitamin D_2 should be discontinued and the patient observed for a year with periodic serum calcium and phosphorus determinations to make certain that the parathyroid function remains adequate. When the serum calcium and phosphorus levels are both low, it is likely that the problem is one of inadequate intake of calcium and phosphorus (i.e., a poor diet) rather than a deficiency of parathyroid hormone. In such instances, the patient should be encouraged to drink more milk, eat more milk products, and be allowed 500 units of vitamin D (commonly in fortified milk) as a vitamin supplement rather than the higher doses required for substitution for parathyroid function. Do not neglect a follow-up over six months to a year after concluding that parathyroid function has returned. The improvement may be transient, and prolonged mild hypoparathyroidism may result in cataracts or other complications (Table 11-2).

MEDULLARY CARCINOMA AND THYROCALCITONIN

Medullary carcinoma, described by Hazard et al. in 1959, is considered a neoplasm of the parafollicular cells of the thyroid which arise from the ultimobranchial bodies probably of the fourth branchial pouch. The cancers which develop are, according to Miller et al., located in the upper one-half of the thyroid gland when the disease is detected in its early stages. Later it may spread to the remainder of the thyroid and to the lymph nodes of the middle neck, inferior to the thyroid, and in superior mediastinal lymph nodes.

Miller et al. in 1972 presented a study of a family comprising nearly 90 members, thus far, with 18 having medullary carcinoma. In 83 of the members who were brought in for study, having no previous evidence of the disease, they found 12 in whom there was an elevation of serum calcitonin or in whom an excessively high serum calcitonin could be produced by the infusion of calcium. One patient with normal serum calcitonin levels was found to have a pheochromocytoma, and 4 of the patients with evidence of medullary carcinoma (an elevation in serum calcitonin) were found to have pheochromocytoma.

In 40% of the family who did not yet have any abnormality of serum calcitonin there was an elevation of serum parathyroid hormone suggesting that parathyroid hyperplasia may be part of the primary and congenital abnormality. Parathyroid hyperplasia, which is often observed in the specimens from these patients, may not be secondary to a lowering in serum calcium levels. Renal calculi were present in 4 members of the family. It is unlikely that there occurred a positive feedback from calcitonin-produced hypocalcemia with production of excessive parathyroid hormone to the point of producing hypercalciuria and calculi. Miller et al. feel that the presence of renal calculi is additional evidence of primary parathyroid hyperplasia. In the discussion of this paper, Cope raised the question as to whether occult carcinomas discovered by screening families of this sort with serum calcitonin assays should be considered in the same vein as other cancers that are discovered after producing symptoms or evidence of metastases. It was mentioned in answer to this question that 8 members in one generation of this large family with medullary carcinoma had already died of their tumors and that 2 others had evidence of liver metastases. With the advent of highly sensitive immunoassay it may be possible to detect and treat these patients with cancer of the thyroid when medullary cancer is in its earliest stages. It is thought that some 3 to 10% of thyroid cancers may fall into this category. This opens up a new area of preventive medicine by selective screening and raises new questions about genetic counseling which may involve the surgeon who accepts his full responsibilities as a physician who operates.

REFERENCES

Ackerman, N. B., and Winder, N.: Evaluation of methods for localizing parathyroid tumors. Amer. J. Surg. *122*:669, 1971.

Albright, F., Bauer, W., Claflin, D., and Cockrill, J. R.: Studies in parathyroid physiology. III. Effect of phosphate ingestion in clinical hyperparathyroidism. J. Clin. Invest. *11*:411, 1932.

Albright, F., and Reifenstein, E. C., Jr.: *The Parathyroid Gland and Metabolic Bone Disease*. Baltimore: Williams & Wilkins, 1948.

Arnaud, C. D., Tsao, H. S., and Littledike, T.: Radioimmunoassay of human parathyroid hormone in serum. J. Clin. Invest. *50*:21, 1971.

Aurback, G. D., Marcus, R., Heersche, J., Marx, S., Niall, H., Tregear, G. W., Keutmann, H. T., and Potts, J. T., Jr.: Hormone and other factors regulating calcium metabolism. Ann. N. Y. Acad. Sci. *185*:386, 1971.

Aurbach, G. D., Marcus, R., Heersche, J., Marx, S., Niall, H., Tregear, J., Keutmann, H. T., Deftos, L. J., and Potts, J. T., Jr.: Hormonal regulation of cyclic 3′,5′-AMP in specific receptor tissues: biological effects of a synthetic N-terminal tetratriacontapeptide of parathyroid hormone. Isr. J. Med. Sci. *7*:341, 1971.

Avioli, L. V.: The diagnosis of primary hyperparathyroidism. Med. Clin. N. Amer. *52*:451, 1968.

Avioli, L. V., Birge, S. J., Scott, S., and Shieber, W.: Role of the thyroid gland during glucagon-induced hypocalcemia in dogs. Amer. J. Physiol. *216*:939, 1969.

Barzel, U. S.: Parathyroid hormone, blood phosphorus, and acid base metabolism. Lancet *1*:1329, 1971.

Barzel, U. S., and Jowsey, J.: The effects of chronic acid and alkali administration on bone turnover in adult rats. Clin. Sci. *36*:517, 1969.

Berson, S. A., and Yalow, R. S.: Parathyroid hormone in plasma in adenomatous hyperparathyroidism, uremia, and bronchogenic carcinoma. Science *154*:907, 1966.

Boquist, L., Bergdahl, L., and Andersson, A.: Parathyroid adenoma complicated by acute hyperparathyroidism: report of a case with particular regard to ultrastructural findings. Ann. Surg. *173*:593, 1971.

Boyd, J. D., Milgram, J. E., and Stearns, G.: Clinical hyperparathyroidism. J.A.M.A. *93*:684, 1929.

Boyle, D. E., and Mason, E. E.: Parathyroid crisis. J. Iowa Med. Soc. *56*:359, 1966.

Breidahl, H. D., and Hamilton, N. T.: Parathyroid intoxication. Aust. New Zeal. J. Surg. *39*:244, 1970.

Breuer, R. I., and LeBauer, J.: Caution in the use of phosphate in the treatment of severe hypercalcemia. J. Clin. Endocr. *27*:695, 1967.

Bronsky, D.: Hyperparathyroidism with Albright's osteodystrophy: case report and a proposed new classification of parathyroid disease. J. Clin. Endocr. *31*:271, 1970.

Brown, J. H., and Kennedy, B. J.: Mithramycin in the treatment of disseminated testicular neoplasms. New Eng. J. Med. *272*:111, 1965.

Buck, B. A., and Robertson, R. D.: Indications for parathyroidectomy in advanced renal disease. Surg. Gynec. Obstet. *133*:218, 1971.

Buckle, R. M.: Hyperparathyroidism in chronic renal failure. Lancet *2*:234, 1970.

Buckwalter, J. A., Soper, R. T., Davies, J., and Mason, E. E.: Postoperative hypoparathyroidism. Surg. Gynec. Obstet. *101*:657, 1955.

Carone, F. A., Epstein, F. H., Beck, D., and Levitin, H.: The effects upon the kidney of transient hypercalcemia induced by parathyroid extract. Amer. J. Path. *36*:77, 1960.

Chakmakjian, Z. H., and Bethune, J. E.: Sodium sulfate treatment of hypercalcemia. New Eng. J. Med. *275*:862, 1966.

Chamberlin, J. A., Nicholas, H. O., and Hanna, E.: Experience with hyperparathyroidism. Surgery *53*:719, 1963.

Coffey, R. J., Potter, J. F., and Canary, J. J.: Diagnosis and surgical control of hyperparathyroidism. Ann. Surg. *161*:732, 1965.

Cope, O.: The story of hyperparathyroidism at the Massachusetts General Hospital. New Eng. J. Med. *274*:1174, 1966.

Cope, O.: Surgery of hyperparathyroidism: the occurrence of parathyroids in anterior mediastinum and the division of the operation into two stages. Ann. Surg. *114*:706, 1941.

Cope, O., Barnes, B. A., Castleman, B., Mueller, G. C. E., and Roth, S. I.: Vicissitudes of parathyroid surgery: trials of diagnosis and management in 51 patients with a variety of disorders. Ann. Surg. *154*:491, 1961.

Cope, O., Culver, P. J., Mixter, C. G., Jr., and Nardi, G. I.: Pancreatitis: a diagnostic clue to hyperparathyroidism. Ann. Surg. *145*:857, 1957.

Copp, D. H.: Discovery of thyrocalcitonin. Proc. Canad. Fed. Biol. Soc. *4*:17, 1961.

Deftos, L. J., Lee, M. R., and Potts, J. T., Jr.: A radioimmunoassay for thyrocalcitonin. Proc. Nat. Acad. Sci. USA, *60*:293, 1968.

Dent, C. E.: Cortisone test for hyperparathyroidism. Brit. Med. J. *1*:230, 1956.

Eilert, J. B., Casey, D., del Greco, F., and Conn, J.: Experience with subtotal parathyroidectomy for "tertiary" hyperparathyroidism. Arch. Surg. (Chicago) *103*:303, 1971.

Eisenberg, E.: Effect of intravenous phosphate on serum strontium and calcium. New Eng. J. Med. *282*:889, 1970.

Elias, E. G., and Evans, J. T.: Hypercalcemic crisis in neoplastic diseases: management with mithramycin. Surgery *71*:631, 1972.

Elias, E. G., Reynoso, G., and Mittelman, A.: Control of hypercalcemia with mithramycin. Ann. Surg. *175*:431, 1972.

Ellison, E. H., and Wilson, S. D.: The Zollinger-Ellison syndrome: re-appraisal and evaluation of 260 registered cases. Ann. Surg. *160*:512, 1964.

Fraser, P., Healy, M., Rose, N., and Watson, L: Discriminant functions in differential diagnosis of hypercalcaemia. Lancet *1*:1314, 1971.

Friderichsen, C., and Rosendal, T.: A 30-year follow-up study of a case of cured hyperparathyroidism. Acta Endocr. *59*:371, 1968.

Frohlich, E. D., Scott, J. B., and Haddy, F. J.: Effect of cations on resistance and responsiveness of renal and forelimb vascular beds. Amer. J. Physiol. *203*:583, 1962.

Goldsmith, R. S., Gall, E. A., Altemeier, W. A., Weinstein, A., and Zalme, E.: Hyperparathyroidism: therapy and response, with a test for assessment of response. Ann. Intern. Med. *75*:395, 1971.

Goldsmith, R. S., and Ingbar, S. H.: Inorganic phosphate treatment of hypercalcemia of diverse etiologies. New Eng. J. Med. *274*:1, 284, 1966.

Goldsmith, R. S., and Ingbar, S. H.: Hyper- to hypocalcemia. New Eng. J. Med. *274*:284, 1966.

Gordon, G. S., Eisenberg, E., Loken, H. G., Gardner, G., and Hayashida, T.: Clinical endocrinology of parathyroid hormone excess. In *Recent Progress in Hormone Research*. Pincus, G. ed. Vol. 18, New York: Academic Press, 1962.

Gordon, G. S., and Roof, B. S.: Laboratory tests for hyperparathyroidism. J.A.M.A. *206*:2729, 1968.

Haddad, J. G., and Avioli, L. V.: Comparative effects of phosphate and thyrocalcitonin on skeletal turnover. Endocrinology *87*:1245, 1970.

Haff, R. C., and Ballinger, W. F.: Causes of recurrent hypercalcemia after parathyroidectomy for primary hyperparathyroidism. Ann. Surg. *173*:884, 1971.

Hanes, F. M.: Hyperparathyroidism due to parathyroid adenoma, with death from parathormone intoxication. Amer. J. Med. Sci. *197*:85, 1939.

Hanna, E. A., Nicholas, H. O., and Chamberlin, J. A.: Nomogram for estimating diffusible serum calcium. Clin. Chem. *10*:235. 1964.

Hazard, J. B., Hawk, W. A., and Crile, J., Jr.: Medullary (solid) carcinoma of the thyroid: a clinicopathological entity. J. Clin. Endocr. *19*:152, 1959.

Heckman, B. A., and Walsh, J. H.: Hypernatremia complicating sodium sulfate therapy for hypercalcemic crisis. New. Eng. J. Med. *276*:1082, 1967.

Hellstrom, J.: Clinical experiences of 21 cases of hyperparathyroidism with special reference to the prognosis following parathyroidectomy. Acta Chir. Scand. *100*:391, 1950.

Henley, R. B.: Management of the parathyroid crisis. Amer. J. Surg. *108*:183, 1964.

Henneman, P. H., Benedict, P. H., Forbes, A. P., and Dudley, H. R.: Idiopathic hypercalciuria. New Eng. J. Med. *259*:802, 1958.

Herbert, L. A., Lemann, J., Jr., Petersen, J. R., and Lennon, E. J.: Studies of the mechanism by which phosphate infusion lowers serum calcium. Clin. Res. *14*:349, 1966.

Hodgkinson, A., Peacock, M., and Nordin, B. E. C.: Asymptomatic hyperparathyroidism. Lancet *2*:49, 1971.

Holmes, E. C., Morton, D. L., and Ketcham, A. S.: Parathyroid carcinoma. Ann. Surg. *169*:631, 1969.

Hume, D. M.: Parathyroid. In *Principles of Surgery*, Schwartz, S. I. ed. New York: McGraw-Hill Book Co., 1969.

Hurvitz, R. J., Hurvitz, J. S., and Morgenstern, L.: "In vivo" staining of the parathyroid glands and pancreas. Arch. Surg. (Chicago) *95*:274, 1967.

Johnson, R. D., and Conn. J. W.: Hyperparathyroidism with a prolonged period of normocalcemia. J.A.M.A. *210*:2063, 1969.

Jowsey, J.: Quantitative microradiography: a new approach in the evaluation of metabolic bone disease (editorial). Amer. J. Med. *40*:485, 1966.

Kahil, M., Orman, B., Gyorkey, F., and Brown, H.: Hypercalcemia. J.A.M.A. *201*: 721, 1967.

Kaplan, E. L., Hill, B. J., Locke, S., and Peskin, G. W.: Acid-base balance and parathyroid function: metabolic alkalosis and hyperparathyroidism. Surgery *70*: 198, 1971.

Katz, A., Kaplan, L., Massry, S. G., Heller, R., Plotmin, D., and Knight, I.: Hyperfunction of parathyroids implicated in hypercalcemia when osseous metastases absent. Arch. Surg. (Chicago) *101*:582, 1970.

Keating, F. R., Jr.: The clinical problem of primary hyperparathyroidism. Med. Clin. N. Amer. *54*:511, 1970.

Kennedy, B. J., Sandberg-Wolheim, M., and Loken, M.: Studies with tritiated mithramycin in C_3H mice. Cancer Res. *27*:1534, 1967.

Knill-Jones, R. P., Buckle, R. M., Parsons, V., Calne, R. Y., and Williams, R.: Hypercalcemia and increased parathyroid-hormone activity in a primary hepatoma. New Eng. J. Med. *282*:704, 1970.

Krementz, E. T., Race, J. L., Sternberg, W. H., and Hawley, W. D.: Parathyroid adenoma: problems in diagnosis and management. Ann. Surg. *165*:681, 1967.

Krull, G. H., Muller, H., Leijnse, B., and Gerbrandy, J.: Venous-compression test in hyperparathyroidism. Lancet *2*:174, 1969.

Lee, C. M., McElhinney, W. T., and Gall, E. A.: Unusual manifestations of parathyroid adenoma. Arch. Surg. (Chicago) *71*:475, 1955.

Leeson, P., and Fourman, P.: Increased sensitivity to vitamin D after vitamin D poisoning. Lancet *1*:1182, 1966.

Ludwig, G. D.: Hyperparathyroidism in relation to pregnancy. New Eng. J. Med. *267*:637, 1962.

Mandl, F.: Therapeutic Versuch bei Ostitis fibrosa generalisata mittels Extirpation eines Epithelkorperchentumors. Wien. Klin. Wchnschr. *38*:1343, 1925.

McMillan, D. E., and Freeman, R. B.: The milk-alkali syndrome: a study of the acute disorder with comments on the development of the chronic condition. Medicine *44*:485, 1965.

Miller, H. H., Melvin, K. E. W., Gibson, I. M., and Tashjian, A. H.: Surgical approach to early familial medullary carcinoma of the thyroid gland. Amer. J. Surg. *123*:438, 1972.

Ohlsson, L.: Renal function in hyperparathyroidism. Acta Endocr. *63*:161, 1970.

Owens, M. P., Sorock, M. L., and Brown, E. M.: The clinical application of in vivo parathyroid staining. Surgery *64*:1049, 1968.

Pak, C. Y. C., Wills, M. R., Smith, G. W., II, and Bartter, F. C.: Treatment with thyrocalcitonin of the hypercalcemia of parathyroid carcinoma. J. Clin. Endocr. *28*:1657, 1968.

Paloyan, E., Lawrence, A. M., Straus, F. H., II, Paloyan, D., Harper, P. V., and Cummings, D.: Alpha cell hyperplasia in calcific pancreatitis associated with hyperparathyroidism. J.A.M.A. *200*:757, 1967.

Paloyan, E., Paloyan, D., and Harper, P. V.: The role of glucagon hypersecretion in the relationship of pancreatitis and hyperparathyroidism. Surgery *62*:167, 1967.

Payne, R. L., and Fitchett, C. W.: Hyperparathyroid crisis: survey of the literature and a report of two additional cases. Ann. Surg. *161*:737, 1965.

Purnell, D. C., Smith, L. H., Scholz, D. A., Elveback, L. R., and Arnaud, C. D.: Primary hyperparathyroidism: a prospective clinical study. Amer. J. Med. *50*:670, 1971.

Raisz, L. G.: Current concepts: the diagnosis of hyperparathyroidism. New Eng. J. Med. *285*:1006, 1971.

Reiss, E.: Primary hyperparathyroidism: a simplified approach to diagnosis. Med. Clin. N. Amer., *54*:131, 1970.

Reiss, E., and Canterbury, J. M.: Primary hyperparathyroidism: application of radioimmunoassay to differentiation of adenoma and hyperplasia and to preoperative localization of hyperfunctioning parathyroid glands. New Eng. J. Med. *280*:1381, 1969.

Riggs, B. L., Arnaud, C. D., Goldsmith, R. S., Taylor, W. F., McCall, J. T., and Sessler, A. D.: Plasma kinetics and acute effects of pharmacologic doses of porcine calcitonin in man. J. Clin. Endocr. Metab. *33*:115, 1971.

Rittel, W., Brugger, M., and Kamber, B.: Thyrocalcitonin. 3. Die synthese des alphathyrocalcitonins. Helv. Clim. Acta *51*:924, 1968.

Salassa, R. M., Jowsey, J., and Arnaud, C. D.: Hypophosphatemic osteomalacia associated with "norendocrine" tumors. New Eng. J. Med. *283*:65, 1970.

Seldin, D. W., and Castleman, B.: Azotemia and bone disease eighteen years after removal of a parathyroid adenoma. New Eng. J. Med. *282*:1028, 1970.

Shackney, S., and Hasson, J.: Precipitous fall in serum calcium, hypotension, and acute renal failure after intravenous phosphate therapy for hypercalcemia. Ann. Intern. Med. *66*:906, 1967.

Shieber, W.: Why hypocalcemia in pancreatitis? Amer. J. Surg. *120*:685, 1970.

Shieber, W., Birge, S. J., Avioli, L. V., and Teitelbaum, S. L.: Normocalcemic hyperparathyroidism with "normal" parathyroid glands. Arch. Surg. (Chicago) *103*:299, 1971.

Slayton, R. E., Shnider, B. I., Elias, E., Horton, J., and Perlia, C. P.: New approach to the treatment of hypercalcemia: the effect of short-term treatment with mithramycin. Clin. Pharm. Thera. *12*:833, 1971.

Smith, L. C., Bradshaw, H. H., and Holleman, I. L., Jr.: Hyperparathyroid crisis: a surgical emergency. Amer. Surg. *29*:761, 1963.

Suki, W. N., Yium, J. J., VonMinden, M., Saller-Hebert, C., Eknoyan, G., and Martinez-Maldonado, M.: Acute treatment of hypercalcemia with furosemide. New Eng. J. Med. *283*:836, 1970.

Turchi, J. J., Flandreau, R. H., Forte, A. L., French, G. N., and Ludwig, G. D.: Hyperparathyroidism and pancreatitis. J.A.M.A. *180*:799, 1962.

Utley, J. R., and Black, W. C.: Hyperparathyroidism: a clinicopathologic evaluation. Amer. J. Surg. *114*:788, 1967.

West, T. E. T., Jofee, M., Sinclair, L., and O'Riordan, J. L. H.: Treatment of hypercalcaemia with calcitonin. Lancet *1*:675, 1971.

Wilder, W. T., Frame, B., and Haubrich, W. S.: Peptic ulcer in primary hyperparathyroidism: an analysis of 52 cases. Ann. Intern. Med., *55*:885, 1961.

Wills, M. R.: Fundamental physiological role of parathyroid hormone in acid-base homeostasis. Lancet *2*:802, 1970.

Wills, M. R., and McGowan, G. K.: Hyperchloraemia as a diagnosis feature in hyperparathyroidism. J. Bone Joint Surg. *45B*:799, 1963.

Wilson, R. E., Bernhard, W. F., Polet, H., and Moore, F. D.: Hyperparathyroidism: the problem of acute parathyroid intoxication. Ann. Surg. *159*:79, 1964.

Wilson, R. E., Hampers, C. L., Bernstein, D. S., Johnson, J. W., and Merrill, J. P.: Subtotal parathyroidectomy in chronic renal failure. Ann. Surg. *174*:640, 1971.

Yeager, R., and Krementz, E.: Toluidine blue in identification of parathyroid glands at operation. Ann. Surg. *169*:829, 1969.

Chapter

12

Fluid Resuscitation of the Burned Patient

C. E. Hartford, M.D.

Burn shock occurs as a consequence of thermal injury and is caused by the translocation of body fluids resulting in hypovolemia, circulatory failure, and renal failure. The administration of fluids to patients with large surface burns prevents death from burn shock, but the mechanism of this salutary effect is imperfectly known. It is the consensus that sodium-containing fluids are necessary, but the issue as to whether colloids are needed or even desirable is unsettled. Many methods, with or without formulas as guides to calculate the volume of fluids required and with or without colloid-containing fluids, have been successfully employed to resuscitate patients with burns, especially with burns of less than 60% of the body surface area (BSA). It is not known which of these methods is best for a given patient. This question, however, is critical among patients with burns of greater than two-thirds BSA and among those with lesser burns who have impairment of function of cardiac, vascular, respiratory, or renal systems, and among those whose fluid resuscitation has been delayed.

There are multiple factors which add to the confusion in this field. First, the sequelae of thermal injury are complex and incompletely understood. Second, such differences as the intensity and duration of heat, its source, the anatomic area of the body exposed, and the premorbid condition and age of the patient all influence the patient's response to the injury and the response to fluid therapy. Third, conclusions derived from experiments conducted among animals cannot definitively be applied to humans. Fourth, both the results of animal research and observations made of burned humans are interpreted differently by different authorities. Fifth, the marriage of an authority to a single technique of fluid therapy and the dogmatic and prolific perpetuation of that concept add to the confusion. Sixth, the strict adherence to any rigid formula in treating a biological disturbance is dangerous.

Seventh, although the *sine qua non* of the scientific method is controlled prospective study, there has only been one published study of this kind in the entire history of fluid resuscitation of patients with burns (Markley). The completed treatise on this subject cannot yet be written.

PHYSIOLOGICAL CONSEQUENCES OF THERMAL INJURY

Heat sufficient to injure cells causes them to lose potassium, acquire sodium (Fox and Baer), and release intracellular enzymes (Fox, Holder, and Malin). In addition, it is probable that biologically active toxic substances are produced in heated tissues. For instance, it has been shown that there is a dialyzable substance that depresses myocardial activity both in vitro and in vivo (Baxter and Shires). Some of these factors and perhaps direct thermal injury contribute to produce a lesion which causes capillaries to become abnormally permeable to colloids (Cotran and Remensnyder). Arturson was able to inhibit the increase in microvascular permeability of the scalded dog paw by the administration of the flavonoid 0-(-hydroxyethyl)-rutoside. As a consequence of the thermal injury, there is an obligatory sequestration of fluid into the area of injury and usually into adjacent uninjured tissues. Among those receiving large quantities of fluids for resuscitation, anasarca may develop. In addition to expansion of the interstitial space, the administered fluid enters cells of injured as well as uninjured tissues. Much of this fluid is inactive in contributing to a normal fluid circulation.

Fox and Baer found that the burned leg of an untreated mouse acquires both sodium and water while it loses potassium. Although higher temperatures caused a similar movement of these cations in the burned leg, the magnitude of the shift was less and there was only scant acquisition of water. Although extracellular sodium and water move in isotonic proportions, Jelenko et al., working with heat contact burns of rabbit skin (rabbit skin is similar in chemical composition to human skin), found that shortly after injury, the cation concentration of the eschar was hyperosmolar; i.e., 254 mEq/l of cation compared to 182 mEq/l of cation of intact skin. This is not explained by heat desiccation because the sodium concentration increased to 26% greater than the concentration of intact skin while, during the same interval, the water content increased by 20%. The mechanism by which sodium moves into the burn independent of water is not known. By 48 hours sufficient water moved into the eschar to yield a sodium concentration equivalent to that of normal skin. Actually, the absolute changes in water and electrolytes of burn eschar are quite small. Theoretically, the absolute gain by the entire eschar of a 70-kg man with a burn of

50% BSA was calculated to be 108 mEq sodium at 8 hours after injury. Therefore, the vast majority of the sodium and fluid given to resuscitate burned patients goes to satisfy the demands of tissues other than eschar.

The movement of proteins is slower than the movement of electrolytes (Fox). This may cause an initial finding of slightly elevated levels of serum proteins. Kilgore et al., by analysis of edema from untreated primates with burns, found a total protein content of 1.2 to 2.8 gm/100 ml with an albumin-globulin ratio which varied between 1:1 and 1.4:1.

The result of this loss of protein-rich fluid from the intravascular space is a decrease in the plasma volume, hemoconcentration, hypovolemia, decrease in the cardiac output, hypotension, poor tissue perfusion, lactic acidemia, and metabolic acidosis. If the patient does not receive adequate treatment or does not respond to the resuscitative effort, acute renal failure supervenes and intravascular thrombi form as blood flow slows. Death ensues.

Determination of the rate of obligatory sequestration of fluid has been based primarily on the rate of fluid administration required to resuscitate humans and animals with burns and is probably maximal soon after injury. The rate of this loss decreases with time, follows a parabolic curve, until 18 to 30 hours after injury when the edema begins to resorb. At that point the fluid requirement becomes less than that required for losses. Pruitt and Mason found by equations derived from the least squares regression technique that the rate of loss of fluid from the plasma volume averaged 4.4 ml/kg/hr during the first 24 hours after injury and was independent of the kind of fluid—plasma, plasmanate, dextran in saline solution, lactated Ringer's solution, or isotonic saline—used in resuscitation. During the second 24 hours there was a small spontaneous increase of plasma volume, and all rates of fluid administration augmented the blood volume. Also, during the second day, colloid-containing solutions resulted in a more effective volume expansion than did fluids that did not contain colloid. The transition from sequestration to augmentation of plasma volume occurring on the second day after injury is presumably due to restoration of microvascular integrity.

Some of the sequestered fluid is lost from the body through the injured surface but the greatest proportion is resorbed into the vascular space and excreted by the kidney. During the period of resorption there is an increase in the active extracellular fluid volume, intravascular volume, cardiac output, and urine. Seldom is there a prompt massive diuresis. The patient returns to water balance in one to two weeks. During resorption of the sequestered fluid there is an increased risk of congestive heart failure and pulmonary edema. Because of this, the risk of death is increased on about the fourth or fifth day, especially among the aged.

Among patients with burns large enough to be biologically significant and whose treatment has not been extensively delayed, there are characteristic findings of the serum electrolytes, blood colloids, and blood gases. Although the serum sodium and potassium are usually in the normal range, the serum chloride is high among those with elevation of blood urea nitrogen (BUN). The low serum bicarbonate reflects metabolic acidosis. Delay in instituting fluid therapy to relieve stagnant hypoxia increases the acidosis. If this is not corrected the myocardium will remain irritable, the likelihood of renal failure is enhanced, and the response to fluid therapy is impaired. Also, because of the stagnant hypoxia, marginally viable cells in the burned skin may die, increasing the depth of injury.

The hematocrit and concentration of hemoglobin are high even though some of the red cells are destroyed by the heat, either directly or indirectly. Usually 15% or less of the red cell mass is destroyed immediately by direct thermal injury. However, among the severely burned, the accumulative loss of red cells may rise to as much as 25% by the end of 48 hours (Muir). Although it is thought by many that blood is not needed during the immediate resuscitative effort, anemia, especially among those with large surface burns, can be anticipated during the latter part of the first week after injury. If, however, the exposure of red cells to injury is prolonged, such as may occur when heat from active chemical agents penetrates into cutaneous or subcutaneous capillaries, destruction of red blood cells may continue.

Hemoglobinemia enhances the risk of renal failure, and it should be cleared rapidly. In the usual instance, the oxygen-carrying capacity of red cells is not affected. However, those patients burned in closed spaces may have an excessive level of carboxyhemoglobin.

The concentrations of serum proteins are usually normal. If the patient is resuscitated with crystalloids alone, or fluid devoid of protein, then serum protein levels are lowered.

Abnormally high admission levels of serum creatinine, even in cases in which treatment has been delayed, usually reflect preexisting renal disease and suggest a poor prognosis. Usually the BUN is normal. Elevation suggests either a prerenal azotemia as with blood in the gastrointestinal tract or impaired renal function. Rising levels of both serum creatinine and BUN, when observed in the course of a seemingly adequate resuscitative effort, indicate a poor prognosis.

A low pH of arterial blood documents the usual metabolic acidosis. The P_{CO_2} of arterial blood is usually below 40 mm Hg, and a normal or elevated Pco_2 suggests either an associated inhalation injury or antecedent pulmonary insufficiency. Either condition worsens the prognosis.

Patients with biologically significant burns are oliguric unless they receive adequate fluid. Urinary output is regarded by many burn therapists as an important index of efficacy of fluid resuscitation. O'Neill et al. found among patients with large burns a depression of renal plasma flow with a slight decrease in glomerular filtration even in the presence of clinically acceptable urine flow. They accounted for these changes on the basis of increased renal vascular peripheral resistance and a decreased cardiac output. As a consequence of depressed renal function and deranged homeostasis, the urine sodium, chloride, and pH are low and the urine potassium is elevated.

FLUID RESUSCITATION OF PATIENTS WITH BURNS—BACKGROUND

There is ample evidence that patients with biologically significant burns will die unless they are treated with sodium-containing fluids. It is probable that the treatment of burn shock was held back for many years because of inadequate techniques for the intravenous delivery of large volumes of fluid. In 1855, Buhl commented on the similiarity between badly burned patients and those suffering from cholera. The latter had been treated with astounding success by Thomas Latta with liberal amounts of a saline solution that contained 60 mEq of sodium chloride and 11 mEq of sodium bicarbonate per liter. Sneve, in 1905 recommended, and Underhill in 1930 re-emphasized, the need for saline solutions to treat burn shock. Underhill recommended that as much as 8 liters or more of intravenously administered saline solution may be needed to offset the large fluid losses which he measured in major burns. Also, he recommended sodium bicarbonate by mouth to correct acidosis. Although Underhill's method of therapy was tried by many physicians, the results he obtained could not be duplicated. Apparently his recommendations for the use of bicarbonate to correct metabolic acidosis were not adhered to. This method was abandoned in favor of the use of blood and plasma as the primary fluids to treat burn shock.

In 1880, Lesser reported a decrease in the recoverable red blood cell mass among severely burned animals and postulated that treatment of burned patients should include whole blood. Robertson introduced the use of citrated whole blood to treat traumatic shock of the wounded of World War I. In Toronto after the war he found that burn shock could also be prevented by the administration of whole blood (Moyer). Stimulated by a report in which

Moyer, Coller, et al. showed a salutary effect of defibrinated blood on burn shock among scalded dogs, Evans and Bigger reported a series of 32 clinical cases in which good results were obtained by giving 500 to 1000 ml of citrated whole blood every 6 hours during the first 48 hours, together with saline and other fluids to maintain a urine output of 50 to 100 ml per hour. Also, with each transfusion an 8-gm dose of sodium bicarbonate was given. These investigators found, by calculation of randomly obtained pretreatment data from 9 severely burned patients, an average red blood cell mass deficit of 40%. Also, when red cell free fluid was administered, recalculation at 72 and 96 hours postburn showed either no change or a slight further decrease in red cell mass. However, by this time a moderate to severe anemia was evident. They found the hematocrit to be valueless in assessing the need for blood transfusions and that it was safe to give whole blood in the face of an elevated hematocrit. When Evans and co-workers published in 1952 their now famous formula, they stated, "Whole blood remains the bulwark of our plan for intravenous therapy for the treatment of shock in the extensively burned patient."

Primarily because of the impact made and the results obtained by those who advocate treating burn shock with crystalloid solutions alone, blood has been used less and less since the 1950s for the immediate treatment of burn shock. It is still recognized that patients with large burns will manifest anemia between the third and seventh day after injury if they are not given blood transfusions during the shock phase. As yet, however, there are no good published comparative clinical studies which show whether whole blood has a salutary effect in the resuscitation of burned patients. Most authors recommend transfusion of blood for the specific indication of anemia. Several recommend giving whole blood to acutely burned patients if poor peripheral tissue perfusion or other evidence of shock cannot be relieved by the administration of other fluids. Hinton et al. found that transfusion sufficient to produce clinical evidence of adequate peripheral tissue perfusion induced an increase in the urinary excretion of sodium. This was interpreted as an indication of restoration of an effective circulation.

In 1881, Tappeiner observed, among patients with large burns, that although the water content of a unit volume of red blood cells was normal, the water content of a unit volume of whole blood was reduced. He therefore concluded that if plasma ever became available, it should be used to treat burn shock. By the late 1930s plasma was in extensive use to treat burn shock.

At the beginning of World War II, formulas for estimating the fluid requirements of burned patients based on the degree of hemoconcentration were in vogue. These formulas failed to take into account continuing losses of plasma fluid when the determination was made early after injury. Therefore, at a conference called by the National Research Council in 1942, it was recommended that a more realistic prediction of the fluid requirement could be made from the extent of the surface area damaged. Cope and Moore made a series of clinical observations of average-sized adults who were given 75 ml of plasma plus 75 ml of physiological saline solution for each per cent body surface area burned at a rate of one-half of the total calculated fluid over the first 8 hours, and the other half over the next 16 hours. It was postulated that these fluids would replace the fluid sequestered and inactive as a result of the thermal injury. These proportions were based on recommendations from the clinical experience of Harkins and the finding that the bleb fluid of a burn contained about one-half to two-thirds the concentration of protein and essentially the same concentration of electrolytes present in plasma. An additional 2000 ml of fluid were given each 24 hours to maintain urine flow.

The principal drawback of this method was the tendency to administer excessive amounts of fluid with an increased risk of pulmonary edema. Cope and Moore concluded that among the severely burned an expansion of the extracellular fluid volume by 50% (from 20% of body weight to approximately 30%) is an important feature of the disordered fluid balance and that therapy must be planned to satisfy but not augment the edema of the wound. From this work evolved a method of calculating the fluid needs which was called "the body-weight burn budget" (Moore). According to this Brigham burn budget, during the first 48 hours the following fluids were recommended: (1) to cover the extracellular fluid expansion, a volume of colloid (plasma, plasmanate, 5% albumin, or dextran with an average molecular weight of 70,000) equal to 10% of the body weight; (2) for renal needs, 2400 ml of 0.45% saline solution; (3) for lung losses, a range of 3000 to 10,000 ml of 5% dextrose in water depending on the clinical condition of the patient (Inhalation injury, fever, dyspnea, and tracheostomy are considered as indications for larger volumes of fluid. Two liters of this fluid are given as 10% mannitol by continuous infusion during the 48 hours as a diuretic to protect the kidney against acute tubular necrosis.); and (4) for skin losses, 2000 to 8000 ml of lactated Ringer's solution (the lesser figure for the drier flame burn and the larger estimate for the wetter scald). Although this guide to the fluid needs of the acutely burned patient has been used for over 20 years "with great ease and effectiveness," and although it is emphasized that the therapist can and should make changes in the budget from careful assessment of the patient's clinical response, there is no evidence to suggest that this relatively complex set of rules for the calculation of fluid for the resuscitation of the acutely burned has any advantage, or is any more rational, than methods to be described.

Evans and co-workers at the Medical College of Virginia in 1952, also dissatisfied with the surface area formula (75 ml plasma plus 75 ml saline for each 1% of burned surface) because of the too frequent occurrence of pulmonary edema, developed the now-famous Evans formula for the fluid resuscitation of burned patients. It was observed in Evans' laboratory that by the sixth hour postburn, a dog with a standard burn lost approximately 1 ml of plasma for each 1% BSA burned for each kilogram of body weight. Also, from analysis of plasma volume data, a similar finding was observed in a series of humans with burns of 20% body surface area.

The Evans formula
First 24 hours:

Colloid (plasma, plasma substitute, and whole blood were recommended originally; now dextran 70 in normal saline is used at the Medical College of Virginia), 1 ml/kg body weight/% body surface area burned.

Crystalloid (0.9% saline solution), 1 ml/kg body weight/% body surface area burned.

Half of the total volume during the first 8 hours and the other half over the next 16 hours.

Maintenance (5% dextrose in water), 2000 ml.

Second 24 hours:

Colloid, 0.5 ml/kg/% BSA burned.
Crystalloid, 0.5 ml/kg/% BSA burned.
Maintenance, 2000 ml.

The restriction was added that burns more extensive than 50% body surface area were to be calculated for fluid needs as if they were 50%.

The use of isotonic saline solution as the crystalloid and the selection of 50% BSA as the upper limit of burn for calculation were both selected empirically. Hutcher and Haynes in 1972 reviewed the case records of 100 consecutive burned patients requiring intravenous fluid resuscitation. They found that the Evans formula predicted accurately the fluid and electrolyte needs of the adult patients; these patients were well resuscitated and fluid overload was not observed. However, among children under 20-kg body weight, the Evans formula underestimated the sodium needs by 50 to 100%. Although 22 deaths among the 100 patients occurred in the first 6 days after injury, only one patient failed to survive 48 hours. The authors contended, even in the face of this high mortality rate, that in no instance was fluid overload a significant complicating factor.

The year following the publication of the Evans formula, Reiss et al. published a modification which is now known as the Brooke formula. These authors were concerned that the 0.9% sodium chloride solution recommended by Evans contained an excess of chloride ion and therefore recommended a "balanced" electrolyte solution (lactated Ringer's [Hartmann's] solution). The bicarbonate made available by metabolism of lactate was to prevent the hyperchloremic acidosis which would occur with use of saline solution. This seemed advisable in view of the tendency towards acidosis frequently observed in the early postburn period. Apparently, based on the reported observation that the increasing plasma protein concentration indicated a more rapid loss of water and electrolytes than of proteins, the authors of the Brooke formula recommended a 3:1 ratio of crystalloid to colloid during the first 24 hours rather than the 1:1 ratio of crystalloid to colloid of the Evans formula. Because of the high risk of hepatitis, they recommended blood, dextran, polyvinal-pyrrolidone, and the gelatins in preference to plasma as the colloid plasma expanders.

The Brooke formula
First 24 hours:
Crystalloid (lactated Ringer's solution), 1.5 ml/kg body weight/% BSA of burn.
Colloid (blood or plasma expander), 0.5 ml/kg body weight/% BSA of burn.
Maintenance (5% glucose in water or lactated Ringer's solution), 2000 ml.
Maximum calculated burn is 50% BSA.
Second 24 hours:
The fluid requirement is quantitatively and qualitatively approximately one-half to three-quarters that of the first 24 hours.

In 1971, Reckler and Mason of the U. S. Army Institute of Surgical Research, Brooke Army Hospital, reviewed the fluid resuscitation of 50 patients aged 15 to 45 years with burns ranging from 2% to 81.5% BSA. Using the Brooke formula as only a guide for planning therapy, they found the total volume of electrolyte- and colloid-containing fluids actually administered during the first 24 hours was parallel to but slightly higher than predicted up to 50% BSA burned. However, beyond 50% BSA burned, the amount of fluid administered increased linearly as the size of the burn increased. The volume of administered colloid was less than predicted by the formula. All 50 of these relatively young adults survived the shock phase. Although there were no instances of renal failure and only one patient developed pulmonary edema on the seventh postburn day, it is well known that young adults are in the most favorable age group for successful resuscitation.

Several investigators have proved the effectiveness of salt solution in treating burn shock in rodents. It is the contention of Fox, Lasker, et al. that the amount of sodium given is the common denominator for successful resuscitation of patients with burns. In Peru, during the 1950s and 1960s, a series of alternate case prospective clinical studies were conducted in an attempt to determine the relative value of saline solutions as compared with solutions containing colloids for the treatment of burn shock. The conclusions of the investigators were reviewed by Markley. Among adults (ages 11 to 73 years): (1) therapy with saline solution (141 mEq Na^+, 114 mEq Cl^-, 28 mEq lactate, and Ca^{++} 1.5 mEq/l) in a dose of 15% body weight was more effective in lowering shock mortality (within 60 hours after injury) than a fluid regimen consisting of plasma plus glucose equivalent to 10% body weight; (2) there was no reduction in the shock mortality from combining plasma with the saline solution; and (3) late mortality was not influenced by these early fluid regimens. Among children (ages 0 to 10 years): (1) addition of adequate amounts of plasma to large amounts of the saline solution significantly decreased shock as well as late mortality; and (2) the addition of albumin to saline solution had no significant effect on mortality whereas the addition of gamma globulin given intramuscularly with saline therapy lowered late mortality and the incidence of septicemia.

Moyer, Margraf, and Monafo, using only lactated Ringer's solution (pH adjust to 8.2) given intravenously and a salt solution (4 gm of sodium chloride and 1.5 gm sodium bicarbonate in 1 liter of ice water) given orally at a rate fast enough to keep the patient comfortably and safely alive, making urine, and oriented, reported the successful resuscitation of 10 patients with burns of 30 to 85% BSA and contended that colloid and blood were not needed for the successful treatment of shock associated with burns covering up to 85% of the body surface of human beings. At the Sixth National Burn Seminar, Baxter reported the results of a study among 221 patients treated with lactated Ringer's solution. The early mortality (within seven days after injury) was high among those with burns of greater than 70% BSA and among those with burns of greater than 50% BSA at the extremes of age.

Baxter (1971) subsequently modified the method advocated by Moyer, Margraf, and Monafo. These modifications were based on the following observations. There is evidence of inactivation of 38 to 50% of the estimated extracellular fluid volume during the first 18 hours after thermal injury. In the dog with 50% BSA flame burn the optimum regimen to maintain a near-normal functional extracellular fluid volume was found by Baxter to average 4 ml of lactated Ringer's solution per kilogram body weight per percent body burn administered in the first 24 hours. Optimally, two-thirds of this volume should be given in the first 8 hours. The colloid content of fluid administered in the first 24 hours does not expand plasma volume. The administration of plasma 24 hours postburn will increase plasma volume by the amount given. Therefore, during the first 24 hours the patient is to receive 4.0 ml of lactated Ringer's solution for each kilogram body weight and each per cent of body surface burned; one-half of this volume in the first 8 hours. When a urine flow of greater than 50 ml per hour has been established, the infusion rate is adjusted to maintain clinical and chemical signs of optimal resuscitation. After 18 to 24 hours, when all of the recommended lactated Ringer's solution has been given, if signs of adequate resuscitation are less than optimal, small amounts of plasma are given slowly.

Using this technique, Baxter reported that death within the first 7 days occurred only in patients with burns exceeding 60% BSA or when there were added factors, such as respiratory insufficiency from inhalation injury, myocardial depression, or an age below 1 year or over 70 years.

Based on the concept that the amount of sodium is the common denominator for successful resuscitation, that colloids are not needed, and that cell injury causes an increase in cellular tonicity, Monafo has advocated using hypertonic lactated saline solution (sodium 300 mEq/l, racemic lactate 200 mEq/l, and chloride 100 mEq/l). This hypertonic solution is designed to reduce the net positive fluid load and thus, theoretically, to reduce the incidence of complications which attend excessive edema. With this technique there is hypernatremia and alkalosis, especially when the burn is greater than 65% BSA. Hypokalemia is a risk of such treatment. Monafo treated 40 patients with a mortality rate of 12.5% during the first 72 hours after injury. He has subsequently changed the ionic concentrations of hypertonic lactated saline solution to sodium 250 mEq/l, chloride 150 mEq/l, and racemic lactate 100 mEq/l. There is no clinical evidence as yet that this approach will be more effective than the use of isotonic solutions.

One of the more impressive records of treatment of burn shock has been accomplished by Stone using a composite solution. This consists of 730 ml of 5% glucose in saline, 20 ml of sodium bicarbonate, and 250 ml of plasma (albumin or plasmanate can be substituted for cross-matched plasma). This solution contains 129.0 mEq of sodium, 101.5 mEq of chloride, 24.5 mEq of bicarbonate, 50.2 gm of glucose, and 15.0 gm protein per liter. The composite solution obviates any decision about the sequence of administration of colloid and crystalloid solutions. This solution was used to treat 231 patients between the ages of 2 months and 85 years with burns ranging from 13% to 98% BSA. There were 9 deaths during the first week after injury. This is an admirable mortality during the shock phase of 3.9%! Even when 7 additional elderly patients who had been considered as having too extensive an area of injury to be treated were added to the shock phase mortality, the mortality rate was only 6.9%.

Hoyle et al. showed that dogs with full thickness scalds of 66% BSA, treated with a solution of 2.5% albumin in lactated Ringer's, required two-thirds less fluid, produced twice as much urine, gained only one-half as much weight, stabilized serum proteins near normal, and maintained higher glomerular filtration rates when compared with similarly injured dogs treated with lactated Ringer's solution alone. Based on this work, Hartford et al. conducted a prospective clinical study comparing the efficacy of lactated Ringer's solution and lactated Ringer's solution with 25 gm albumin added* (2.3% albumin) for fluid resuscitation of 29 patients with burns greater than 30% BSA. The fluid was given intravenously at such a rate as to maintain a urine flow of 30 to 50 ml per hour for adults and a correspondingly lesser amount for children. No formula for preliminary calculation of fluid need was used. During the first 24 hours children (ages 2 to 12 years) were given significantly more of either kind of fluid than were adults (ages 13 to 59 years) for the same extent of injury (Table 12-1). Among both adults and children those treated with the albumin-containing solution required one-third less volume and one-third less sodium (Table 12-1). These findings are statistically significant at the 95% level of confidence. There was no difference in acute phase (up to 7 days after injury) or subsequent mortality of either children or adults. There was a lower incidence of acute phase complications among those adults (age 13 to 59 years) treated with the colloid-containing solution. Although none of the patients above the age of 60 survived complications arising in the acute phase regardless of which fluid was used, it might be argued that the lower risk of acute phase complications noted among young adults is an indication that the use of colloid-containing solutions will ultimately prove to be the preferred approach.

---

*Lactated Ringer's solution—1000 cc

Sodium	135.0 mEq
Potassium	4.0 mEq
Calcium	2.7 mEq
Chloride	109.7 mEq
Lactate	27.0 mEq

Lactated Ringer's, albumin (2.3%) solution—1100 cc

Albumin	25.0 gm
Sodium	148.5 mEq
Potassium	4.0 mEq
Calcium	2.7 mEq
Chloride	109.7 mEq
Lactate	27.0 mEq

TABLE 12-1

a) Average Volumes of Fluid Given First 24 Hours

Age Years	Lactated Ringer's ml/kg/% burn	Lactated Ringer's + Albumin ml/kg/% burn
2-12	5.2	3.4
13-59	2.9	2.0

b) Average Amount of Sodium Given First 24 Hours

Age Years	Lactated Ringer's mEq/kg/% burn	Lactated Ringer's + Albumin mEq/kg/% burn
2-12	0.66	0.46
13-59	0.40	0.27

There is a limit as to how much can be accomplished by using fluids of any kind to resuscitate acutely burned patients. Most investigators admit to difficulty in resuscitating patients with burns of greater than 60% BSA, and among infants and the aged with even lesser extents of injury. It may be that other supportive measures are needed among those whose mortality is predictably high. It has been suggested that positive pressure ventilation, large doses of steroids, heparin, cardiac augmentation, and hemodialysis are methods which might be tried by investigators to decrease the morbidity and mortality during the first week after injury.

CONSIDERATIONS FOR FLUID RESUSCITATION

In most instances children and adults with burns of less than 10% and 15% BSA respectively do not require intravenously administered fluids to prevent burn shock. It is clear that most older children and relatively young adults, if premorbid health was good, with burns of less than two-thirds of the body surface can be successfully resuscitated with relative ease by one of a variety of fluid resuscitation techniques. There is general agreement that sodium-containing fluids are necessary. To date, the most rational kind of solution is a "balanced" saline solution, isotonic with extracellular fluid such as lactated Ringer's solution. If a decrease in the amount of sodium or net positive fluid load is thought to be desirable then a colloid should be included. It is my contention that the use of colloids does reduce the incidence of complications related to edema and subsequently the complications associated with fluid overload during mobilization of inactivated fluid. This can be albumin, plasmanate, or plasma. Plasma has the disadvantage of a predictable incidence of hepatitis. Dextran, although advocated by some authors, may interfere with the cross-matching of blood and coagulation. There is a limit to the amount which can be given safely. It is recommended that the colloid be given simultaneously with the electrolyte solution so that there is temporal quantitative and qualitative correspondence between replacement and sequestration.

Since there is no evidence that blood has a salutary effect in the treatment or prevention of burn shock, blood is usually given only for the correction of anemia. However, transfusion may be tried if shock is not relieved by treatment with other fluids.

All the existing formulas for predicting the quantity of fluid necessary for treatment of burned patients are only guides; and in most instances, poor guides at best. The central theme of most authors, regardless of which techniques they advocate, is careful, thorough, intelligent, and repeated assessment of the patient and his response to therapy throughout the resuscitation period. Those physicians who take this attitude will have the best results. To encompass that time during which the "lost" fluid is being remobilized and the risk of cardiopulmonary overload is high, the resuscitation period should be considered as lasting about one week.

MANAGEMENT OF THE PATIENT

When a patient with burns is first seen, a rapid assessment should be made to determine the overall condition of the patient and whether or not fluid therapy is needed. A large-bore intravenous cannula should be placed, even through burned tissue if no other practical site is available. Blood should be obtained for laboratory examination and for cross-matching of blood and/or plasma. Then the fluid for resuscitation should be selected. For young children, for those over 50 years of age and for all patients with burns greater than 30% BSA we use lactated Ringer's solution with 25 gm of albumin added to each liter. To the initial fluid is added 44.7 mEq sodium bicarbonate (1 ampule) to start correction of the inevitable metabolic acidosis. Young healthy adults with burns less than 30% BSA are usually given lactated Ringer's solution unless there are complicating circumstances. We do not use any electrolyte-free fluid for insensible loss and urine replacement during the first 24 hours.

The urinary bladder is catheterized, and the tubing connected to a system from which urine output can be measured each hour. Also a nasogastric tube is inserted to obviate the risk of acute gastric dilatation and vomiting until effective gastrointestinal function is restored. Temporary ileus is a frequent consequence of large surface thermal injury, especially if it is accompanied by shock.

The fluid chosen is administered rapidly until urine flow occurs, then the infusion is adjusted to maintain a urine outflow of 30 to 50 ml per hour. The initial rate of fluid administration required will usually exceed 4.4 ml per kilogram body weight per hour to keep pace with the rate at which the administered fluid is sequestered. The rate of fluid administration will gradually decline, following a parabolic curve, until 18 to 30 hours after injury at which time the fluid required to maintain the desired urine flow will be less than losses. At this time, the risk of shock solely from the burn is virtually nil. Excessive amounts of fluid administered will only increase the edema and increase the risk of cardiopulmonary failure.

EXAMINATION OF THE PATIENT

The physician responsible should attend the patient continuously until it has been determined whether or not the patient is going to develop acute renal insufficiency. The manipulation of fluids should not be left to the discretion of any other person, no matter how well trained. After the initial measures for resuscitation have been started, a detailed history and physical examination should be recorded.

At least once each hour, the patient's clinical condition should be evaluated, observing carefully the patient's level of consciousness, respiratory rate, the ease or difficulty of breathing, the pulse or heart rate and rhythm, the urine output and its specific gravity and pH, the blood pressure if measurable, and the condition of the patient's extremities. From these observations, changes in colloid and electrolyte composition and rate of administration of fluid should be made, and also the necessity of obtaining additional laboratory studies. As the condition of the patient stabilizes, the frequency of bedside examination can be reduced.

LABORATORY TESTS

While balanced salt solutions are being used, the concentrations of sodium, potassium, and chloride in serum are usually in the normal range.

Serum Bicarbonate

Because of the presence of metabolic acidosis on admission, the level of bicarbonate in the serum is invariably low. Therefore, sodium bicarbonate is added to the initial resuscitation fluid. When the pH of arterial blood and level of bicarbonate in the serum become normal, there is no need for additional bicarbonate in the fluids being given intravenously.

Serum Creatinine and BUN

Even in the most severe thermal injury, it is unusual for the initially measured levels of BUN and creatinine in the serum to be abnormally elevated unless treatment has been delayed. If the serum creatinine is elevated and rises progressively in the face of fluid therapy, the patient's prognosis is poor. An elevated BUN may indicate gastrointestinal bleeding from gastritis or less frequently from a stress ulcer.

Blood Gases

Initially the pH of arterial blood is usually low, consistent with the level of metabolic acidosis. As resuscitation measures succeed, the pH will move into the normal range or even indicate an alkalosis.

In most instances, the patient's PO_2 is normal on admission. As resuscitation progresses it tends to be lowered, especially among those with severe thermal injury. This is usually due to either an increase in the interstitial fluid of the lung or an associated inhalation injury. In both situations, modification of the treatment is necessary, and if clinically indicated the patient should be given positive pressure ventilation. As with other conditions in which positive pressure ventilation is used, there is usually a decreased fluid requirement. A dense unyielding eschar of a full thickness burn around the torso may inhibit respiratory excursions. If this is present, the restriction should be relieved by escharotomy.

The PCO_2 of arterial blood after thermal injury is usually normal or low. The latter instance reflects compensation for the metabolic acidosis. Retention of carbon dioxide indicates pre-existing pulmonary insufficiency or the occurrence of inhalation injury or both and worsens the prognosis.

The carbon monoxide level of the blood may be elevated, especially in instances in which the injury was sustained in a closed space fire. In hospitals where carboxyhemoglobin levels can be measured, it should be routinely done. A pink or cherry skin in the face of a low arterial PO_2 invariably means the patient has a biologically significant level of carboxyhemoglobin.

Hemoglobin and Hematocrit

These are usually elevated on admission, reflecting hemoconcentration. If they are not elevated, pre-existing anemia was probably present. As resuscitation progresses, the levels of hemoglobin and hematocrit fall. If clinically indicated, the patient should be transfused. Appearance of the first signs of anemia after a burn is frequently between the third and seventh day.

Excessive sampling of blood undoubtedly contributes to the development of anemia.

Blood Pressure

Measurement of blood pressure by auscultation is impractical in many instances among the severely burned. In the usual instance, arterial lines are not necessary, and if one is placed in a burned extremity, it may add to vascular compromise. The use of the Doppler technique to measure blood pressure shows promise in such patients.

In most instances, with a urine flow of greater than 30 ml per hour, the blood pressure will be normal. The danger, of course, occurs in instances in which the patient excretes 30 ml of urine in a 15- to 30-minute segment of an hour but is hypotensive, oliguric, and in need of additional intravenous fluid to maintain circulation for the remaining 30 to 45 minutes of that particular hour.

Urine

On admission the urinary bladder should be emptied. Subsequently, while the risk of shock is great, the urine flow should be measured each hour. The rate of urine flow is a highly regarded sign of success or failure of resuscitation among burned patients. Urine flows which we recommend as an index of adequate resuscitation and those volumes which indicate oliguria are shown in Table 12-2. If the patient is oliguric he should be given a test load of fluid intravenously, the volume to exceed 4.4 ml per kilogram of body weight over the next hour. Central venous pressure (CVP) and blood pressure should be monitored. If oliguria con-

TABLE 12-2. GUIDE TO OLIGURIA AND DESIRED URINE VOLUMES PER HOUR

Admission body weight, kg	Desired (more than), ml	Oliguria (less than), ml
45 and above	35	20
40	35	18
35	35	16
30	35	15
25	35	14
20	33	13
15	28	11
10	20	8
5	10	4

tinues in the face of a low or normal CVP, the rate of fluid administration is maintained in excess of 4.4 ml per kilogram of body weight per hour and 100 ml of 18% mannitol are infused slowly by a hand-driven syringe. If this fails to produce a satisfactory urine flow, the patient is given 40 mg of furosemide intravenously. At that point if satisfactory urine flow is not re-established, the likelihood of occurrence of acute renal failure is high. Subsequent therapeutic maneuvers including the administration of additional fluids must be carefully weighed with the knowledge that matters may be made worse in the face of acute tubular necrosis.

The presence of hemoglobinuria increases the risk of acute renal failure, and the usual measures to rapidly clear free hemoglobin from the blood should be taken.

In most instances the concentration of urine is above 1.020 and usually between 1.025 and 1.030. Isosthenuria must be regarded with suspicion. In instances in which the likelihood of acute renal failure is high, urine sodium, potassium, and osmolarity may help in diagnosis.

Body Weight

The patient should be weighed soon after admission. The subsequent monitoring of body weight during the shock phase, as advocated by some, to help adjust fluid therapy has not been particularly useful in our hands.

Sedation

By the time most severely burned patients reach the hospital they are virtually free of pain. Most patients feel relatively well and do not understand why all the fuss is made about their condition. Restlessness is a sign of shock or hypoxia and should not be treated with narcotics. If the patient does have pain, he should be given small doses of morphine intravenously to obtain the desired effect. Hypodermic administration of narcotics is not recommended because of the slow and inconsistent absorption.

Digitalis

Whether digitalis has a salutary effect on burn shock is not known. If there is evidence of congestive heart failure, it should be used.

Ending Intravenous Fluid Therapy

Between 18 and 30 hours after injury the patient should be carefully evaluated for adequacy of resuscitation. Fluids administered after 18 hours should be carefully weighed against the risk of increasing the complications of overload.

Oral alimentation should be started as soon as there is evidence that the ileus has resolved. The intravenous cannulas and urinary bladder catheters should be removed as soon as possible to prevent the occurrence of infection.

BIOLOGICAL DANGERS OF TOPICALLY APPLIED SUBSTANCES CURRENTLY IN USE

There are several topical antibacterial agents which are currently in vogue for treatment of burns. Of these, 0.5% silver nitrate and mafenide (Sulfamylon) can produce metabolic disturbances which are dangerous.

One-half per cent silver nitrate is hypotonic, 29.4 mEq/l. As a consequence, salt loss and water gain across the wound can cause serious disturbances. We have found that as long as the patient receives balanced electrolyte solutions intravenously no electrolyte disturbances occur. When, however, the balanced electrolyte solution is stopped, hyponatremia and hypokalemia will occur rapidly unless sodium and potassium supplements are given. Bicarbonate supplementation should also be given. For adults the starting dose by mouth for sodium chloride is in the range of 9 to 12 gm per day; for potassium gluconate, 40 to 80 mEq per day; and for sodium bicarbonate, 3 to 4 gm per day; corresponding but lesser amounts for children. Adjustments are made from results of analysis of the patient's serum and urine electrolytes. For patients with large burns who will have a prolonged convalescence, some burn therapists also supply calcium. If it is not given as a matter of routine, the patient should be observed for signs of hypocalcemia and the serum calcium measured periodically.

Mafenide diffuses through the eschar and is absorbed into the body. It is a strong carbonic anhydrase inhibitor and causes a bicarbonate diuresis. To maintain normal body pH, carbon dioxide must be blown off through the lungs. Therefore, patients treated with mafenide have hyperpnea. This does not cause difficulty unless a pulmonary complication supervenes (e.g., inhalation injury, atelectasis, or pneumonia) which causes retention of carbon dioxide. A fatal degree of acidosis may develop unless the mafenide is stopped and the pulmonary complication vigorously treated.

Most burn therapists recommend that the patient have a tub bath at least once each day. This bath should be limited to a maximum of 20 minutes, because there is diffusion of water across the wound into the body, and water intoxication may occur if prolonged immersion is allowed.

REFERENCES

Arturson, G.: Effects of 0-(-hydroxyethyl)-rutosides (HR) on the increased microvascular permeability in experimental skin burns: preliminary report. Acta Chir. Scand. *138*:111, 1972.

Baxter, C. R.: Therapy of burns. Sixth National Burn Seminar, Chicago. J. Trauma *7*:69, 1967.

Baxter, C. R.: Crystalloid resuscitation of burn shock. In *Contemporary Burn Management*. Polk, H. C., Jr., and Stone, H. H., eds. Boston: Little, Brown and Co. 1971.

Baxter, C. R., and Shires, G. T.: Physiological response to crystalloid resuscitation of severe burns. Ann. N. Y. Acad. Sci. *150*:874, 1968.

Buhl: Mittheilungen aus der pfeuferschen klinik, epidemische cholera. Z. Rationelle Med. *6*:1, 1855.

Cope, O., and Moore, F. D.: The redistribution of body water and fluid therapy of the burned patient. Ann. Surg. *126*:1010, 1947.

Cotran, R. S., and Remensnyder, J. P.: The structural basis of increased vascular permeability after graded thermal injury—light and electron microscopic studies. Ann. N. Y. Acad. Sci. *150*:495, 1968.

Evans, E. I., and Bigger, I. A.: The rationale of whole blood therapy in severe burns. Ann. Surg. *122*:693, 1945.

Evans, E. I., Purnell, O. J., Robinett, P. W., Batchelor, A., and Martin, M.: Fluid and electrolyte requirements in severe burns. Ann. Surg. *135*:804, 1952.

Fox, C. L., Jr.: Systemic therapy for resuscitation in severe burns. Modern Treatment *4*:1203, 1967.

Fox, C. L., Jr., and Baer, H.: Redistribution of potassium, sodium and water in burns and trauma, and its relation to the phenomena of shock. Amer. J. Physiol. *151*:155, 1947.

Fox, C. L., Jr., Holder, I. A., and Malin, L. L.: Toxic, thromboplastic extracts of skin—potential role in thermal injury. J.A.M.A. *187*:655, 1964.

Fox, C. L., Jr., Lasker, S. E., Winfield, J. M., Mersheiner, W. L., and Silverstein, M. E.: Observations on the effects of blood, plasma and sodium salt solutions in the treatment of extensive burns. Amer. J. Surg. *89*:730, 1955.

Hartford, C. E., Recinos, P. R., and Ziffren, S. E.: Fluid resuscitation of burn patients comparing a crystalloid with a colloid containing solution: a prospective study. To be published.

Hinton, P., Allison, S. P., Farrow, S., Littlejohn, S., and Lloyd, J.: Blood-volume changes and transfusion requirements of burned patients after the shock phase of injury. Lancet *1*:913, 1972.

Hoyle, C. L., McCall, D. C., Danford, R. O., Desuto-Nagy, G. I., and Hays, M. A.: Renal function during the early post-burn period: a comparison of colloid versus non-colloid containing balanced salt solution. Ann. Surg. *169*:404, 1969.

Hutcher, N., and Haynes, B. W., Jr.: The Evans formula revisited. J. Trauma *12*:453, 1972.

Jelenko, C., III, Ginsburg, J. M., Anderson, A. P., and Wheeler, M. L.: Studies in burns. IX. Sodium, potassium and water content of skin and burn eschar. Ann. Surg. *38*:364, 1972.

Kilgore, H. E., Baxter, C. R., and Shires, G. T.: Changes in body fluid compartments in full thickness burns. Surg. Forum *16*:29, 1965.

Latta, T.: Letter from Dr. Latta to the Secretary of the Central Board of Health, London, affording a view of the rationale and results of his practice in the treatment of cholera by aqueous and saline injections. Lancet *2*:274, 1832.

vonLesser, L.: Ueber Todesursachen bei verbrennungen. Virchow Arch. Path. Anat. *79*:248, 1880.

Markley, K.: Comparison of sodium salts and plasma therapy in burned patients in Peru. Ann. N. Y. Acad. Sci. *150*:845, 1968.

Monafo, W. W.: Hypertonic lactated saline solution in the treatment of burn shock. In *Research in Burns*. Matter, P., Barclay, T. L., and Koníčková, Z., eds. Bern: Hans Huber Publishers, 1970.

Moore, F. D.: The body-weight burn budget: basic fluid therapy for the early burn. Surg. Clin. N. Amer. *50:*1249, 1970.

Moyer, C. A.: The treatment of burn shock. In *On Burns*. Womack, N. A., ed. Springfield, Ill.: Charles C Thomas, 1953.

Moyer, C. A., Coller, F. A., Iob, V., Vaugh, H. H., and Marty, D.: A study of the interrelationship of salt solutions, serum and defibrinated blood in the treatment of severely scalded, anesthetized dogs. Ann. Surg. *120:*367, 1944.

Moyer, C. A., Margraf, H. W., and Monafo, W. W., Jr.: Burn shock and extravascular sodium deficiency: treatment with Ringer's solutions with lactate. Arch. Surg. (Chicago) *90:*799, 1965.

Muir, I. F. K.: Red cell destruction in burns, with particular reference to the shock period. Brit. J. Plast. Surg. *14:*273, 1961.

O'Neill, J. A., Jr., Pruitt, B. A., and Moncrief, J. A.: Studies of renal function during the early post burn period. In *Research in Burns*. Matter, P., Barclay, T. L., and Koníčková, Z., eds. Bern: Hans Huber Publishers, 1971.

Pruitt, B. A., Jr., and Mason, A. D., Jr.: Hemodynamic studies of burned patients during resuscitation. In *Research in Burns*. Matter, P., Barclay, T. L., and Koníčková, Z., eds. Bern: Hans Huber Publishers, 1971.

Reckler, J. M., and Mason, A. D., Jr.: A critical evaluation of fluid resuscitation in the burned patient. Ann. Surg. *174:*115, 1971.

Reiss, E., Stirman, J. A., Artz, C. P., Davis, J. H., and Amspacher, W. H.: Fluid and electrolyte balance in burns. J.A.M.A. *152:*1309, 1953.

Sneve, H.: The treatment of burns and skin grafting. J.A.M.A. *45:*1, 1905.

Stone, H. H.: The composite burn solution. In *Contemporary Burn Management*. Polk, H. C., Jr., and Stone, H. H., eds. Boston: Little, Brown and Co., 1971.

vonTappeiner, H.: Ueber veranderungen des blutes und der muskeln nach ausgedehnten hautverbrennungen. Centralbl. Med. Wissenschaften *31:*385, 1881.

Underhill, F. P.: The significance of anhydremia in extensive superficial burns. J.A.M.A. *95:*852, 1930.

Index

Page numbers in italic refer to figures; those followed by *t* refer to tables